METHODS IN MOLECULAR BIOLOGY

Series Editor
John M. Walker
School of Life and Medical Sciences
University of Hertfordshire
Hatfield, Hertfordshire, AL10 9AB, UK

For further volumes:
http://www.springer.com/series/7651

Biomarkers for Alzheimer's Disease Drug Development

Edited by

Robert Perneczky

Department of Psychiatry and Psychotherapy, Ludwig-Maximilians-Universität München, Munich, Germany

German Center for Neurodegenerative Diseases (DZNE) Munich, Munich, Germany

Neuroepidemiology and Ageing Research Unit, School of Public Health, The Imperial College of Science, Technology and Medicine, London, UK

West London Mental Health NHS Trust, London, UK

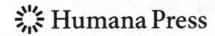 Humana Press

Editor
Robert Perneczky
Department of Psychiatry and Psychotherapy
Ludwig-Maximilians-Universität München
Munich, Germany

German Center for Neurodegenerative Diseases (DZNE) Munich
Munich, Germany

Neuroepidemiology and Ageing Research Unit, School of Public Health
The Imperial College of Science, Technology and Medicine
London, UK

West London Mental Health NHS Trust
London, UK

ISSN 1064-3745   ISSN 1940-6029   (electronic)
Methods in Molecular Biology
ISBN 978-1-4939-7703-1   (hardcover)   ISBN 978-1-4939-7704-8   (eBook)
ISBN 978-1-4939-9262-1   (softcover)
https://doi.org/10.1007/978-1-4939-7704-8

Library of Congress Control Number: 2018932034

Printed on acid-free paper

This Humana Press imprint is published by Springer Nature
The registered company is Springer Science+Business Media, LLC
The registered company address is: 233 Spring Street, New York, NY 10013, U.S.A.

Preface

The prevalence of Alzheimer's disease and its healthcare and socioeconomic impact are exploding worldwide, and drug development success rates need to be improved urgently; the traditional linear model of pharmaceutical R&D has become outdated and virtually all new drugs have failed since the cholinesterase inhibitors were introduced to the markets two decades ago. Drug development has been more successful in other fields of medicine such as infectious diseases and cancer, in which translational models are applied, linking population-based cohorts and genetic data with potential drug targets and study endpoints. This powerful translational approach is fuelled by technology platforms such as neuroimaging, -omics, and fluid biomarkers. The Alzheimer's disease field requires a significant cultural change to discover and develop effective disease-modifying treatment options (until 2025, as postulated at the 2013 G8 Dementia Summit).

The main objective of this book is to bridge and converge population, -omics, and imaging sciences (typically owned by academia) with R&D approaches for new technologies and novel, effective drugs (the traditional remit of industry). The book will help building a new generation of experts with a broader understanding of key topics to initiate the disruptive innovation required to make real progress. Given the high complexity and multifactorial disease nature related to dementias, a precision/personalized medicine approach in designing the next generation R&D strategies is now urgently required.

This publication comprises nine parts: In Part I (Chapters 1–3) we explain why Alzheimer's disease is one of the major challenges for the global societies and healthcare systems, and how population-based and systems biology approaches can be leveraged to develop more effective treatments. In Part II (Chapters 4–6) we present innovative approaches to the discovery of novel biomarkers in cerebrospinal fluid, whereas in Part III (Chapters 7–9) innovation in blood-based biomarkers is discussed. Part IV (Chapters 10–12) and Part V (Chapters 13–16) provide a comprehensive overview of magnetic resonance imaging and molecular imaging approaches and their value for developing drugs for Alzheimer's disease, respectively. In Part VI (Chapters 17 and 18) cutting-edge developments in neuropathology and their relevance for Alzheimer's disease trials are presented. Part VII (Chapters 19–21) covers novel genomic strategies for biomarker development. Part VIII (Chapters 22 and 23) highlights the contribution of preclinical research to the development of novel biomarkers and drugs. Finally, in Part IX (Chapters 24 and 25), we consider relevant related topics including neuropsychological testing and advanced analytical methods.

The book is targeted at individuals with an interest in the use of advanced biomarker strategies to accelerate the development of effective, disease-modifying drugs for Alzheimer's disease. This includes researchers, clinicians, and those interested in regulatory and medical affairs, both from academia and industry. We wish to present biomarker development approaches as a strategy for the study of Alzheimer's disease with the hope and expectation that the results will translate into more effective treatments. We expect this book to complement other excellent volumes and monographs on Alzheimer's disease that cover basic science or clinical aspects of the disease.

Munich, Germany   *Robert Perneczky*

Contents

Contributors

AHMED ABDULKADIR · *University Hospital of Old Age Psychiatry and Psychotherapy Bern, Bern, Switzerland*

M. ARFAN IKRAM · *Departments of Epidemiology, Radiology, Neurology, Erasmus University Medical Center Rotterdam, Rotterdam, The Netherlands*

GIUSEPPE ASTARITA · *Department of Biochemistry and Molecular and Cellular Biology, Georgetown University, Washington, DC, USA*

FILIPPO BALDACCI · *AXA Research Fund & UPMC Chair, Paris, France; Sorbonne Université, AP-HP, GRC n° 21, Alzheimer Precision Medicine (APM), Hôpital de la Pitié-Salpêtrière, Boulevard de l'hôpital, Paris, France; Institut du Cerveau et de la Moelle Épinière (ICM), INSERM U 1127, CNRS UMR 7225, Boulevard de l'hôpital, Paris, France; Institut de la Mémoire et de la Maladie d'Alzheimer (IM2A), Département de Neurologie, Hôpital de la Pitié-Salpêtrière, AP-HP, Boulevard de l'hôpital, Paris, France; Department of Clinical and Experimental Medicine, University of Pisa, Pisa, Italy*

RITA BARONE · *CNR, Istituto per i Polimeri, Compositi e i Biomateriali Catania, Catania, Italy; Pediatric Neurology Unit, Department of Pediatrics, University of Catania, Catania, Italy*

MATTEO BAUCKNEHT · *Nuclear Medicine Unit, Polyclinic San Martino Hospital, Genova, Italy; Department of Health Sciences, University of Genoa, Genoa, Italy*

BART N.M. VAN BERCKEL · *Department of Radiology and Nuclear Medicine, Neuroscience Campus Amsterdam, VU University Medical Center, Amsterdam, The Netherlands*

ROSARIA ORNELLA BUA · *CNR, Istituto per i Polimeri, Compositi e i Biomateriali Catania, Catania, Italy*

MARC AUREL BUSCHE · *Department of Neurology, Massachusetts General Hospital, Harvard Medical School, MassGeneral Institute for Neurodegenerative Disease, Charlestown, MA, USA; Department of Psychiatry and Psychotherapy, Technical University of Munich, Munich, Germany; Munich Cluster for Systems Neurology, Munich, Germany*

ANA L. CARDOSO · *Center for Neuroscience and Cell Biology, University of Coimbra, Coimbra, Portugal*

JUAN I. CASTRILLO · *Genetadi Biotech S.L. Parque Tecnológico de Bizkaia, Derio, Bizkaia, Spain*

ROBERTO CERAVOLO · *Department of Clinical and Experimental Medicine, University of Pisa, Pisa, Italy*

JOHANNES DENK · *Department of Psychiatry and Psychotherapy, University Medical Center Hamburg-Eppendorf, Hamburg, Germany*

CORNELIUS K. DONAT · *Division of Brain Sciences, Imperial College London, Hammersmith Hospital, London, UK*

JUERGEN DUKART · *F. Hoffmann-La Roche, Pharma Research Early Development, Roche Innovation Centre Basel, Basel, Switzerland; Roche Pharmaceutical Research and Early Development, Neuroscience, Ophthalmology and Rare Diseases, Discovery and Translational Area, Roche Innovation Center Basel, Basel, Switzerland*

PAUL EDISON · *Division of Brain Sciences, Imperial College London, Hammersmith Hospital, London, UK*

CARLES FALCON · *Barcelonaβeta Brain Research Center, Pasqual Maragall Foundation, Barcelona, Spain; Centro de Investigación Biomédica en Red de Bioingeniería, Biomateriales y Nanomedicina (CIBER-BBN), Madrid, Spain*

ÁNGELES FERNÁNDEZ-RECAMALES · *Department of Chemistry, Faculty of Experimental Sciences, University of Huelva, Huelva, Spain; International Campus of Excellence CeiA3, University of Huelva, Huelva, Spain*

GIOVANNI B. FRISONI · *Faculty of Medicine, Nuclear Medicine Department, Geneva University Medical Center, University of Geneva, Geneva, Switzerland; Department of Internal Medicine, Geneva University Hospitals, Geneva, Switzerland*

VALENTINA GARIBOTTO · *Division of Nuclear Medicine and Molecular Imaging, Geneva University Hospitals, Geneva, Switzerland; Faculty of Medicine, Nuclear Medicine Department, Geneva University Medical Center, University of Geneva, Geneva, Switzerland*

DOMENICO GAROZZO · *CNR, Istituto per i Polimeri, Compositi e i Biomateriali Catania, Catania, Italy*

STEVE GENTLEMAN · *Division of Brain Sciences, Department of Medicine, Imperial College London, London, UK*

JUAN DOMINGO GISPERT · *Barcelonaβeta Brain Research Center, Pasqual Maragall Foundation, Barcelona, Spain; Centro de Investigación Biomédica en Red de Bioingeniería, Biomateriales y Nanomedicina (CIBER-BBN), Madrid, Spain*

RAÚL GONZÁLEZ-DOMÍNGUEZ · *Department of Chemistry, Faculty of Experimental Sciences, University of Huelva, Huelva, Spain; International Campus of Excellence CeiA3, University of Huelva, Huelva, Spain*

ÁLVARO GONZÁLEZ-DOMÍNGUEZ · *Department of Chemistry, Faculty of Experimental Sciences, University of Huelva, Huelva, Spain; International Campus of Excellence CeiA3, University of Huelva, Huelva, Spain*

JOANA R. GUEDES · *Center for Neuroscience and Cell Biology, University of Coimbra, Coimbra, Portugal*

SARA HÄGG · *Department of Medical Epidemiology and Biostatistics, Karolinska Institutet, Stockholm, Sweden*

HARALD HAMPEL · *AXA Research Fund & UPMC Chair, Paris, France; Sorbonne Université, AP-HP, GRC n° 21, Alzheimer Precision Medicine (APM), Hôpital de la Pitié-Salpêtrière, Boulevard de l'hôpital, Paris, France; Institut du Cerveau et de la Moelle Épinière (ICM), INSERM U 1127, CNRS UMR 7225, Boulevard de l'hôpital, Paris, France; Institut de la Mémoire et de la Maladie d'Alzheimer (IM2A), Département de Neurologie, Hôpital de la Pitié-Salpêtrière, AP-HP, Boulevard de l'hôpital, Paris, France*

STEFAN HOLIGA · *F. Hoffmann-La Roche, pharma Research Early Development, Roche Innovation Centre Basel, Basel, Switzerland*

HOLGER JAHN · *Department of Psychiatry and Psychotherapy, University Medical Center Hamburg-Eppendorf, Hamburg, Germany*

HANS W. KLAFKI · *Department of Psychiatry and Psychotherapy, University Medical Center Goettingen, Georg-August-University, Goettingen, Germany*

STEFAN KLÖPPEL · *University Hospital of Old Age Psychiatry and Psychotherapy Bern, Bern, Switzerland*

ADRIAAN A. LAMMERTSMA · *Department of Radiology and Nuclear Medicine, Neuroscience Campus Amsterdam, VU University Medical Center, Amsterdam, The Netherlands*

RUI LI · *Alibaba, Hangzhou, Zhejiang, China*

SIMONE LISTA · *AXA Research Fund & UPMC Chair, Paris, France; Sorbonne Université, AP-HP, GRC n° 21, Alzheimer Precision Medicine (APM), Hôpital de la Pitié-Salpêtrière, Boulevard de l'hôpital, Paris, France; Institut du Cerveau et de la Moelle Épinière (ICM), INSERM U 1127, CNRS UMR 7225, Boulevard de l'hôpital, Paris, France; Institut de la Mémoire et de la Maladie d'Alzheimer (IM2A), Département de Neurologie, Hôpital de la Pitié-Salpêtrière, AP-HP, Boulevard de l'hôpital, Paris, France*

ALAN KING LUN LIU · *Division of Brain Sciences, Department of Medicine, Imperial College London, London, UK*

ISMINI C. MAINTA · *Division of Nuclear Medicine and Molecular Imaging, Geneva University Hospitals, Geneva, Switzerland; Faculty of Medicine, Nuclear Medicine Department, Geneva University Medical Center, University of Geneva, Geneva, Switzerland*

ANGELA MESSINA · *CNR, Istituto per i Polimeri, Compositi e i Biomateriali Catania, Catania, Italy*

NAZANIN MIRZAEI · *Division of Brain Sciences, Imperial College London, Hammersmith Hospital, London, UK*

JOSÉ LUIS MOLINUEVO · *Barcelonaβeta Brain Research Center, Pasqual Maragall Foundation, Barcelona, Spain; CIBER Fragilidad y Envejecimiento Saludable (CIBERFES), Madrid, Spain*

SILVIA MORBELLI · *Nuclear Medicine Unit, Polyclinic San Martino Hospital, Genova, Italy; Department of Health Sciences, University of Genoa, Genoa, Italy*

AGNETA NORDBERG · *Division of Translational Alzheimer Neurobiology, Center for Alzheimer Research, Department of Neurobiology, Care Sciences and Society, Karolinska Institutet, Stockholm, Sweden; Department of Geriatric Medicine, Karolinska University Hospital Huddinge, Stockholm, Sweden*

SID E. O'BRYANT · *Institute for Healthy Aging, University of North Texas Health Science Center, Fort Worth, TX, USA*

GRÉGORY OPERTO · *Barcelonaβeta Brain Research Center, Pasqual Maragall Foundation, Barcelona, Spain*

MARION M. ORTNER · *Department of Psychiatry and Psychotherapy, Klinikum rechts der Isar, Technische Universität München, Munich, Germany*

RIK OSSENKOPPELE · *Department of Neurology and Alzheimer Center, Neuroscience Campus Amsterdam, VU University Medical Center, Amsterdam, The Netherlands; Department of Radiology and Nuclear Medicine, Neuroscience Campus Amsterdam, VU University Medical Center, Amsterdam, The Netherlands*

GIUSEPPE PAGLIA · *EURAC Institute for Biomedicine, Institute for Biomedicine, European Academy of Bolzano/Bozen, Bolzano, Italy*

ANGELO PALMIGIANO · *CNR, Istituto per i Polimeri, Compositi e i Biomateriali Catania, Catania, Italy*

ROBERT PERNECZKY · *Department of Psychiatry and Psychotherapy, Ludwig-Maximilians-Universität München, Munich, Germany; German Center for Neurodegenerative Diseases (DZNE) Munich, Munich, Germany; Neuroepidemiology and Ageing Research Unit, School of Public Health, The Imperial College of Science, Technology and Medicine, London, UK; West London Mental Health NHS Trust, London, UK*

GERAINT PRICE · *Faculty of Medicine, Neuroepidemiology and Ageing Research Unit, School of Public Health, The Imperial College of Science Technology and Medicine, London, UK*

CRAIG W. RITCHIE · *Centre for Clinical Brain Sciences, University of Edinburgh, Edinburgh, UK*

ELENA RODRIGUEZ-VIEITEZ · *Division of Translational Alzheimer Neurobiology, Center for Alzheimer Research, Department of Neurobiology, Care Sciences and Society, Karolinska Institutet, Stockholm, Sweden*

MAGDALENA SASTRE · *Division of Brain Sciences, Imperial College London, Hammersmith Hospital, London, UK*

ANA SAYAGO · *Department of Chemistry, Faculty of Experimental Sciences, University of Huelva, Huelva, Spain; International Campus of Excellence CeiA3, University of Huelva, Huelva, Spain*

MATTEO STOCCHERO · *Department of Women's and Children's Health, University of Padova, Padova, Italy*

LUISA STURIALE · *CNR, Istituto per i Polimeri, Compositi e i Biomateriali Catania, Catania, Italy*

PETROS TAKOUSIS · *Neuroepidemiology and Ageing Research Unit, School of Public Health, Imperial College, London, UK*

SAC-PHARM TANG · *Imanova Limited, London, UK*

TESSA TIMMERS · *Department of Neurology and Alzheimer Center, Neuroscience Campus Amsterdam, VU University Medical Center, Amsterdam, The Netherlands; Department of Radiology and Nuclear Medicine, Neuroscience Campus Amsterdam, VU University Medical Center, Amsterdam, The Netherlands*

NICOLA TOSCHI · *Department of Biomedicine and Prevention, University of Rome "Tor Vergata", Rome, Italy; Department of Radiology "Athinoula A. Martinos", Center for Biomedical Imaging, Boston, MA, USA; Harvard Medical School, Boston, MA, USA*

SARA TROMBELLA · *Faculty of Medicine, Nuclear Medicine Department, Geneva University Medical Center, University of Geneva, Geneva, Switzerland*

PAUL G. UNSCHULD · *Institute for Regenerative Medicine and Hospital for Psychogeriatric Medicine, University of Zurich, Zurich, Switzerland*

MARIA I. VARGAS · *Faculty of Medicine, Nuclear Medicine Department, Geneva University Medical Center, University of Geneva, Geneva, Switzerland; Division of Neuroradiology, Geneva University Hospitals, Geneva, Switzerland*

JONATHAN VOGELGSANG · *Department of Psychiatry and Psychotherapy, University Medical Center Goettingen, Georg-August-University, Goettingen, Germany*

JENS WILTFANG · *Department of Psychiatry and Psychotherapy, University Medical Center Goettingen, Georg-August-University, Goettingen, Germany; German Center for Neurodegenerative Diseases (DZNE), Goettingen, Germany; Medical Sciences Department, iBiMED, University of Aveiro, Aveiro, Portugal*

FRANK J. WOLTERS · *Department of Epidemiology, Erasmus Medical Centre, Rotterdam, The Netherlands*

RANDALL L. WOLTJER · *Department of Neurology, Oregon Health Science University and Portland VA Medical Center, Portland, OR, USA*

PAUL L. WOOD · *Metabolomics Unit, College of Veterinary Medicine, Lincoln Memorial University, Harrogate, TN, USA*

MARIO ZAPPIA · *Section of Neurosciences, Department of GF Ingrassia, University of Catania, Catania, Italy*

YIQIANG ZHAN · *Department of Medical Epidemiology and Biostatistics, Karolinska Institutet, Stockholm, Sweden*

Part I

The Need for Alzheimer's Disease Biomarkers

Chapter 1

Epidemiology of Dementia: The Burden on Society, the Challenges for Research

Frank J. Wolters and M. Arfan Ikram

Abstract

Dementia is among the leading causes of death and disability. Due to the ageing population, its prevalence is expected to nearly triple worldwide by 2050, urging the development of preventive and curative interventions. Various modifiable risk factors have been identified in community-based cohort studies, but insight into the underlying pathophysiological mechanisms is lacking. Clinical trials have thus far failed in the development of disease-modifying therapy in patients with dementia, thereby triggering a shift of focus toward the presymptomatic phase of disease. The extensive preclinical disease course of Alzheimer's disease warrants reliable, easily obtainable biomarkers to aid in timely application of preventive strategies, selecting participants for neuroprotective trials, and disease monitoring in trials and clinical practice. Biomarker and drug discovery may yield the fruits from technology-driven developments in the field of genomics, epigenetics, metabolomics, and brain imaging. In that context, bridging the gap between translational and population research may well prove a giant leap toward development of successful preventive and curative interventions against dementia.

Key words Dementia, Alzheimer's disease, Epidemiology, Population-based, Omics, Prevention, Genetics, Imaging

1 Introduction: The Burden of Disease

At present, 48 million people worldwide are suffering from dementia, and this number is projected to increase to 131 million by 2050 [1]. The enormous burden this poses on patients, their caregivers, and society as a whole is only in part reflected by the estimated $818 billion per annum needed for dementia care worldwide. Costs for dementia already exceed those for any other disease [2, 3], and as the number of patients with dementia grows the annual health expenditure is projected to reach one trillion dollars as soon as 2018 [1]. Every year, nearly ten million people develop dementia, with a median age at diagnosis of around 80 years (Fig. 1). Similar to other disorders with steeply increasing prevalence at higher ages, the burden of dementia arises predominantly from disability rather than mortality. In industrialized countries, 80% of those in care homes

Robert Perneczky (ed.), *Biomarkers for Alzheimer's Disease Drug Development*, Methods in Molecular Biology, vol. 1750, https://doi.org/10.1007/978-1-4939-7704-8_1, © Springer Science+Business Media, LLC 2018

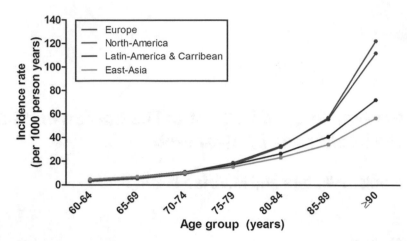

Fig. 1 Age-specific incidence of dementia per geographic area. Data source: World Alzheimer Report, 2015

have dementia or significant cognitive problems, and despite good care less than half experience a good quality of life [4]. Prior to institutionalization, caregivers alleviate much of the burden of disease, but often at the cost of their own well-being [5].

Meanwhile, health expenditure continues to fall short in anticipating long-term care costs. A 2012 study in the UK found that every £10 of health and social care costs attributable to dementia are counterbalanced by only £0.08 for dementia research [6]. This is particularly striking, as investments in long-term prevention are projected to result in cost-effective gains in quality-adjusted life years in the population [7]. Driven by the projections of the burden on public health, governments have only recently designated dementia as a major public health threat, and started to prioritize research in their federal budgets accordingly. This will undoubtedly spark advances in research and clinical care, but time is not on our side. Subclinical alterations in brain health are thought to occur decades before diagnosis of dementia [8], and the social and economic burden of dementia will thus increase enormously, unless curative and preventive measures can be rapidly established.

As the burden of dementia grows across the globe, the largest increase will occur in low- and middle-income countries, such that by 2050 roughly two-thirds of people with dementia will live in these regions (Fig. 2). Yet, only a minority of patients receive (extensive) investigation or a formal diagnosis, particularly in settings poor in resources [9, 10]. Together with differences in patient care, the low rate of diagnoses accounts for a stark contrast in global healthcare expenditure, where over 90% of current dementia care costs are incurred in high-income countries [11]. It shows above all that wide availability and accessibility of diagnostics, preventive measures, and feature disease-modifying agents will be vital to control the global dementia epidemic.

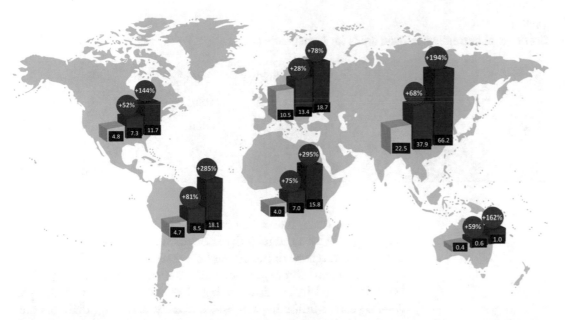

Fig. 2 The numbers of people living with dementia in millions (black box) per geographic area in 2015 (light grey), with projections for 2030 (dark blue) and 2050 (dark grey). Corresponding percentage increase compared to 2015 is depicted in red labels. Data source: World Alzheimer Report, 2015

In this chapter, we shall provide a brief overview of the current state of affairs in preventive and curative medicine, and highlight the main challenges and opportunities encountered in etiological research and drug development.

2   Preventive and Curative Efforts: Small Successes in the Light of Failure

The urgency for new drugs is reflected in a steep increase in the number of trials registered for drugs against Alzheimer's disease. Over the past 20 years, hundreds of registered trials set out to determine the efficacy of potential drugs for dementia, but this has resulted in only four drugs offering limited symptom relief (Table 1), while thus far no disease-modifying therapies are available. The cost of these trials culminates to billions of euros. Of 244 compounds that were assessed in 413 trials in the past decade, none have made it to the market since the approval of *memantine* for symptom relief in 2003 [12]. Of every 100 compounds entering phase 1 trials for Alzheimer's disease, 28% make it to phase 2, in which 8% succeed [12]. For comparison, success rates of phase 1 and phase 2 trials for infectious disease are 70% and 43%, respectively, while for cardiovascular disease these percentages are 59% and 24% [13]. As of 2016, another large phase 3 Alzheimer trial, assessing the efficacy of amyloid antibody *solanezumab*, has joined the long list of unsuccessful intervention for (mild) Alzheimer's disease, along with the 5-HT6 antagonist *idalopirdine* that was aimed

Table 1
Overview of currently approved drugs for Alzheimer's disease

Generic drug (brand name)	Approval for disease stage	Year of approval	Indication
Donepezil (Aricept)	All stages	1996	Symptom relief
Rivastigmine (Exelon)	All stages	2000	Symptom relief
Galantamine (Razadyne)	Mild-moderate	2001	Symptom relief
Memantine (Namenda)	Moderate-severe	2003	Symptom relief

at symptom relief. Nevertheless, over 20 phase 3 trials are currently ongoing, of which the majority is directed against amyloid, either by antibodies, vaccines, or inhibiting beta-secretase 1 (BACE).

With regard to prevention, various modifiable risk factors have been identified in community-based cohort studies over the past 20–30 years. Midlife hypertension, obesity, smoking, diabetes mellitus, low educational attainment, and physical activity are consistently associated with an increased risk of disease, and account for about 25% of all cases of dementia [14, 15]. As these risk factors are largely shared with other (cardiovascular) diseases, improvements in cardiovascular risk management may have had positive effects on dementia risk over the past decades also. In fact, multiple reports now suggest a decline in the incidence of dementia in industrialized countries by about 20% per decade since the 1970s [16–18]. However, the precise causes of this trend have not been accounted for, data from low- and middle-income countries are not available, and even if the current trend continues it will not suffice to offset the effects of a rapidly ageing population on the number of patients with dementia. In addition, trials assessing the efficacy of specific preventive interventions for lowering the risk of dementia have thus far been largely unsuccessful [19]. Following the failures of these dementia prevention trials in the late 1990s and early 2000s, subsequent trials have determined the effect of interventions on cognition as a more sensitive outcome measure than dementia, with more positive results in particular for trials assessing the efficacy of physical activity and multi-domain interventions [19]. For example, the Scandinavian FINGER trial (a multi-domain intervention involving diet, exercise, vascular risk monitoring, and cognitive training) has shown benefit on cognitive function [20], and participants continue to be surveyed for the incidence of dementia. Despite generally modest effect sizes at the individual level, these preventive efforts could greatly reduce the burden of disease at the population level. If preventive efforts succeed in delaying the onset of dementia by merely 5 years, this could reduce the incidence of dementia by as much as 50% over the next decades [3]. Yet again, in an unselected population of elderly Dutch people (the preDIVA trial), multidomain vascular care intervention did not significantly lower dementia incidence, and the French Multi-domain Alzheimer Prevention Trial (MAPT—testing similar interventions plus omega-3 supplements) found no significant benefit on cognitive decline over a 3-year period [21, 22]. These inconsistencies across trials employing closely aligned interventions emphasize that much work remains to be done to understand the specific pathways underlying successes and failures of these preventive trials.

Summarizing the small successes and many disappointing past attempts to halt dementia at any stage of disease, the question rises why so many efforts have thus far failed. What are the difficulties medical research faces in developing treatments against dementia and specifically Alzheimer's disease, while successful battles have been fought against many other similarly common and age-related diseases? The next section will therefore focus on the challenges and opportunities in striving to improve the process and outcomes of drug discovery.

3   Challenges in Clinical Trials

Part of the lagging behind of dementia treatments, compared to improvements in treatment of cardiovascular disease and cancer, could be linked to lack of research funding [6]. Every £10 of health and social care costs attributable to dementia are counterbalanced by £0.08 for dementia research in the UK, compared with £1.08 for cancer and £0.65 for heart disease [6]. This 8–14-fold difference in research investment may reflect the differences in disease perception and heterogeneous nature of cancer as a disease entity, as well as less direct effects of preventive measures for dementia, compared to acute vascular events. Today's intervention might prevent tomorrow's myocardial infarction, whereas the long preclinical phase of dementia precludes return of investment within several years from initiation of preventive measures. Nevertheless, a Swedish-Finnish study that modeled cost and utilities of such investments suggests that long-term prevention can in fact result in a cost-effective gain in quality-adjusted life years in the population [7], emphasizing the necessity of prioritizing dementia research funding.

Other challenges in dementia research pertain to the disease course and impairment of dementia itself, which make it different from other diseases that medicine has successfully engaged. These include high attrition rates in trials, insensitive or inaccurate outcome assessments [23], and—perhaps foremost—a long and variable presymptomatic disease phase that has repeatedly been put forward as an explanation for why so many clinical trials have failed. By the time of diagnosis, the brain of patients with dementia shows high degrees of degeneration that vary greatly across patients and are unlikely to be ameliorated by treatment. Moreover, markers for risk of neurodegeneration may arise years before diagnosis of dementia [8], and intervention at the time of disease may consequently be too late. Trials have therefore moved from including patients in any stage of disease to those with mild dementia only, and, driven by yet again disappointing results, ongoing trials now focus on presymptomatic individuals. As such, the Alzheimer Prevention Initiative's A4 trial currently enrols cognitively healthy individuals in the USA, Canada, and Australia for 39 months of treatment with intravenous *solanezumab* or placebo (ClinicalTrials.gov Identifier NCT02008357). However, when targeting earlier, presymptomatic stages of the disease, enrichment of people at highest risk of developing the disease is vital for the trial to be sufficiently powered. Strategies for enrichment include targeting individuals who are at increased genetic risk, and several studies now focus exclusively on genetically high-risk individuals, such as *crenezumab* for preclinical PSEN1 mutation carriers of Colombian kindred (ClinicalTrials.gov Identifier NCT01998841), and the Generation Study for individuals aged 60–75 years who carry two copies of the apolipoprotein E epsilon 4 allele (ClinicalTrials.gov Identifier NCT02565511). Although this might in part circumvent the problem of eleventh-hour interventions, it could render results less applicable to the large population at risk due to the strong selection on relatively rare genetic variants. In addition, time to event in these preventive trials remains prolonged, making them costly and unable to provide rapid answers to urgent questions. The feasibility of future trials will therefore depend on the ability to either recruit (representative) individuals at risk of developing disease during the trial period or develop reliable biomarkers that can serve as surrogate endpoints for preventive trials.

4   Biomarkers and Treatment Targets: The Search Continues

Risk stratification of individuals for a certain disease generally starts with easily obtainable demographics and details about personal history. This approach has been highly effective in predicting for instance long-term risk of cardiovascular disease in the community [24], short-term risk of stroke in patients with transient ischemic attack [25], or odds of having pulmonary embolism [26]. However, for dementia, such simple models using demographics and personal history have thus far proven of limited predictive value in the general population [27]. Of potential predictors, educational attainment, a positive family history, and subjective memory complaints appear most informative, but their incremental value over merely age and gender is limited. In the setting of memory clinics, additional, more advanced tools are generally available for diagnosis. Biomarker levels of (phosphorylated) tau and β-amyloid in cerebrospinal fluid are consistently associated with a diagnosis of dementia or mild cognitive impairment due to AD [28], but this does not automatically translate into improved diagnostic accuracy above and beyond clinical observations [29]. Similarly, prediction of conversion from mild cognitive impairment to dementia might be improved by advanced (PET) imaging, but currently available data are deemed insufficient to recommend these expensive investigations for routine use in clinical setting [30]. Regardless, the stage at which patients present at memory clinics may be too late in the disease process to initiate a prevention trial, because those patients are symptomatic per definition. Standardization of any marker will be vital to prevent the large inter-site variability in measurements that currently hampers definition of prediction rules across clinical sites [31]. Moreover, diagnostic value cannot simply be inferred from association studies, and diagnostic accuracy strongly depends on the screening strategy and setting [32]. For example a biomarker with high sensitivity and low specificity can be very useful as a first screening phase in primary care, while it will likely not be very helpful in clinical setting. Similarly, a biomarker that is more reflective of late-state disease can be very useful in the monitoring disease course, whereas it will be of limited value in risk stratification in asymptomatic individuals. Screening strategy and setting will also largely affect cost-effectiveness, which should be taken into account in the development of any biomarker. While investigations in memory clinics generally include state-of-the-art brain imaging and cerebrospinal fluid samples, screening strategies in the general population, by contrast, should rely on more readily attainable measures from for instance blood, urine, or saliva. In any case, high intra-individual reliability is essential for disease monitoring, and for these tests to be applied in clinical trials. Given the multifactorial nature of dementia, incremental value of biomarkers for the prediction of dementia, or even Alzheimer's disease, is likely to be found only by the combination of multiple entities, rather than individual markers. Lastly, any candidate (set of) biomarker(s) will require validation in independent samples to confirm and establish their predictive value.

Similar to biomarker development, identification and validation of potential treatment targets is an important combined task for population, clinical, and translational medicine. As highlighted above, many modifiable risk factors for dementia have been identified, but lack of understanding of their biological underpinning has long hampered drug development. Amyloid has been the major target for drug interventions, but the string of negative trial results has led to fierce criticism in the field that amyloid might be a downstream result of changes leading to Alzheimer's disease [33]. The challenge for alternative theories is to explain why amyloid accumulates in the brain if it is not causing neurodegeneration while proposing reasonable alternative mechanisms for neurodegeneration in Alzheimer's disease. Alternatives that have been put forward include (but are not limited to) mechanisms related to microvascular function and neurovascular coupling, inflammation, angiogenesis, and lipid or iron metabolism. While these ideas frequently originate from observations in clinical or population studies, identification of the biological underpinning of these mechanisms relies on translational medicine. Yet, also at the preclinical stage, models in the past decades have been mostly aimed at overexpression of amyloid or tau, thereby overlooking a range of important determinants of dementia in population studies. Animal models are generally built on rare familial types of Alzheimer's disease, and may therefore not reflect the pathology of the common late onset, in which for example vascular disease and diabetes are prominent features. Although therapeutic targets may produce desired effects in transgenic mouse models, current animal studies have not been able to aid discovery of Alzheimer therapy, and have consequently faced criticism about questionable validity to reflect human disease [34]. At the same time, limitations to in vivo imaging of amyloid and tau have long precluded etiological research of amyloid and tau in humans, and still the required tracers at a price of around €1500 per acquired brain scan are generally beyond the scope of (large) population studies. Aside efforts to incorporate these types of research on a population level, the matching of findings from preclinical models to observations in clinical and population studies is vital to unravel pathophysiological mechanisms. It is this translation of group differences to the individual variation that is the biological underpinning of the disease. Understanding the interindividual differences in pathology and clinical presentation is the step forward to developing and electing proper treatments for very individual (future) patient.

5 Big Data and Precision Medicine

"Doctors have always recognized that every patient is unique, and doctors have always tried to tailor their treatments as best they can to individuals. You can match a blood transfusion to a blood type – that was an important discovery. What if matching a cancer cure to our genetic code was just as easy, just as standard? What if figuring out the right dose of medicine was as simple as taking our temperature?" With these words US President Barack Obama kicked of the Precision Medicine Initiative in early 2015. Aside short-term goals for personalizing cancer care, the long-term ambitions of the program focus on all areas of health, including neurological disease. And given the multifactorial and complex pathophysiological nature of dementia, a personalized approach in the development of interventions may benefit dementia as much as cancer therapy.

Over the past decades, the quest for unraveling the etiology of common diseases has led to instigation of multiple large studies in the general population. These studies' sizes range from 10,000 to 15,000 participants for community-based cohorts like the Framingham Heart Study and the Rotterdam Study [35, 36] to an intended 500,000 subjects examined for the UK Biobank and

1,000,000 for the US Precision Medicine Initiative. Already, these types of studies have shown to be valuable in identifying genetic risk alleles and imaging markers predisposing for dementia. Since the first genome-wide association studies in the early 2000s, increasingly large quantities of genetic data have revolutionized the way aforementioned research questions can be addressed. Together with epigenetics and proteomics, genomics and neuroimaging have yielded previously unimagined opportunities to obtain rich information about the influence of an individual's biological sketch and the environment on virtually any phenotype. But big data does not just allude to large quantity. More than sheer numbers, it is the opportunities presented by the combination of aforementioned modalities that allows hypothesis free research of the -omics data. Also, the linkage of these cohort data to potential drug targets holds promise for drug development, as is increasingly acknowledged among researchers, funding agencies (e.g., the U.S. National Institutes of Health BD2K project), pharmaceutical industry, and consultant companies alike. By no means does such an approach substitute detailed study about disease pathways and singular treatment targets. On the contrary, sometimes this may lead directly to development of new drugs, such as for *PCSK9* inhibitors [37–39], while arguably more often (genetic) data could be applied to increase success rate of drug development by selecting genetically supported drug targets from potential candidates [40, 41]. Also for Alzheimer's disease, genomics approaches have recently shown interest in identifying disease-relevant tissues, variants, and regulators [42].

At the same time, the diverse and often complex methods pose new challenges of their own. Data harmonization, storage, access and sharing, and analysis are some of the main hurdles to large-scale analyses and collaborations that can be taken only by international standardization, improvements in infrastructure for collaboration, and advanced technology for data acquisition, storage, and analyses. In addition, unlike genetic studies, application of proteomics and epigenetics is vulnerable to selection bias, confounding, and other biases that traditionally hamper research [43]. For example, while the UK Biobank achieves its intended 10% response rate [44], this is far lower than the response rates of about 60–80% in population-based cohort studies. Sufficient response rates are important to avoid selection bias and guarantee generalizability of findings to a larger population. Similarly, other fundamentals of epidemiology need to be upheld, such as avoidance of attrition, accuracy of outcome assessment, and accounting for potential biases. These methodological challenges cannot be counterbalanced by quantity, and warrant careful study design and choice of appropriate methods for data analysis. If, and only if, these hurdles can be overcome, the combination of powerful computational methods and large-scale -omics data with biological information about the disease from translational models has the potential to boost drug discovery and biomarker development. It may well be the bridge between observations in large-scale population data and (molecular) biology of a disease that can transform the -omics era into that of precision medicine, with Alzheimer's disease as one of its primary targets.

6   Concluding Remarks

The increasingly heavy burden of dementia on society poses one of the greatest challenges for modern medicine. Despite our best efforts, to date no disease-modifying treatments have evolved from identification of various risk factors in (clinical) populations. It is therefore not simply an option, but a necessity to combine insights and approaches in laboratory, clinics, and population setting toward the development of biomarkers and treatments for dementia. Science presents us with an increasing number of research tools to this aim. In the coming years, we are to use these tools inventively and in compliance with fundamental epidemiological principles, if we are to fulfil the potential for the development of preventive and curative interventions that these approaches hold.

References

1. Alzheimer's Disease International (2016) World Alzheimer Report 2016 alz.co.uk

2. Kelley AS, McGarry K, Gorges R, Skinner JS (2015) The burden of health care costs for patients with dementia in the last 5 years of life. Ann Intern Med 163:729–736

3. Winblad B, Amouyel P, Andrieu S, Ballard C, Brayne C, Brodaty H, Cedazo-Minguez A, Dubois B, Edvardsson D, Feldman H, Fratiglioni L, Frisoni GB, Gauthier S, Georges J, Graff C, Iqbal K, Jessen F, Johansson G, Jönsson L, Kivipelto M, Knapp M, Mangialasche F, Melis R, Nordberg A, Rikkert MO, Qiu C, Sakmar TP, Scheltens P, Schneider LS, Sperling R, Tjernberg LO, Waldemar G, Wimo A, Zetterberg H (2016) Defeating Alzheimer's disease and other dementias: a priority for European science and society. Lancet Neurol 15:455–532

4. Alzheimer's Society UK (2013) Low expectations. Attitudes on choice, care and community for people with dementia in care homes, 2013 edn. alzheimers.org.uk

5. Etters L, Goodall D, Harrison BE (2008) Caregiver burden among dementia patient caregivers: a review of the literature. J Am Acad Nurse Pract 20:423–428

6. Luengo-Fernandez R, Leal J, Gray A (2015) UK research spend in 2008 and 2012: comparing stroke, cancer, coronary heart disease and dementia. BMJ Open 5:e006648

7. Zhang Y, Kivipelto M, Solomon A, Wimo A (2011) Cost-effectiveness of a health intervention program with risk reductions for getting demented: results of a Markov model in a Swedish/Finnish setting. J Alzheimers Dis 26:735–744

8. Jack CR, Knopman DS, Jagust WJ, Petersen RC, Weiner MW, Aisen PS, Shaw LM, Vemuri P, Wiste HJ, Weigand SD, Lesnick TG, Pankratz VS, Donohue MC, Trojanowski JQ (2013) Tracking pathophysiological processes in Alzheimer's disease: an updated hypothetical model of dynamic biomarkers. Lancet Neurol 12:207–216

9. Jitapunkul S, Chansirikanjana S, Thamarpirat J (2009) Undiagnosed dementia and value of serial cognitive impairment screening in developing countries: a population-based study. Geriatr Gerontol Int 9:47–53

10. Savva GM, Arthur A (2015) Who has undiagnosed dementia? A cross-sectional analysis of participants of the Aging, Demographics and Memory Study. Age Ageing 44:642–647

11. Anonymous (2015) A global assessment of dementia, now and in the future. Lancet 386:931

12. Cummings JL, Morstorf T, Zhong K (2014) Alzheimer's disease drug-development

pipeline: few candidates, frequent failures. Alzheimers Res Ther 6:37

13. Biotechnology Innovation Organization, Biomedtracker, Amplion Clinical Development Success Rates 2006–2015, 2016 edn. bio.org

14. de Bruijn RFAG, Bos MJ, Portegies MLP, Hofman A, Franco OH, Koudstaal PJ, Ikram MA (2015) The potential for prevention of dementia across two decades: the prospective, population-based Rotterdam Study. BMC Med 13:132

15. Norton S, Matthews FE, Barnes DE, Yaffe K, Brayne C (2014) Potential for primary prevention of Alzheimer's disease: an analysis of population-based data. Lancet Neurol 13:788–794

16. Matthews FE, Stephan BCM, Robinson L, Jagger C, Barnes LE, Arthur A, Brayne C, Collaboration CFaASC (2016) A two decade dementia incidence comparison from the Cognitive Function and Ageing Studies I and II. Nat Commun 7:11398

17. Satizabal CL, Beiser AS, Chouraki V, Chêne G, Dufouil C, Seshadri S (2016) Incidence of dementia over three decades in the Framingham Heart Study. N Engl J Med 374:523–532

18. Schrijvers EMC, Verhaaren BFJ, Koudstaal PJ, Hofman A, Ikram MA, Breteler MMB (2012) Is dementia incidence declining? Trends in dementia incidence since 1990 in the Rotterdam Study. Neurology 78:1456–1463

19. Andrieu S, Coley N, Lovestone S, Aisen PS, Vellas B (2015) Prevention of sporadic Alzheimer's disease: lessons learned from clinical trials and future directions. Lancet Neurol 14:926–944

20. Ngandu T, Lehtisalo J, Solomon A, Levälahti E, Ahtiluoto S, Antikainen R, Bäckman L, Hänninen T, Jula A, Laatikainen T, Lindström J, Mangialasche F, Paajanen T, Pajala S, Peltonen M, Rauramaa R, Stigsdotter-Neely A, Strandberg T, Tuomilehto J, Soininen H, Kivipelto M (2015) A 2 year multidomain intervention of diet, exercise, cognitive training, and vascular risk monitoring versus control to prevent cognitive decline in at-risk. elderly people (FINGER): a randomised controlled trial. Lancet 385(9984):2255–2263

21. Andrieu S, Guyonnet S, Coley N, Cantet C, Bonnefoy M, Bordes S, Bories L, Cufi M-N, Dantoine T, Dartigues J-F, Desclaux F, Gabelle A, Gasnier Y, Pesce A, Sudres K, Touchon J, Robert P, Rouaud O, Legrand P, Payoux P, Caubere J-P, Weiner M, Carrié I, Ousset P-J, Vellas B, Group MS (2017) Effect of long-term omega 3 polyunsaturated fatty acid supplementation with or without multidomain intervention on cognitive function in elderly adults with memory complaints (MAPT): a randomised, placebo-controlled trial. Lancet Neurol 16:377–389

22. Moll van Charante EP, Richard E, Eurelings LS, van Dalen J-W, Ligthart SA, van Bussel EF, Hoevenaar-Blom MP, Vermeulen M, van Gool WA (2016) Effectiveness of a 6-year multidomain vascular care intervention to prevent dementia (preDIVA): a cluster-randomised controlled trial. Lancet 388:797–805

23. Knopman DS (2008) Clinical trial design issues in mild to moderate Alzheimer disease. Cogn Behav Neurol 21:197–201

24. Wilson PW, D'Agostino RB, Levy D, Belanger AM, Silbershatz H, Kannel WB (1998) Prediction of coronary heart disease using risk factor categories. Circulation 97:1837–1847

25. Rothwell PM, Giles MF, Flossmann E, Lovelock CE, Redgrave JNE, Warlow CP, Mehta Z (2005) A simple score (ABCD) to identify individuals at high early risk of stroke after transient ischaemic attack. Lancet 366:29–36

26. Wells PS, Anderson DR, Rodger M, Stiell I, Dreyer JF, Barnes D, Forgie M, Kovacs G, Ward J, Kovacs MJ (2001) Excluding pulmonary embolism at the bedside without diagnostic imaging: management of patients with suspected pulmonary embolism presenting to the emergency department by using a simple clinical model and d-dimer. Ann Intern Med 135:98–107

27. Tang EYH, Harrison SL, Errington L, Gordon MF, Visser PJ, Novak G, Dufouil C, Brayne C, Robinson L, Launer LJ, Stephan BCM (2015) Current developments in dementia risk prediction modelling: an updated systematic review. PLoS One 10:e0136181

28. Olsson B, Lautner R, Andreasson U, Öhrfelt A, Portelius E, Bjerke M, Hölttä M, Rosén C, Olsson C, Strobel G, Wu E, Dakin K, Petzold M, Blennow K, Zetterberg H (2016) CSF and blood biomarkers for the diagnosis of Alzheimer's disease: a systematic review and meta-analysis. Lancet Neurol 15:673–684

29. Ritchie C, Smailagic N, Noel-Storr AH, Takwoingi Y, Flicker L, Mason SE, McShane R (2014) Plasma and cerebrospinal fluid amyloid beta for the diagnosis of Alzheimer's disease dementia and other dementias in people with mild cognitive impairment (MCI). Cochrane Database Syst Rev (6):CD008782

30. Zhang S, Smailagic N, Hyde C, Noel-Storr AH, Takwoingi Y, McShane R, Feng J (2014) (11)C-PIB-PET for the early diagnosis of Alzheimer's disease dementia and other dementias in people with mild cognitive impairment (MCI). Cochrane Database Syst Rev (7):CD010386

31. Mattsson N, Andreasson U, Persson S, Carrillo MC, Collins S, Chalbot S, Cutler N, Dufour-Rainfray D, Fagan AM, Heegaard NHH, Robin Hsiung G-Y, Hyman B, Iqbal K, Kaeser SA, Käser SA, Lachno DR, Lleó A, Lewczuk P, Molinuevo JL, Parchi P, Regeniter A, Rissman RA, Rissman R, Rosenmann H, Sancesario G, Schröder J, Shaw LM, Teunissen CE, Trojanowski JQ, Vanderstichele H, Vandijck M, Verbeek MM, Zetterberg H, Blennow K, Group AAQPW (2013) CSF biomarker variability in the Alzheimer's Association quality control program. Alzheimers Dement 9:251–261

32. Sackett DL, Haynes RB (2002) The architecture of diagnostic research. BMJ 324:539–541

33. Drachman DA (2014) The amyloid hypothesis, time to move on: amyloid is the downstream result, not cause, of Alzheimer's disease. Alzheimers Dement 10:372–380

34. Saito T, Matsuba Y, Mihira N, Takano J, Nilsson P, Itohara S, Iwata N, Saido TC (2014) Single App knock-in mouse models of Alzheimer's disease. Nat Neurosci 17:661–663

35. Feinleib M, Kannel WB, Garrison RJ, McNamara PM, Castelli WP (1975) The Framingham Offspring Study. Design and preliminary data. Prev Med 4:518–525

36. Hofman A, Brusselle GGO, Darwish Murad S, van Duijn CM, Franco OH, Goedegebure A, Ikram MA, Klaver CCW, Nijsten TEC, Peeters RP, Stricker BHC, Tiemeier HW, Uitterlinden AG, Vernooij MW (2015) The Rotterdam Study: 2016 objectives and design update. Eur J Epidemiol 30:661–708

37. Robinson JG, Farnier M, Krempf M, Bergeron J, Luc G, Averna M, Stroes ES, Langslet G, Raal FJ, El Shahawy M, Koren MJ, Lepor NE, Lorenzato C, Pordy R, Chaudhari U, Kastelein JJP, Investigators OLT (2015) Efficacy and safety of alirocumab in reducing lipids and cardiovascular events. N Engl J Med 372:1489–1499

38. Sabatine MS, Giugliano RP, Wiviott SD, Raal FJ, Blom DJ, Robinson J, Ballantyne CM, Somaratne R, Legg J, Wasserman SM, Scott R, Koren MJ, Stein EA, Investigators O-LSoL-TEaLCO (2015) Efficacy and safety of evolocumab in reducing lipids and cardiovascular events. N Engl J Med 372:1500–1509

39. Willer CJ, Sanna S, Jackson AU, Scuteri A, Bonnycastle LL, Clarke R, Heath SC, Timpson NJ, Najjar SS, Stringham HM, Strait J, Duren WL, Maschio A, Busonero F, Mulas A, Albai G, Swift AJ, Morken MA, Narisu N, Bennett D, Parish S, Shen H, Galan P, Meneton P, Hercberg S, Zelenika D, Chen W-M, Li Y, Scott LJ, Scheet PA, Sundvall J, Watanabe RM, Nagaraja R, Ebrahim S, Lawlor DA, Ben-Shlomo Y, Davey-Smith G, Shuldiner AR, Collins R, Bergman RN, Uda M, Tuomilehto J, Cao A, Collins FS, Lakatta E, Lathrop GM, Boehnke M, Schlessinger D, Mohlke KL, Abecasis GR (2008) Newly identified loci that influence lipid concentrations and risk of coronary artery disease. Nat Genet 40:161–169

40. Nelson MR, Tipney H, Painter JL, Shen J, Nicoletti P, Shen Y, Floratos A, Sham PC, Li MJ, Wang J, Cardon LR, Whittaker JC, Sanseau P (2015) The support of human genetic evidence for approved drug indications. Nat Genet 47:856–860

41. Patel MN, Halling-Brown MD, Tym JE, Workman P, Al-Lazikani B (2013) Objective assessment of cancer genes for drug discovery. Nat Rev Drug Discov 12:35–50

42. Gjoneska E, Pfenning AR, Mathys H, Quon G, Kundaje A, Tsai L-H, Kellis M (2015) Conserved epigenomic signals in mice and humans reveal immune basis of Alzheimer's disease. Nature 518:365–369

43. Ikram MA (2015) Molecular pathological epidemiology: the role of epidemiology in the omics-era. Eur J Epidemiol 30:1077–1078

44. Watts G (2007) UK Biobank gets 10% response rate as it starts recruiting volunteers. BMJ 334:659

Chapter 2

Population-Based Approaches to Alzheimer's Disease Prevention

Robert Perneczky

Abstract

Progress in prevention and treatment of Alzheimer's disease (AD) and dementia is hampered by the restricted understanding of the biological and environmental causes underlying pathophysiology. It is widely accepted that certain genetic factors are associated with AD and a number of lifestyle and other environmental characteristics have also been linked to dementia risk. However, interactions between genes and the environment are not yet well understood, and coordinated global action is required to utilize existing cohorts and other resources effectively and efficiently to identify new avenues for dementia prevention. This chapter provides a brief summary of current research on risk and protective factors and opportunities and challenges in relation to population-based approaches are discussed.

Key words Alzheimer's disease, Dementia, Drug development, Population-based, Cohort studies, Lifestyle, Environment, Genetics

1 Introduction

The traditional linear model of pharmaceutical research and development has become outdated and attrition rates have almost been 100% over the last two decades in the field of Alzheimer's disease (AD). At the same time the prevalence of AD and its healthcare and socioeconomic impact are exploding worldwide and drug development success rates need to be improved urgently. Successful drug discovery and development in other fields of medicine, such as cancer and infectious diseases, have shown that translational models linking epidemiological cohort and genetic data to potential drug targets and study end points can lead to success [1]. Technology platforms such as neuroimaging, -omics, and biomarkers have been shown to be powerful tools in this translational process. A significant cultural change has to be initiated to discover and develop novel disease-modifying treatments in the dementia field until 2025, as postulated at the 2013 G8 Dementia Summit [2].

Robert Perneczky (ed.), *Biomarkers for Alzheimer's Disease Drug Development*, Methods in Molecular Biology, vol. 1750, https://doi.org/10.1007/978-1-4939-7704-8_2, © Springer Science+Business Media, LLC 2018

Increased life expectancy is a major achievement of modern society, which however comes at the price of a growing prevalence of age-associated disorders with severe consequences for the global healthcare systems. Within the next 30–40 years, the number of people affected by late-onset neurodegenerative disorders such as AD and Parkinson's disease will globally be three to four times higher than today [3]. The individual risk for these disorders is highly variable and the development of effective preventive and therapeutic strategies is hindered by the still incomplete knowledge about factors influencing the vulnerability to neurodegeneration. There is emerging academic consensus that an individual's susceptibility to AD is determined by both biological and environmental factors, which has important implications for the development of effective treatment options [4]. Even though AD has a significant heritability, monogenic familial forms caused by clearly pathogenic mutations in certain genes are extremely rare; the vast majority of AD cases are likely to be caused by an interplay between common genetic variants and other factors. The biological mechanisms by which genes influence the individual vulnerability to AD are still largely unknown, but recently identified risk genes point to the involvement of certain biological pathways such as immune response and lipid processing [5].

1.1 A Multicausal Model of Alzheimer's Disease

As with most complex diseases, an individual's vulnerability to AD is not exclusively defined by genetic factors, but also by nongenetic determinants such as the environment and epigenetic mechanisms. Genetic susceptibility is innate but risk associated with certain environmental factors may be modifiable and changes in lifestyle may offer a chance to prevent or treat AD. Many of the known environmental risk factors are related to obesity, diabetes mellitus, and vascular disease, all of which can potentially be modified; the impact of protective environmental factors such as Mediterranean diet and cognitive and physical activity can also be actively strengthened. An individual's personality and inherent beliefs affect their behavior and therefore have an important impact on their lifestyle choices and the associated dementia risk [6]. Furthermore, factors outside an individual's control also influence their chronic disease risk, such as the current healthcare system, air pollution, and wider economy (Fig. 1).

2   Epidemiological Approaches to Alzheimer's Disease Research

While the link between AD risk and certain environmental and lifestyle factors seems well established, the biological mechanisms underlying these associations are not yet well understood. The application of high-throughput "omics" technologies to prospective cohort studies with stored biospecimens offers a unique opportunity to phenotype individuals at the molecular level. Cutting-edge

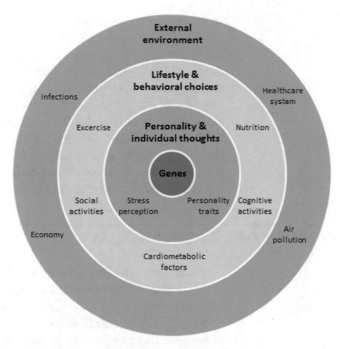

Fig. 1 A multicausal model of Alzheimer's disease

technologies such as epigenomics and metabolomics can be applied to pre-diagnostic biosamples for the detection of early disease markers. Etiological research combining epidemiologic and molecular data, with a focus on gene-environment interactions, can pave the way to the identification of etiopathogenetic pathways via systems biology approaches.

2.1 The Value of Established Global Infrastructures

Worldwide, several large-scale prospective cohort studies on ageing and neurodegenerative disease have been established in the past decades (for a comprehensive listing of European cohorts *see* [7]); the studies have collected detailed dietary, lifestyle, and clinical information, and in some cases biological samples and neuroimaging data, from very large numbers of participants at various points in life. The continued follow-up of these existing infrastructure and a collection of repeated and additional detailed information from these ageing populations is a highly efficient strategy to address the existing knowledge gaps. However, data analysis has so far mostly been restricted to individual cohorts due to differences in assessment procedures and applied methods between countries. Concerted action is therefore urgently required to facilitate the comprehensive analysis of large datasets and to increase knowledge transfer between experts in different countries. It is crucial to achieve standardized data analysis across global ageing and neurodegeneration cohorts and effective networking activities between researchers in the field. The main aims of such networking activities would be to develop harmonized measures for the key outcomes used in the different cohort studies (e.g., genome-wide data, environmental exposures, neuroimaging data, blood and cerebrospinal fluid proteins) and to facilitate knowledge transfer and expert exchanges between countries and institutions, including the best possible training and career opportunities for early-stage researchers. Examples of large-scale initiatives to effectively integrate information from diverse cohorts include the Dementias Platform UK (http://www.dementiasplatform.uk/) and the EU Joint Program for Neurodegenerative Disease Research (JPND) longitudinal cohort studies action group [7].

3   Gene-Environment Interaction Analyses

There is growing consensus that AD and other forms of dementia are the result of both genetic and environmental exposures and their interactions [8, 9]. Subtle differences in DNA sequence composition (e.g., different allele status at polymorphic sites) cause people to respond differently to the same environmental exposure. This at least partly explains why some individuals have a fairly low risk of developing the disease because of an environmental insult, while others are much more vulnerable. For example, not all carriers of the *APOE* ε4 risk allele, the by far most substantial genetic risk factor, develop AD or dementia even very late in life [10]. The presence of unknown gene-environment patterns may also explain the difficulties in detecting other major genetic effects in addition to *APOE*.

All population-based studies so far have consistently shown that 40–50% of people who reach the age of 90 are free of dementia, suggesting that dementia is not an unavoidable event when people are getting older [11]. However, several important questions have yet to be answered, including why certain individuals escape dementia and which genetic and/or environmental features distinguish them from those who develop dementia. Epidemiological studies have already provided some answers to these questions, but the picture lacks several pieces, especially related to the interactions among different factors acting at different times in life.

Previous studies suggested interactions between genes and several environmental factors. Gene-diet interactions for example have been found between the *APOE* gene and nutrients including *n*-3 polyunsaturated fatty acids, vitamin E, and total fat and energy intake in relation to the risk of AD and dementia [12]. Emerging evidence also suggests that vascular changes exacerbate preexistent amyloid-β (Aβ) pathology, thereby leading to a higher risk of AD and dementia; vascular pathology seems to strengthen the risk of AD exerted by the *APOE* ε4 allele [13] and *APOE* ε4 also seems to influence how certain life habits modify cognitive trajectories. For example, the protective effect of regular leisure time physical activity against AD and dementia seems to be more pronounced among *APOE* risk allele carriers [14]. Also, a low vascular burden and a healthy lifestyle seem to modulate the genetic susceptibility [10]. However, evidence on gene-environment interactions beyond *APOE* is scarce.

3.1 Diet and Nutrition

Diet is a major environmental factor that acts during the entire life. In AD, the neurodegenerative process is accompanied by exacerbated inflammation and oxidative stress that could partially be alleviated by several classes of nutrients. Epidemiological studies showed that higher intake or blood levels of several components of the diet were associated with slower cognitive decline or lower risk of AD and dementia, including long-chain *n*-3 polyunsaturated fatty acids [15], antioxidant vitamins C and E, carotenoids, polyphenols, and vitamins B and D [16, 17]. The potential role of fatty acids in AD was emphasized by the discovery of a set of phospholipids measured in peripheral blood that was able to predict the risk of amnestic mild cognitive impairment (MCI) or AD over a 2- to 3-year period with an accuracy of 90% [18]; however, the predictive validity of these biomarkers has yet to be reproduced over a longer follow-up to rule out reverse causality.

Healthy diets that provide combinations of the mentioned nutrients, such as the Mediterranean diet, have also been linked to a lower risk of dementia or cognitive decline [19], which is supported by evidence from a limited number of controlled trials [20, 21]; however, so far most intervention studies with dietary supplements (e.g., *n*-3 polyunsaturated fatty acids, antioxidants, B vitamins) were unsuccessful [22]. Among the many different reasons to explain this failure, it is possible that those studies did not adequately target individuals according to their genetic susceptibility to AD or to genetic characteristics linked to nutrient metabolism [9].

Although few epidemiological studies have investigated this domain, the most widely documented AD gene-diet interaction is related to the *APOE* genotype with *n*-3 polyunsaturated fatty acids (including a controlled trial [23], *see* [12] for a review), vitamin E [24], and total fat and energy intake [25]. These studies yielded conflicting results, showing a protective effect of diet in *APOE* ε4 noncarriers only or in *APOE* ε4 carriers only or no effect at all. However, modest sample sizes in the studies have limited the ability to accurately investigate these nutrient-*APOE* interactions. More recently discovered genetic polymorphisms implied in the risk of AD in large genome-wide association studies (GWAS; e.g., *CLU*, *CR1*, *BIN1*, *PICALM*, or *ABCA7*) could be involved as well but their interaction with diet has yet to be investigated.

There is biological plausibility for interactions between diet and several AD genes, based on their involvement in common pathways. For example, dietary intake of nutrients with antioxidant properties such as vitamins C and E, carotenoids, and polyphenols influences the oxidative status of the body, whereas total antioxidant status and glutathione peroxidase activity are reduced in individuals carrying the *APOE* ε4 allele, suggesting reduced antioxidant defense mechanisms [26]. Furthermore, *n*-3 polyunsaturated fatty acids may modulate systemic inflammation, whereas *CR1*, a novel locus for AD risk, encodes the main receptor of the protein complement C3b, which is involved in inflammatory processes [27]. Some AD genes might also interact with diet, based on their role in nutrient bioavailability, in particular with lipids; for example, *APOE* and *CLU* genes encode the APOE and clusterin (APOJ) apolipoproteins, respectively, which are the most abundantly expressed apolipoproteins in the central nervous system and important regulators of lipid metabolism in the brain. Both APOE and CLU apolipoproteins are involved in the transport of cholesterol and phospholipids [28].

Healthy diets such as the Mediterranean diet and the Dietary Approaches to Stop Hypertension (DASH) provide combinations of nutrients that may impact the inflammatory, metabolic, and oxidative status. Interactions between some of the novel loci associated with AD and the Mediterranean diet on cognitive function have been reported in a subsample from a recent intervention study [29] and these interactions need replication in larger samples. Other potential candidate genes for gene-diet interactions in AD and dementia include variants associated with the metabolism of the most promising candidate nutrients for dementia prevention, as these variants likely impact the bioavailability of the nutrients to the bloodstream and the brain. For example, *FADS1/FADS2* [30] and *ELOVL2* encode fatty acid desaturases and elongases, respectively, which modify plasma levels of long-chain polyunsaturated fatty acids [31] and *BCMO1* encodes beta-carotene 15′-monooxygenase-1 which impacts blood levels of carotenoids [32]; it is thus possible that these genes modify the relation of diet and AD risk. Finally, genes related to more general pathways linking diet to health, such as cholesterol or homocysteine metabolism [33, 34], might also be interesting modulators of the association between diet and AD.

3.2 Physical Activity and Other Active Lifestyles

Active lifestyles, which include physical, cognitive, and social activities, are known to promote good overall and vascular health, and increase functional capacity and quality of life in all age groups. Epidemiological studies indicate that midlife [14] or late-life [35] physical activity is associated with a reduced risk of cognitive impairment, AD, and dementia. Staying physically active, or becoming more active, after midlife also contributes to lowering dementia risk, especially in people who are overweight or obese in midlife. These findings suggest that the window of opportunity for physical activity interventions to prevent dementia may extend from midlife to older ages [36]. Regular leisure time physical activity with at least moderate intensity was associated with a reduced risk for AD and dementia but in some studies even less intensive physical activity (e.g., walking) was protective.

Participation in cognitively stimulating activities [37, 38] and engagement in social activities [39] are linked to lower AD and dementia risk. Education and occupational status were shown to be important determinants of later life cognitive performance [40–42]. Many activities, occupational exposures, and hobbies include several active lifestyle domains (i.e., dancing has physical, mental, and social components) and it is important to explore further their relative importance and interactions. Also, there is regular co-occurrence with life habits and other lifestyle-related and psychosocial risk factors (e.g., unhealthy nutrition, smoking, and stress) and further work using large, long-term studies is needed to understand the interplay between these factors.

The cognitive reserve hypothesis (i.e., the capacity of the brain to cope with pathology to minimize or postpone the clinical expression of AD pathophysiology) was proposed to explain the disjunction between the degree of brain damage and its clinical presentation. Epidemiological studies suggest that lifelong experiences, including educational and occupational attainment, and leisure activities in later life are associated with a higher reserve [43]. However, several mechanisms may mediate the protective effect of an active lifestyle against dementia. Previous experimental studies suggested that physical activity can influence the ageing brain through several mechanisms such as impact on Aβ burden, improving cerebral perfusion, increasing neurogenesis, induction of several gene transcripts, as well as central and peripheral growth factors such as brain-derived neurotrophic factor, which are relevant for the maintenance of cognitive functions [44–46]. Also, physical activity and engagement in cognitive and social activities were associated with both structural and functional brain changes [45].

There is only limited evidence about interactions between active lifestyles and genetic variants. It was reported that the protective effect of regular leisure time physical activity against AD and dementia may be more pronounced among *APOE* ε4 carriers vs. noncarriers [10, 14]. The protective effect of higher education was also reported to be more pronounced in carriers of the *APOE* risk allele [47], and lifetime cognitive activity moderated the *APOE* genotype effect such that cortical Aβ pathology in positron-emission tomography was lower in ε4 carriers that reported higher cognitive activity [48].

APOE has been linked to all the major features in AD pathogenesis including Aβ generation and clearance, neurofibrillary tangle formation, oxidative stress, apoptosis, dysfunction in lipid transport and homeostasis, modulation of intracellular signaling, and synaptic plasticity. In all cases, the presence of the *APOE* ε4 allele has been shown to exacerbate these disturbances, in contrast to the protection seen with other *APOE* isoforms. Because of this and the relatively high frequency of the ε4 allele in the general population, possible *APOE*-lifestyle interactions may have a relevance for dementia prevention (e.g., targeted/tailored interventions for the *APOE* risk allele carriers) [49].

Some evidence also exists for AD risk genes other than *APOE*. It was suggested that individuals at a high genetic risk (estimated by an integration of risk alleles within *PICALM*, *BIN1*, and *CLU*) who maintain a physically active lifestyle show selective benefits in episodic memory performance [50]. However, these findings need to be validated in larger studies and more research is needed to clarify potential gene-physical activity interactions.

3.3 Psychosocial Factors

There is increasing evidence that the development and clinical manifestation of AD in old age is not determined during a restricted period (e.g., old age) but that it is a result of complex interactions between biological factors and environmental exposures over the life course. Psychosocial factors, defined as factors relating to the interrelationships of social variables and individual thoughts and behaviors, as determinants of dementia have recently emerged from several longitudinal population-based studies. There is growing evidence supporting the hypothesis that stress-related psychosocial factors experienced across the life course, such as negative life events during early life, midlife occupational stress, and late-life depression, sleep problems, and perception of psychological stress, play a role in the development of neuropsychiatric disorders such as AD and dementia [39].

The timing of a stressor may determine how much of an impact it will have on the brain. Experience of stress is thought to have a detrimental effect on the brain especially during stages of life when the brain undergoes major changes (e.g., development in early life and deterioration in late life) [51, 52]. Although only few studies have investigated such long-term associations, it was reported that people who experienced two or more stressful life events in early life had significantly smaller amygdala and hippocampal volumes in later life, and those who experienced a late-life event had significantly larger amygdala volumes. In line with these findings, other studies have also shown that history of early parental death or other negative events increases dementia risk [53].

Although the brain is more mature and stable in midlife and therefore should be less vulnerable to environmental insults, stress may still cause a number of physiological reactions in the central nervous, endocrine, immune, and cardiovascular systems, and all of these factors may exacerbate cognitive deficits leading to dementia. Consistent with this notion, midlife occupation-related stress (low control at work and low job demands) was shown to be related to an increased dementia risk [54]. High job strain was related to an increased risk of late-life AD and dementia over a 6-year follow-up period [39]. In addition, it was reported that women who experienced midlife negative life events were at higher risk of AD and dementia over a 38-year follow-up period [55]. These findings suggest that midlife occupational stressors are relevant for AD and dementia risk, and that there may be gender differences in terms of vulnerability to psychological stress from life events experienced in midlife.

During the ageing process the brain loses its plasticity, which is crucial to post-stress dendritic atrophy. Life after retirement may be viewed as a calm period when stressors such as work load and family responsibilities are no longer present; however, old age also encompasses powerful stressors due to important life changes, such as the loss of loved ones and the occurrence of new health problems. Therefore, these stressors and accompanying stress responses may affect functioning due to reduced plasticity of the ageing brain [56]. To date, evidence on late-life stress in relation to the risk of AD and dementia is limited. Late-life depressive symptoms, stress-prone personality traits (high neuroticism in combination with low extraversion) [57], sleep problems [58], and stressful life events [59] were related to an increased risk of dementia.

Several genes were implicated in stress response and stress-related disorders, including *IGF-1R*, *COMT*, *BDNF*, and *IDE*. However, it has not been sufficiently explored so far if these genes interact with the known stressors and how they impact on the related increased AD and dementia risk. For example, individuals carrying the *APOE* ε4 allele may have less effective neural protection and repair mechanisms, and therefore they may be more vulnerable to the effects of environmental factors on cognitive function. Because of the common mechanisms shared by psychosocial factors and *APOE* ε4, it is plausible to hypothesize that these factors have interactive effects on the risk of AD and dementia.

3.4 Cardiometabolic Factors

It is well established that cardiovascular and metabolic pathology affects AD and dementia risk, with various studies showing an association with hypertension [60], arterial stiffness [61], diabetes mellitus [62], smoking [63], hypercholesterolemia [64], and cardiac diseases [65]. Importantly, this link is not only reported with vascular dementia, but also with AD. Cardiometabolic factors have a direct effect on this association as well as serve as mediators for other factors, such as lifestyle and nutrition. For instance, physical activity leads to lower stiffness of the vasculature, better glycemic control, and less cardiac disease. Therefore, physical activity may lower the risk of dementia directly (e.g., via better brain perfusion or improved neurogenesis), but may also exert its effect through any of the three mentioned cardiometabolic factors, all of which affect AD and dementia risk. Similarly, dietary factors can directly affect brain metabolism, and diet may also influence the cardiovascular system, which in turn can affect the brain.

Although cardiometabolic factors have been implicated in the development of all-cause dementia and AD, few studies have examined the association between subclinical atherosclerosis markers and prospective risk of dementia. High values of carotid intima-media thickness were associated with a significantly increased risk of dementia and AD during a 5-year follow-up [66]. Similarly, over a median follow-up of 9 years, the highest quintile of carotid intima-media thickness was related to prospective AD and dementia risk [67]. During up to 14 years of follow-up, multiple measures of carotid atherosclerosis were associated with a significant risk of AD and dementia [68]. All these findings suggest the possibility that early intervention to reduce atherosclerosis may help delay or prevent dementia onset.

Only few studies have evaluated the association between MRI markers of cerebrovascular disease and prospective risk of AD and dementia. Recent MRI studies found that, compared with healthy controls, subjects with AD and MCI show white matter volumetric abnormalities suggestive of reduced white matter integrity [69]. These changes affect complex networks relevant to episodic memory and other cognitive processes, which characterize cognitive impairment and dementia. White matter abnormalities are also associated with an increased risk of progression from MCI to dementia [70]. Overall, the severity of white matter degeneration appears to be higher in advanced clinical stages of dementia, supporting the construct that these abnormalities are part of the relevant pathophysiological processes. Again, these findings may have relevant therapeutic implications because white matter lesions can be prevented through appropriate control of cardiometabolic factors.

Even though the association between cardiometabolic factors, alone or clustered within the concept of metabolic syndrome [71], and risk of AD and dementia is well established, it remains largely unclear how cardiometabolic pathology leads to cognitive impairment. There is evidence suggesting that this effect is at least partly exerted through interaction of cardiometabolic pathology with genetic factors. For instance, many studies have shown that vascular pathology and *APOE* ε4 have a multiplicative rather than an additive effect with regard to risk of AD and dementia [72]. Similar findings were reported with regard to MRI markers of vascular disease and *APOE* ε4. Carriers of the ε4 allele, for example, have more subclinical brain lesions if they suffer from hypertension as well, which could reflect a diminished capacity of neuronal repair in the risk allele carrier group [73]. Conversely, several novel genes recently identified for AD are postulated to be involved in pathways that involve lipid processing and vascular disease [5]. *ABCA7*, a member of a superfamily of cholesterol and phospholipid transporters, is one of several loci involved in both lipid homeostasis and AD risk [74]. This superfamily was shown not only to influence lipids, but also to affect the vessel wall directly [75]. However, putative interactions between cardiometabolic and genetic risk factors of AD and dementia largely remain to be investigated.

4   Conclusions

Developing more effective, ideally disease-modifying, treatment options for AD is a major societal priority, and the integration of existing cohort resources with advanced gene-environment analytical approaches may be an effective means to achieve this goal. After decades of intensive research on AD and other types of dementia, in the past few years disease concepts with a stronger biological focus compared to the traditional clinically oriented classification systems have emerged; consensus regarding these concepts is increasing among specialists in the field. Epidemiological research has shown that AD and dementia are predominantly disorders of older individuals; this means that ageing and dementia are closely related processes, and both are related to lifelong accumulation of biological alterations and organ damage.

Although AD is the most common pathology underlying dementia in adults aged 65 years and older, recent studies suggest that the relationship between AD pathology and expression of dementia is attenuated in the oldest old [76]. The traditional diagnosis of dementia subtypes has been challenged by neuropathological and neuroimaging studies. Those studies have revealed that AD-related lesions are often present in the brain of older adults with intact cognition, and that more than half of the people with a clinical diagnosis of AD at autopsy have other neurodegenerative alterations and cerebrovascular injuries [77]. Moreover, epidemiological research strongly supports a relevant role of lifestyle and cardiovascular risk factors in the development of dementia. Most of these factors are especially relevant if present during middle age, and many of them are also related to cardiovascular disease [78]. Several studies report a decreasing trend of dementia incidence in Europe, possibly due to the decreased vascular burden during the last two to three decades [79, 80]. It is likely that after the age of 75 years, the majority of dementia cases are due to both vascular and neurodegenerative disease of different types. In order to improve dementia prevention worldwide, a closer collaboration of existing and planned population-based studies is required, and associations between biological and external factors should be scrutinized.

Acknowledgments

The author would like to thank the following individuals for their valuable contribution to the chapter: Profs Lefkos Middleton (Imperial College London, UK); Miia Kivipelto and Laura Fratiglioni (Karolinska Institutet Stockholm, Sweden); M. Arfan Ikram (Erasmus University Medical Center Rotterdam, The Netherlands); and Pascale Barberger-Gateau and Cécilia Samieri (Inserm U1219 and Bordeaux University, France).

References

1. Hutter CM, Mechanic LE, Chatterjee N et al (2013) Gene-environment interactions in cancer epidemiology: a National Cancer Institute Think Tank report. Genet Epidemiol 37(7):643–657. https://doi.org/10.1002/gepi.21756
2. The Lancet Neurology (2014) G8 dementia summit: a chance for united action. Lancet Neurol 13(1):1. https://doi.org/10.1016/S1474-4422(13)70275-8
3. Prince M, Wimo A, Guerchet M et al. (2015) World Alzheimer Report 2015—The Global Impact of Dementia: an analysis of prevalence, incidence, cost and trend. London, UK: Alzheimer's Disease International
4. Scheltens P, Blennow K, Breteler MM et al (2016) Alzheimer's disease. Lancet 388(10043):505–517. https://doi.org/10.1016/S0140-6736(15)01124-1
5. Lambert JC, Ibrahim-Verbaas CA, Harold D et al (2013) Meta-analysis of 74,046 individuals identifies 11 new susceptibility loci for Alzheimer's disease. Nat Genet 45(12):1452–1458. https://doi.org/10.1038/ng.2802
6. Terracciano A, Sutin AR, An Y et al (2014) Personality and risk of Alzheimer's disease: new data and meta-analysis. Alzheimers Dement 10(2):179–186. https://doi.org/10.1016/j.jalz.2013.03.002
7. JPND. Longitudinal cohort studies in neurodegeneration research. Report of the JPND Action Group (2013)
8. Elbaz A, Dufouil C, Alperovitch A (2007) Interaction between genes and environment in neurodegenerative diseases. C R Biol 330(4):318–328. https://doi.org/10.1016/j.crvi.2007.02.018
9. Barberger-Gateau P, Lambert JC, Feart C et al (2013) From genetics to dietetics: the contribution of epidemiology to understanding Alzheimer's disease. J Alzheimers Dis 33(Suppl 1):S457–S463. https://doi.org/10.3233/JAD-2012-129019
10. Ferrari C, WL X, Wang HX et al (2013) How can elderly apolipoprotein E epsilon4 carriers remain free from dementia? Neurobiol Aging 34(1):13–21. https://doi.org/10.1016/j.neurobiolaging.2012.03.003
11. Yang Z, Slavin MJ, Sachdev PS (2013) Dementia in the oldest old. Nat Rev Neurol 9(7):382–393. https://doi.org/10.1038/nrneurol.2013.105
12. Barberger-Gateau P, Samieri C, Feart C et al (2011) Dietary omega 3 polyunsaturated fatty acids and Alzheimer's disease: interaction with apolipoprotein E genotype. Curr Alzheimer Res 8(5):479–491
13. Hofman A, Ott A, Breteler MM et al (1997) Atherosclerosis, apolipoprotein E, and prevalence of dementia and Alzheimer's disease in the Rotterdam Study. Lancet 349(9046):151–154. https://doi.org/10.1016/S0140-6736(96)09328-2
14. Rovio S, Kareholt I, Helkala EL et al (2005) Leisure-time physical activity at midlife and the risk of dementia and Alzheimer's disease. Lancet Neurol 4(11):705–711. https://doi.org/10.1016/S1474-4422(05)70198-8
15. Cunnane SC, Plourde M, Pifferi F et al (2009) Fish, docosahexaenoic acid and Alzheimer's disease. Prog Lipid Res 48(5):239–256. https://doi.org/10.1016/j.plipres.2009.04.001
16. Clarke RJ, Bennett DA (2008) B vitamins for prevention of cognitive decline: insufficient evidence to justify treatment. JAMA 300(15):1819–1821. https://doi.org/10.1001/jama.300.15.1819
17. Annweiler C, Montero-Odasso M, Llewellyn DJ et al (2013) Meta-analysis of memory and executive dysfunctions in relation to vitamin D. Journal Alzheimers Dis 37(1):147–171. https://doi.org/10.3233/JAD-130452
18. Mapstone M, Cheema AK, Fiandaca MS et al (2014) Plasma phospholipids identify antecedent memory impairment in older adults. Nat Med 20(4):415–418. https://doi.org/10.1038/nm.3466
19. Feart C, Samieri C, Alles B et al (2013) Potential benefits of adherence to the Mediterranean diet on cognitive health. Proc Nutr Soc 72(1):140–152. https://doi.org/10.1017/S0029665112002959
20. Martinez-Lapiscina EH, Clavero P, Toledo E et al (2013) Virgin olive oil supplementation and long-term cognition: the PREDIMED-NAVARRA randomized, trial. J Nutr Health Aging 17(6):544–552. https://doi.org/10.1007/s12603-013-0027-6
21. Scheltens P, Twisk JW, Blesa R et al (2012) Efficacy of Souvenaid in mild Alzheimer's disease: results from a randomized, controlled trial. J Alzheimers Dis 31(1):225–236. https://doi.org/10.3233/JAD-2012-121189
22. Barberger-Gateau P, Feart C, Samieri C et al (2013) Dietary patterns and dementia. In: Yaffe K (ed) Chronic medical disease and cognitive aging: toward a healthy body and brain. Oxford University Press, New York, pp 197–224
23. Quinn JF, Raman R, Thomas RG et al (2010) Docosahexaenoic acid supplementation and cognitive decline in Alzheimer disease: a randomized trial. JAMA 304(17):1903–1911. https://doi.org/10.1001/jama.2010.1510

24. Morris MC, Evans DA, Bienias JL et al (2002) Dietary intake of antioxidant nutrients and the risk of incident Alzheimer disease in a biracial community study. JAMA 287(24):3230–3237

25. Luchsinger JA, Tang MX, Shea S et al (2002) Caloric intake and the risk of Alzheimer disease. Arch Neurol 59(8):1258–1263

26. Kharrazi H, Vaisi-Raygani A, Rahimi Z et al (2008) Association between enzymatic and non-enzymatic antioxidant defense mechanism with apolipoprotein E genotypes in Alzheimer disease. Clin Biochem 41(12):932–936. https://doi.org/10.1016/j.clinbiochem.2008.05.001

27. Lambert JC, Heath S, Even G et al (2009) Genome-wide association study identifies variants at CLU and CR1 associated with Alzheimer's disease. Nat Genet 41(10):1094–1099. https://doi.org/10.1038/ng.439

28. Sleegers K, Lambert JC, Bertram L et al (2010) The pursuit of susceptibility genes for Alzheimer's disease: progress and prospects. Trends Genet 26(2):84–93. https://doi.org/10.1016/j.tig.2009.12.004

29. Martinez-Lapiscina EH, Galbete C, Corella D et al (2014) Genotype patterns at CLU, CR1, PICALM and APOE, cognition and Mediterranean diet: the PREDIMED-NAVARRA trial. Genes Nutr 9(3):393. https://doi.org/10.1007/s12263-014-0393-7

30. Harslof LB, Larsen LH, Ritz C et al (2013) FADS genotype and diet are important determinants of DHA status: a cross-sectional study in Danish infants. Am J Clin Nutr 97(6):1403–1410. https://doi.org/10.3945/ajcn.113.058685

31. Lemaitre RN, Tanaka T, Tang W et al (2011) Genetic loci associated with plasma phospholipid n-3 fatty acids: a meta-analysis of genome-wide association studies from the CHARGE Consortium. PLoS Genet 7(7):e1002193. https://doi.org/10.1371/journal.pgen.1002193

32. Ferrucci L, Perry JR, Matteini A et al (2009) Common variation in the beta-carotene 15,15'-monooxygenase 1 gene affects circulating levels of carotenoids: a genome-wide association study. Am J Hum Genet 84(2):123–133. https://doi.org/10.1016/j.ajhg.2008.12.019

33. Kathiresan S, Willer CJ, Peloso GM et al (2009) Common variants at 30 loci contribute to polygenic dyslipidemia. Nat Genet 41(1):56–65. https://doi.org/10.1038/ng.291

34. van Meurs JB, Pare G, Schwartz SM et al (2013) Common genetic loci influencing plasma homocysteine concentrations and their effect on risk of coronary artery disease. Am J Clin Nutr 98(3):668–676. https://doi.org/10.3945/ajcn.112.044545

35. Scarmeas N, Luchsinger JA, Schupf N et al (2009) Physical activity, diet, and risk of Alzheimer disease. JAMA 302(6):627–637. https://doi.org/10.1001/jama.2009.1144

36. Tolppanen AM, Solomon A, Kulmala J et al (2015) Leisure-time physical activity from mid- to late life, body mass index, and risk of dementia. Alzheimers Dement 11(4):434–443.e6. https://doi.org/10.1016/j.jalz.2014.01.008

37. Wilson RS, Mendes De Leon CF, Barnes LL et al (2002) Participation in cognitively stimulating activities and risk of incident Alzheimer disease. JAMA 287(6):742–748

38. Stern Y, Gurland B, Tatemichi TK et al (1994) Influence of education and occupation on the incidence of Alzheimer's disease. JAMA 271(13):1004–1010

39. Paillard-Borg S, Fratiglioni L, Xu W et al (2012) An active lifestyle postpones dementia onset by more than one year in very old adults. J Alzheimers Dis 31(4):835–842. https://doi.org/10.3233/JAD-2012-120724

40. Liu Y, Julkunen V, Paajanen T et al (2012) Education increases reserve against Alzheimer's disease—evidence from structural MRI analysis. Neuroradiology 54(9):929–938. https://doi.org/10.1007/s00234-012-1005-0

41. Finkel D, Andel R, Gatz M et al (2009) The role of occupational complexity in trajectories of cognitive aging before and after retirement. Psychol Aging 24(3):563–573. https://doi.org/10.1037/a0015511

42. Karp A, Andel R, Parker MG et al (2009) Mentally stimulating activities at work during midlife and dementia risk after age 75: follow-up study from the Kungsholmen Project. Am J Geriatr Psychiatry 17(3):227–236. https://doi.org/10.1097/JGP.0b013e318190b691

43. Stern Y (2012) Cognitive reserve in ageing and Alzheimer's disease. Lancet Neurol 11(11):1006–1012. https://doi.org/10.1016/S1474-4422(12)70191-6

44. Cotman CW, Berchtold NC (2002) Exercise: a behavioral intervention to enhance brain health and plasticity. Trends Neurosci 25(6):295–301

45. Rovio S, Spulber G, Nieminen LJ et al (2010) The effect of midlife physical activity on structural brain changes in the elderly. Neurobiol Aging 31(11):1927–1936. https://doi.org/10.1016/j.neurobiolaging.2008.10.007

46. Komulainen P, Pedersen M, Hanninen T et al (2008) BDNF is a novel marker of cognitive function in ageing women: the DR's EXTRA Study. Neurobiol Learn Mem 90(4):596–603. https://doi.org/10.1016/j.nlm.2008.07.014

47. Wang HX, Gustafson DR, Kivipelto M et al (2012) Education halves the risk of dementia due to apolipoprotein epsilon4 allele: a collaborative study from the Swedish brain power initiative. Neurobiol Aging 33(5):1007.e1–1007.e7. https://doi.org/10.1016/j.neurobiolaging.2011.10.003

48. Wirth M, Villeneuve S, La Joie R et al (2014) Gene-environment interactions: lifetime cognitive activity, APOE genotype, and beta-amyloid burden. J Neurosci 34(25):8612–8617. https://doi.org/10.1523/JNEUROSCI.4612-13.2014

49. Maioli S, Puerta E, Merino-Serrais P et al (2012) Combination of apolipoprotein E4 and high carbohydrate diet reduces hippocampal BDNF and arc levels and impairs memory in young mice. J Alzheimers Dis 32(2):341–355. https://doi.org/10.3233/JAD-2012-120697

50. Ferencz B, Laukka EJ, Welmer AK et al (2014) The benefits of staying active in old age: physical activity counteracts the negative influence of PICALM, BIN1, and CLU risk alleles on episodic memory functioning. Psychol Aging 29(2):440–449. https://doi.org/10.1037/a0035465

51. Cohen RA, Grieve S, Hoth KF et al (2006) Early life stress and morphometry of the adult anterior cingulate cortex and caudate nuclei. Biol Psychiatry 59(10):975–982. https://doi.org/10.1016/j.biopsych.2005.12.016

52. Wolkowitz OM, Epel ES, Reus VI et al (2010) Depression gets old fast: do stress and depression accelerate cell aging? Depress Anxiety 27(4):327–338. https://doi.org/10.1002/da.20686

53. Savva GM, Wharton SB, Ince PG et al (2009) Age, neuropathology, and dementia. N Engl J Med 360(22):2302–2309. https://doi.org/10.1056/NEJMoa0806142

54. Seidler A, Nienhaus A, Bernhardt T et al (2004) Psychosocial work factors and dementia. Occup Environ Med 61(12):962–971. https://doi.org/10.1136/oem.2003.012153

55. Fratiglioni L, Qiu C (2011) Prevention of cognitive decline in ageing: dementia as the target, delayed onset as the goal. Lancet Neurol 10(9):778–779. https://doi.org/10.1016/S1474-4422(11)70145-4

56. McEwen BS, Morrison JH (2013) The brain on stress: vulnerability and plasticity of the prefrontal cortex over the life course. Neuron 79(1):16–29. https://doi.org/10.1016/j.neuron.2013.06.028

57. Wang HX, Karp A, Herlitz A et al (2009) Personality and lifestyle in relation to dementia incidence. Neurology 72(3):253–259. https://doi.org/10.1212/01.wnl.0000339485.39246.87

58. Hahn EA, Wang HX, Andel R et al (2014) A change in sleep pattern may predict Alzheimer disease. Am J Geriatr Psychiatry 22(11):1262–1271. https://doi.org/10.1016/j.jagp.2013.04.015

59. Barnes DE, Yaffe K (2011) The projected effect of risk factor reduction on Alzheimer's disease prevalence. Lancet Neurol 10(9):819–828. https://doi.org/10.1016/S1474-4422(11)70072-2

60. Skoog I, Lernfelt B, Landahl S et al (1996) 15-year longitudinal study of blood pressure and dementia. Lancet 347(9009):1141–1145

61. Hanon O, Haulon S, Lenoir H et al (2005) Relationship between arterial stiffness and cognitive function in elderly subjects with complaints of memory loss. Stroke 36(10):2193–2197. https://doi.org/10.1161/01.STR.0000181771.82518.1c

62. Ott A, Stolk RP, van Harskamp F et al (1999) Diabetes mellitus and the risk of dementia: the Rotterdam Study. Neurology 53(9):1937–1942

63. Anstey KJ, von Sanden C, Salim A et al (2007) Smoking as a risk factor for dementia and cognitive decline: a meta-analysis of prospective studies. Am J Epidemiol 166(4):367–378. https://doi.org/10.1093/aje/kwm116

64. Anstey KJ, Lipnicki DM, Low LF (2008) Cholesterol as a risk factor for dementia and cognitive decline: a systematic review of prospective studies with meta-analysis. Am J Geriatr Psychiatry 16(5):343–354. https://doi.org/10.1097/JGP.0b013e31816b72d4

65. de la Torre JC (2006) How do heart disease and stroke become risk factors for Alzheimer's disease? Neurol Res 28(6):637–644. https://doi.org/10.1179/016164106X130362

66. Newman AB, Fitzpatrick AL, Lopez O et al (2005) Dementia and Alzheimer's disease incidence in relationship to cardiovascular disease in the Cardiovascular Health Study cohort. J Am Geriatr Soc 53(7):1101–1107. https://doi.org/10.1111/j.1532-5415.2005.53360.x

67. van Oijen M, de Jong FJ, Witteman JC et al (2007) Atherosclerosis and risk for dementia. Ann Neurol 61(5):403–410. https://doi.org/10.1002/ana.21073

68. Wendell CR, Waldstein SR, Ferrucci L et al (2012) Carotid atherosclerosis and prospective risk of dementia. Stroke 43(12):3319–3324. https://doi.org/10.1161/STROKEAHA.112.672527

69. Radanovic M, Pereira FR, Stella F et al (2013) White matter abnormalities associated with Alzheimer's disease and mild cognitive impairment: a critical review of MRI studies. Expert Rev Neurother 13(5):483–493. https://doi.org/10.1586/ern.13.45

70. de Bruijn RF, Akoudad S, Cremers LG et al (2014) Determinants, MRI correlates, and prognosis of mild cognitive impairment: the

Rotterdam study. J Alzheimers Dis 42(Suppl 3):S239–S249. https://doi.org/10.3233/JAD-132558

71. Eckel RH, Grundy SM, Zimmet PZ (2005) The metabolic syndrome. Lancet 365(9468):1415–1428. https://doi.org/10.1016/S0140-6736(05)66378-7

72. Skoog I, Kalaria RN, Breteler MM (1999) Vascular factors and Alzheimer disease. Alzheimer Dis Assoc Disord 13(Suppl 3):S106–S114

73. de Leeuw FE, Richard F, de Groot JC et al (2004) Interaction between hypertension, apoE, and cerebral white matter lesions. Stroke 35(5):1057–1060. https://doi.org/10.1161/01.STR.0000125859.71051.83

74. Hollingworth P, Harold D, Sims R et al (2011) Common variants at ABCA7, MS4A6A/MS4A4E, EPHA1, CD33 and CD2AP are associated with Alzheimer's disease. Nat Genet 43(5):429–435. https://doi.org/10.1038/ng.803

75. Hovingh GK, Van Wijland MJ, Brownlie A et al (2003) The role of the ABCA1 transporter and cholesterol efflux in familial hypoalphalipoproteinemia. J Lipid Res 44(6):1251–1255. https://doi.org/10.1194/jlr.M300080-JLR200

76. Imhof A, Kovari E, von Gunten A et al (2007) Morphological substrates of cognitive decline in nonagenarians and centenarians: a new paradigm? J Neurol Sci 257(1-2):72–79. https://doi.org/10.1016/j.jns.2007.01.025

77. Serrano-Pozo A, Frosch MP, Masliah E et al (2011) Neuropathological alterations in Alzheimer disease. Cold Spring Harb Perspect Med 1(1):a006189. https://doi.org/10.1101/cshperspect.a006189

78. Qiu C, Kivipelto M, von Strauss E (2009) Epidemiology of Alzheimer's disease: occurrence, determinants, and strategies toward intervention. Dialogues Clin Neurosci 11(2):111–128

79. Matthews FE, Arthur A, Barnes LE et al (2013) A two-decade comparison of prevalence of dementia in individuals aged 65 years and older from three geographical areas of England: results of the Cognitive Function and Ageing Study I and II. Lancet 382(9902):1405–1412. https://doi.org/10.1016/S0140-6736(13)61570-6

80. Qiu C, von Strauss E, Backman L et al (2013) Twenty-year changes in dementia occurrence suggest decreasing incidence in central Stockholm, Sweden. Neurology 80(20):1888–1894. https://doi.org/10.1212/WNL.0b013e318292a2f9

Chapter 3

Systems Biology Methods for Alzheimer's Disease Research Toward Molecular Signatures, Subtypes, and Stages and Precision Medicine: Application in Cohort Studies and Trials

Juan I. Castrillo, Simone Lista, Harald Hampel, and Craig W. Ritchie

Abstract

Alzheimer's disease (AD) is a complex multifactorial disease, involving a combination of genomic, interactome, and environmental factors, with essential participation of (a) intrinsic genomic susceptibility and (b) a constant dynamic interplay between impaired pathways and central homeostatic networks of nerve cells. The proper investigation of the complexity of AD requires new holistic systems-level approaches, at both the experimental and computational level. Systems biology methods offer the potential to unveil new fundamental insights, basic mechanisms, and networks and their interplay. These may lead to the characterization of mechanism-based molecular signatures, and AD hallmarks at the earliest molecular and cellular levels (and beyond), for characterization of AD subtypes and stages, toward targeted interventions according to the evolving precision medicine paradigm. In this work, an update on advanced systems biology methods and strategies for holistic studies of multifactorial diseases—particularly AD—is presented. This includes next-generation genomics, neuroimaging and multi-omics methods, experimental and computational approaches, relevant disease models, and latest genome editing and single-cell technologies. Their progressive incorporation into basic research, cohort studies, and trials is beginning to provide novel insights into AD essential mechanisms, molecular signatures, and markers toward mechanism-based classification and staging, and tailored interventions. Selected methods which can be applied in cohort studies and trials, with the European Prevention of Alzheimer's Dementia (EPAD) project as a reference example, are presented and discussed.

Key words Alzheimer's disease (AD), Systems biology, Omics, Interactomes, Networks, APP, Amyloid-β (Aβ), Tau, Proteinopathy, Homeostasis networks, Proteostasis, Experimental systems biology, Next-generation genomics, Neuroimaging, Next-generation omics techniques, Computational systems biology, Network biology, Molecular biomarkers, Standardization, Validation, Risk classification, Staging, AD subtypes, AD stages, Tailored treatments, Clinical trials, European Prevention of Alzheimer's Dementia project, EPAD, Precision medicine

Robert Perneczky (ed.), *Biomarkers for Alzheimer's Disease Drug Development*, Methods in Molecular Biology, vol. 1750, https://doi.org/10.1007/978-1-4939-7704-8_3, © Springer Science+Business Media, LLC 2018

1 Alzheimer's Disease (AD), a Polygenic Multifactorial Disease with Genomic, Interactomes, and Environmental Contributions: Need for Holistic Systems Biology Methods

Alzheimer's disease (AD) and many other clinically heterogeneous diseases (including diabetes, other neurodegenerative diseases (NDs), and most cancers) are complex multifactorial diseases involving genomic, interactome, and environmental factors. Next-generation molecular and high-throughput techniques are shedding new light on the mechanisms and networks underlying these complex diseases [1–6]. These are due to continued progress toward new molecular signatures, comprehensive risk classification, and translational (directly applicable to patient) targeted interventions according to the precision medicine paradigm [7–13]. The precision medicine strategy is supposed to enable a paradigm shift from the traditional "one-treatment-fits-all" approach in drug discovery toward biomarker-guided "tailored" therapies, i.e., targeted interventions adapted to the biological profile of individual patients. In this context, the U.S. Precision Medicine Initiative (PMI) [14] and the U.S. "All of Us Research Program" have been effectively developed. As is the case in most fields of medicine, important progresses in detecting, treating, and preventing AD are anticipated to evolve from the implementation of a systematic precision medicine strategy. This approach will likely be founded on the success from more advanced research fields, such as oncology. Therefore, after more than a decade of failed therapy trials and one of the lowest success rates in drug development in medicine, the time has come to launch an international Alzheimer PMI (APMI) and link it with the US PMI and other associated worldwide initiatives [13, 14].

First, a new "genomics in medicine revolution" is already in progress, with genome sequencing (whole-genome sequencing (WGS)) and screening of individuals' sequences, copy number variants (CNVs), and structural rearrangements, candidate pathogenic or protective, projected to permeate clinical practice as a routine procedure in the upcoming 5–10 years (Illumina's executive chairman Jat Flatley speaks of genomic sequencing future. June 20, 2016; http://www.sandiegouniontribune.com/news/2016/jun/20/jay-flatley-illumina-innovation/). Next-generation genomics technologies are already being utilized for both diagnostic and treatment purposes in diseases with a clear genetic component (e.g., Mendelian and, as yet, uncharacterized diseases) ([2] and references therein, [15]). However, AD and many other clinically heterogeneous diseases (e.g., diabetes, other NDs, and most cancers) are far too complex to have a single cause or to rely on genomic variations alone. Such complex diseases are characterized by the following features: (1) multifactorial nature, i.e., involving a combination of genomic, epigenomic, interactomic, and environmental factors; (2) being primarily the result of "altered networks," affecting essential modules and interactomes; (3) being fundamentally dynamic, with a fine interplay between impaired networks and homeostatic defense mechanisms ([2] and references therein, [16]). For these multifactorial diseases, comprehensive holistic, systems-level approaches are necessary (*see* below).

Systems biology aims at deciphering the genotype–phenotype relationships and mechanisms at the following levels: genome/epigenome, transcripts (RNAs), peptides, proteins, metabolites, interactomes, and environmental factors participating in complex cellular networks. Systems biology is not so much concerned with inventories of working parts but rather aimed at investigating (1) how those parts interact to produce working units of biological organization whose properties are much greater than the sum of their parts, (2) what makes complex networks and systems sustainable and viable, and (3) how complex diseases—including AD—can arise from "altered network states" whose mechanisms and dynamics can ideally be investigated using integrative, systems-level methods (experimental and computational), with the ultimate goal to reveal specific molecular signatures and candidate-tailored interventions according to the precision medicine paradigm ([1, 2] and references therein, [5, 6, 12, 13, 17–19]).

Accumulated evidence from studies of multifactorial diseases (e.g., several cancers and NDs) is showing that the standard "one-treatment-fits-all" approach may be too simplistic in some cases. As a consequence, some patients and groups of patients may benefit from mechanism-based targeted interventions directed to specific subgroups or subtypes at different stages of the disease (*see* next sections). In order to unveil the underlying mechanisms, regulatory networks, candidate molecular markers and targets, which treatments may be applicable to specific subgroups or stages, and which ones are applicable to a broader group of patients, holistic systems biology methods in advanced studies and trials should be implemented [2, 3, 12]. At present, considerable advances in terms of discovery, development, and validation of mechanism-related AD biomarkers have allowed to enter the novel era of multimodal investigations integrating different biofluids and modalities [20–25]. In particular, they may result from neurogenetics [26–28], neurochemistry via biofluids [29] including cerebrospinal fluid [30–33] and blood (plasma/serum) [34–38], and structural/functional/metabolic neuroimaging as well as neurophysiology [39, 40].

The application of systems biology methods to AD toward the paradigm of precision medicine is presented in Fig. 1. Comprehensive screenings of individuals, groups, and subgroups should start with advanced next-generation genomics methods (1), to reveal specific variants and genomic signatures for basic risk assessment at the genomic level (i.e., intrinsic susceptibility to disease). These techniques will allow the detection of individuals at high genomic risk. Subsequently, new comprehensive systems-level analyses, including systems biology neuroimaging and multi-omics methods (experimental and computational) (2), should be implemented [2, 3, 12].

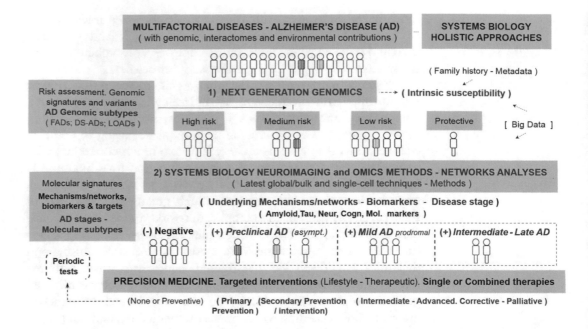

Fig. 1 Systems biology holistic approaches and methods applied to multifactorial diseases. Alzheimer's disease (AD). From systems biology methods to precision medicine. Pipeline: Multifactorial diseases involve genomic, interactomic, and environmental contributions, for which systems biology approaches are necessary. Comprehensive screenings of individuals, groups, and subgroups should start with advanced next-generation genomics methods (1), to unveil specific variants and genomic signatures for basic risk assessment at the genomic level (i.e., intrinsic susceptibility to disease). These techniques will be able to detect individuals at high genomic risk (in red). At this point, for complex multifactorial diseases such as AD, new comprehensive systems-level analyses, including systems biology neuroimaging and multi-omics methods (experimental and computational), (2) are necessary [2, 3, 12, 13]. These advanced methods, with incorporation of standardized techniques and guidelines, will allow to reveal specific molecular signatures and biomarkers at different disease stages, different subgroups and/or subtypes, the underlying mechanisms, and actual disease risk, toward mechanism-based, tailored interventions and precision medicine. These may include primary or secondary prevention strategies, and intermediate, corrective, or palliative treatments (at lifestyle and/or therapeutic levels) [2, 12]. Abbreviations: *FAD* familial Alzheimer's disease, *DS-AD* Alzheimer's disease in Down syndrome individuals, *LOAD* late-onset Alzheimer's disease. Disease stages: *Preclinical AD*. Early AD stage, asymptomatic, subject of exhaustive investigation (e.g., search for molecular and pathophysiological biomarkers and signatures characteristic of different subgroups or subtypes during this stage) [204, 205]; *mild AD* (prodromal), when early signs and symptoms appear but not yet clinically specific nor severe; *intermediate AD* and *late AD*. Illness periods with clear symptoms, worsening from intermediate to advanced, acute/severe stages (Amyloid, Tau, Neur, Cogn, Mol. markers): Amyloid deposition, tauopathy, neurological, cognitive and molecular biomarkers for advanced subtype classification and staging

The application of such advanced methods in cohort studies and trials is aimed to reveal specific molecular signatures and biomarkers (e.g., amyloid deposition, tauopathy, neurological, cognitive and molecular biomarkers) and could guide in the classification/stratification of different subtypes, groups, and subgroups at the different stages of the disease (preclinical AD (asymptomatic); mild AD (prodromal); intermediate-late AD), the underlying mechanisms, and actual disease risk, toward mechanism-based, affordable, tailored treatments and precision medicine [2, 3, 12, 13]. These may include primary or secondary prevention strategies, and intermediate, corrective, or palliative interventions (at lifestyle and/or therapeutic levels) [2, 12].

The main objective of this work is to present an update on advanced systems biology and studies applied to AD and multifactorial diseases. There is an urgent need to summarize the current knowledge in the field and make it available to experts and researchers [3, 41]. These will include next-generation genomics, neuroimaging, and multi-omics methods, and experimental and computational, bulk and single-cell technologies at the molecular and cellular levels (and beyond). Such techniques will be hopefully improved and refined in the upcoming years. Their progressive incorporation into new cohort studies and trials will be the next essential step (*see* below), to provide new insights into molecular signatures/markers toward mechanism-based classification and staging, and tailored interventions (single or combined therapies applicable to specific subtypes, groups of patients at different stages) (Fig. 1). The take-home message is the following: "For comprehensive, mechanisms-based Precision Medicine strategies of multifactorial diseases to succeed, holistic systems-level methods are necessary" [2, 3, 12].

2   Systems Biology Methods for AD Research, Including Next-Generation Genomics, Neuroimaging, and Multi-Omics Approaches: Advanced Studies in Disease Models, Genome Editing, Bulk and Single-Cell Technologies

This section aims to provide an up-to-date review of advanced systems biology methods and strategies for holistic studies of multifactorial diseases, with a special focus on AD. For a comprehensive analysis modeled on the schematic representation displayed in Fig. 1, next-generation genomics methods will be presented first, with the latest neuroimaging and rest of systems biology methods and studies thereafter.

Subheading 2.1 will thus include (1) next-generation genomics methods: from classic to next-generation genomics approaches and studies to unveil genomic subtypes and intrinsic susceptibility to disease. Selected examples will be presented and discussed. Subheading 2.2 will focus on the latest neuroimaging and rest of advanced systems biology methods and approaches. These will include (2) neuroimaging methods: physiological and phenotypic advances toward unified AD diagnosis and characterization of subtypes and stages; (3) methods for the study of mechanisms, pathways/networks underlying AD; (4) experimental systems biology. Omics levels, interactomes, and networks involved in AD, including next-generation molecular and high-throughput omics methods; (5) computational systems biology. Next-generation computational and integrative network biology approaches for the study of modules, pathways, and networks; (6) specific approaches using disease models recapitulating AD features to characterize underlying mechanisms; (7) next-generation genome editing methods for AD studies; (8) new single-cell technologies for single-cell functional analysis. All of these topics will be presented in Subheading 2.2. Selected examples of methods and strategies which may be applied in next-generation cohort studies and trials will be discussed.

2.1 Next-Generation Genomics: From Classic to Next-Generation Genomics Methods to Unveil Intrinsic Genomic Susceptibility—Latest Personal Genomics Sequencing and Advanced Methods

Although AD is characterized by clear histological features and patterns of progression [42–44], families and groups of individuals exhibit marked differences and heterogeneity which are revealing distinct contributions of genomic/epigenomic and environmental factors in different cases. First, only approximately <1% of the AD cases are familial forms of autosomal dominant inheritance, which are generally characterized by an onset before 65 years of age. This form of the disease is known as autosomal dominant Alzheimer's disease (ADAD) [45]. Most of the autosomal dominant ADs can be attributed to mutations in one of the three genes: those encoding amyloid precursor protein (APP) and presenilins 1 and 2 [46, 47] which points to a relevant role of impairment of APP processing pathways and abnormal amyloid-β (Aβ) species in these cases. Some of these pathways may also be responsible for the reported high risk of developing AD in individuals with Down syndrome (DS-AD). This high risk has been linked in part to the presence of an extra copy of the APP gene in chromosome 21, with the additional involvement of other specific mechanisms and networks ([2] and references therein).

Apart from these, the reality is that most cases of AD do not exhibit autosomal dominant inheritance or high genomic risk and are termed "sporadic" or late-onset AD (LOAD). In such cases, both genetic and environmental differences act as risk factors. LOAD is the most common form of AD, accounting for >90% of cases, with overt symptoms usually occurring after 65 years of age ([2] and references therein, [48]).

Studies on genetic susceptibility have identified several genes that may be associated with LOAD (AlzGene database (http://www.alzgene.org/). Each of them appears to contribute only to a limited extent, or only confer a small, slightly increased risk of developing LOAD. The best known genetic risk factor is the inheritance of the ε4 allele of the apolipoprotein E (APOE) gene [49]. Here it is important to note that the mere detection of one LOAD mutation or variant does not necessarily imply that one individual will develop LOAD. More comprehensive studies on the contributions of genomic-environmental interactions and the interplay of pathways and networks are necessary ([2] and references therein).

At the genomic level, next-generation genomics methods need to address the study of not only gene sequences (with mutations occurring in both coding and noncoding regions), but also genomic alterations (including copy number variations (CNVs), structural rearrangements, aneuploidies, and others) which can affect the regulation of pathways and networks underlying disease susceptibility. New advances in our understanding of missing heritability, genomic sequences' interactions, and intrinsic susceptibility are being obtained from classic genomic studies, CNV analyses, and next-generation sequencing (NGS) methods. Additional insights and discoveries are eagerly expected from the latest long-read sequencing tools, new genome assembly techniques for the determination of diploid genome sequences and de novo genome sequencing (which is becoming progressively more affordable), new advanced tools to analyze the impact of structural variants (SVs), and new tools to unveil functional elements in noncoding and coding regions in individual genomes. A perspective of latest classic and next-generation genomics methods to identify novel genomic contributions to multifactorial diseases (with a particular focus on AD) is presented in Table 1 [50–80]. Most relevant advances are the following:

1. Classic genomics studies and advanced methods leading to essential discoveries on AD genomic susceptibility, genetic risk factors, and missing heritability [50–58] included in well-annotated and curated databases, repositories, and projects including Alzforum, AlzGene database, National Institute of Ageing (NIA), and the Alzheimer's Disease Sequencing Project (ADSP) (*see also* [2] and references therein).

2. Next-generation sequencing methods applied to AD [59].

3. New genome-wide methods for elucidation of candidate CNVs in AD [61].

4. Whole-exome sequencing (WES) coupled with longitudinal electronic health record (EHR) phenotype data to identify rare variants [62].

5. Next-generation whole-genome sequencing (WGS) to investigate the full spectrum of human genetic variation and structural variations. Long-read sequencing and de novo assembly of an individual genome [63–65].

6. Direct determination of diploid genome sequences [66].

7. 3D chromosome conformation capture genome assembly method to assemble an organism's genetic material from scratch. Sequencing a patient's genome using 3D assembly comparable in cost to a magnetic resonance imaging (MRI) scan [67–69].

8. New discoveries changing the personal genomics field. When a mutation doesn't spell disease. The Exome Aggregation Consortium (ExAC) turning human genetics upside down. Genome robustness [70–72].

9. Next-generation genomics advances and beyond. New high-throughput screening techniques (e.g., CRISPR-Cas9 epigenome and RNA-Seq) for the discovery and analysis of functional regulatory elements in coding and noncoding regions [73, 76].

Table 1
Next-generation genomics

Description of method/study	References
Classic and next-generation genomics methods to study genomic contributions to multifactorial diseases. Alzheimer's disease (AD) intrinsic susceptibility. New discoveries changing the genomics field	
Classic genomics studies and advanced methods	
Relevant discoveries on AD genomic susceptibility, genetic and genomic risk factors, and missing heritability AlzGene database (http://www.alzgene.org/)	[2] and refs. therein; [50–58]
Next generation genomics. Methods	
Relevant studies on new genomic risk factors and missing heritability using latest techniques such as next-generation sequencing (NGS) and latest studies, databases, and curated repositories. Alzheimer's disease sequencing project (ADSP) (https://www.niagads.org/adsp/). Toward risk classification/stratification of stages and subtypes	
Next-generation sequencing in Alzheimer's disease	[59]
Pooled DNA sequencing for new genomic risk factors, rare variants underlying AD	[60]
New genome-wide methods for elucidation of candidate copy number variations (CNVs)	[61]
Whole-exome sequencing (WES) coupled with longitudinal electronic health record (EHR) phenotype data to identify rare variants, linking human genetic variation with phenotypic traits (http://www.the-scientist.com/?articles.view/articleNo/47848/title/Exome-Study-Reveals-Novel-Disease-Linked-Alleles/)	[62]
Next-generation whole-genome sequencing (WGS) to investigate the full spectrum of human genetic variation. Structural variations. From genotype to phenotype and disease	
Long-read haploid genome sequencing. Structural variation studies	[63]
Long-read single-molecule real-time (SRMT) sequencing. De novo assembly and phasing of a human genome	[64]
The impact of structural variation on human gene expression. Structural variants (SVs)	[65]
The pangenome concept to describe all the genetic variation within a species (http://www.the-scientist.com/?articles.view/articleNo/47510/title/The-Pangenome--Are-Single-Reference-Genomes-Dead-/)	

Direct determination of diploid genome sequences	[66]
Hi-C (3D high-resolution chromosome conformation capture interaction mapping) genome assembly method to make it easier and cheaper to assemble all of an organism's genetic material (short/long reads) from scratch. Sequencing a patient's genome using 3D assembly comparable in cost to an MRI (https://www.bcm.edu/news/genome-sequencing/scientist-assemble-genome-of-zika-virus); (https://www.theatlantic.com/science/archive/2017/03/the-game-changing-technique-that-cracked-the-zika-mosquito-genome/521190/?utm_source=twb); (http://www.the-scientist.com/?articles.view/articleNo/48992/title/Aedes-aegypti-Genome-Assembled-From-Scratch/)	[67–69]
New discoveries changing the personal genomics field. A radical revision of human genetics	
When a mutation doesn't spell disease. Genome robustness	[70, 71]
The exome aggregation consortium (ExAC) turning human genetics upside down (http://exac.broadinstitute.org/) (http://www.nature.com/news/the-flip-side-of-personal-genomics-when-a-mutation-doesn-t-spell-disease-1.20986)	[72]
Next-generation genomics advances and beyond	
New high-throughput screening techniques for the discovery and analysis of functional regulatory elements in the human genome (CRISPR-Cas9 epigenome method; *see also* Table 2, below). Probing the regulatory roles of specific noncoding DNA sequences (http://www.the-scientist.com/?articles.view/articleNo/49055/title/CRISPR-Screen-Detects-Functional-Gene-Regulation/)	[76]
RNA-Seq advanced studies to unveil genetic disorder-causing mutations in coding and noncoding regions (http://www.the-scientist.com/?articles.view/articleNo/49236/title/RNA-Seq-Reveals-Previously-Hidden--Genetic-Disorder-Causing-Mutations/)	[73]
Latest next-generation genomic studies for classification, stratification of AD types/subtypes, stages	[78, 79]
Single-cell genomic techniques (*see also* Table 2) to study somatic mutations and their relevance in neuropsychiatric disorders. The brain somatic mosaicism network (BSMN)	[77]
Next-generation genomics resources and initiatives offering genomics services to investigate complex diseases and big data integration	
FDA (April 6, 2017) allows marketing of first direct-to-consumer 23andMe personal genome service genetic health risk (GHR) tests for certain diseases, including late-onset AD (LOAD) (note: these informative tests are only intended to provide genetic risk information, but cannot determine a person's overall risk of developing a disease; results should not be used for diagnosis or to inform treatment decisions; users should consult a healthcare professional) (https://www.fda.gov/NewsEvents/Newsroom/PressAnnouncements/ucm551185.htm?source=govdelivery&utm_medium=email&utm_source=govdelivery)	

(continued)

Table 1
(continued)

Description of method/study	References
New York genome Center (NYGC), including genomics research on neurodegenerative diseases (NDs) (http://www.bio-itworld.com/2017/1/20/whole-genome-sequencing-testing-is-available-at-the-new-york-genome-center.aspx; http://www.nygenome.org/lab-groups-overview/center-genomics-neurodegenerative-disease-phatnani-lab/)	
National Institute of Mental Health (NIMH) genomic resources for the study of neuropsychiatric disorders	[80]
New global initiatives such as the Global Alliance for Genomics and Health (GA4GH) to enable large-scale sharing of genomics data and clinical outcomes ("big data"), to investigate molecular patterns underlying disease and health (http://genomicsandhealth.org/)	
Beyond the genome. Need to incorporate holistic, systems biology methods to unveil disease susceptibility, mechanisms, and networks for advanced AD staging (stages and subtypes) (*see* Fig. 1, Table 2, and text)	
Beyond the genome (http://www.nature.com/news/beyond-the-genome-1.16929)	
Latest studies unveiling the influence/role of APOE isoforms (http://www.alzforum.org/news/research-news/apoe-risk-explained-isoform-dependent-boost-app-expression-uncovered)	[74, 75]

Latest next-generation genomics methods including next-generation sequencing (NGS), whole-exome (WES) and whole-genome sequencing (WGS), and genome assembly techniques for the determination of diploid genome sequences and de novo genome sequencing, new methods to study the impact of structural variants (SVs) and advanced tools to unveil functional elements in noncoding and coding regions. New discoveries changing the personal genomics field and human genetics. Next-generation genomics applied to the study of genomic contributions to multifactorial diseases (e.g., neurodegenerative diseases, cancers) coupled with large-scale sharing of genomics and health data ("Big Data"). Alzheimer's disease (AD) intrinsic susceptibility and beyond

10. Latest next-generation genomic studies for classifying AD into specific subtypes and stages [78, 79].

11. Next-generation genomics resources and initiatives offering genomics services to investigate complex diseases and big data integration. As relevant examples: (1) FDA allows marketing of first direct-to-consumer personal genome genetic health risk tests for certain diseases, including LOAD (note: these are only intended to provide genetic risk information, but cannot determine a person's overall risk of developing a disease. Results should not be used for diagnosis or to inform treatment decisions); (2) National Institute of Mental Health (NIMH) genomic resources for the study of neuropsychiatric disorders [80]; (3) Global Alliance for Genomics and Health (GA4GH) to enable large-scale sharing of genomics data and clinical, to investigate molecular patterns underlying disease and health (http://genomicsandhealth.org/).

At this point, it is becoming increasingly clear that the progressive implementation of next-generation standard methods (e.g., genomics, neuroimaging, multi-omics methods, and others—*see* below) will result in a massive generation of high-quality data ("Big Data"). First, clear rules for use and sharing of personal data need to be implemented [81]. After this, since not all datasets will be directly comparable (e.g., obtained from different subjects, subtypes, cohort studies or trials, utilizing several methods or under different conditions), there is a clear risk that a careless use (for example, merging or pooling data from independent studies) may inadvertently introduce spurious bias or noise, ultimately hampering the extraction of solid conclusions. There is an increasing consensus on the need for developing initiatives promoting strict guidelines for standardization, proper curation, harmonization, and storage of big data in health research, in appropriate databases and repositories, together with their associated metadata [82, 83]. Relevant initiatives toward this goal, being applied to multifactorial diseases and AD, include the Global Alliance for Genomics and Health (GA4GH) (http://genomicsandhealth.org/), the European Medical Information Framework for AD (EMIF-AD), Global Alzheimer's Association Interactive Network (GAAIN) (http://www.alzforum.org/news/research-news/emif-gaain-online-gateways-reams-alzheimers-data), and the AMP-AD Knowledge Portal, the latter distributing data, analysis results, analytical methodology, and research tools generated through multiple National Institute of Aging (NIA) programs (https://www.nia.nih.gov/alzheimers/amp-ad).

Next-generation genomics methods represent the first step to investigate intrinsic susceptibility to disease (Fig. 1). Their goal is to decipher disease-associated functional elements in personal genomes, candidate mechanisms, and pathways contributing to disease, and to help in the initial classification of individuals, groups, and subgroups based on their intrinsic genomic risk. However, in multifactorial diseases such as AD, with genomic, interactomic, and environmental contributions responsible for the observed clinical heterogeneity, with a broad spectrum of AD patterns, ages of onset, and rates of progression (*see* [2] and references therein and [78]), this calls for the necessity to go *beyond the genome*, that is, to incorporate comprehensive holistic studies, integrative neuroimaging, and systems biology methods to investigate the actual state and interplay of AD pathways and networks in groups or subgroups of individuals. These methods and studies are beginning to deliver key insights into the role of specific mechanisms and pathways including impaired APP processing and tau networks, inflammation, and homeostatic networks (*see* [2, 3] and references therein). The final goal will always be to unveil essential molecular mechanisms, pathways, and networks and molecular signatures, as well as candidate combined biomarkers that may characterize different subtypes, for proper classification and staging toward mechanism-based tailored interventions.

2.2 Advanced Systems Biology Neuroimaging and Multi-Omics Methods for AD Research: Experimental and Computational Advanced Studies in Disease Models— Latest Bulk and Single-Cell Methods

Most advanced holistic, systems biology neuroimaging and multi-omics methods are summarized in Table 2 [84–178]. These include (a) latest neuroimaging, physiological and phenotypic advances toward unified AD diagnosis, and characterization of stages and subtypes; (b) relevant methods for the study of mechanisms, pathways, and networks underlying AD; (c) experimental systems biology methods. Omics levels, interactomes, and networks: Next-generation molecular and high-throughput omics methods for the study of disease susceptibility and network dynamics in multifactorial diseases and AD; (d) computational systems biology. Network biology methods: Next-generation computational and integrative network biology approaches for the study of modules, network dynamics, and their interplay in multifactorial diseases and AD; (e) specific approaches and discoveries using disease models recapitulating AD features to characterize underlying mechanisms and subtypes: from cellular models to human; (f) next-generation genome editing methods and their application to AD; (g) new single-cell technologies for single-cell functional analysis. Selected methods and studies leading to new discoveries and advances are highlighted below. For a more exhaustive review, the reader can refer to all methods and studies included in Table 2.

2.2.1 Neuroimaging Methods: Physiological and Phenotypic Advances Toward Unified AD Diagnosis, Characterization of Stages and Subtypes, and New Discoveries

These include (a) advances in neuroimaging, physiological, and phenotypic biomarkers toward unified AD diagnostic criteria; (b) most relevant advances in new neuroimaging tracers and methods toward characterization of AD stages and subtypes and new discoveries; (c) new advances in studies of vascular impairment in neurodegenerative diseases and AD; and many others (Table 2, section II).

Table 2
Advanced systems biology methods to investigate mechanisms and networks underlying multifactorial diseases

Description of method/study	References
I. Next-generation genomics methods (*see* Table 1)	
II. Neuroimaging, physiological, and phenotypic advances toward unified AD diagnosis and characterization of AD stages and subtypes	
Advances in neuroimaging, physiological, and phenotypic biomarkers toward unified criteria	
Advancing research diagnostic criteria for Alzheimer's disease	[84]
Fitting epidemiology and neuropathology features at AD early stages	[85]
Proposed unbiased A/T/N biomarker system ("A" for β-amyloid biomarkers, "T," for tau, and "N," for biomarkers of neurodegeneration or neuronal injury)	[86, 87]
Toward a definition of the "preclinical AD stage" (asymptomatic, with presence of molecular and/or pathophysiological signatures)	[204, 205]
Advanced neuroimaging methods toward characterization of AD stages and subtypes. Best practices	[84, 88–92]
Emerging multitracer technologies (e.g., amyloid, tau) for in vivo imaging revealing hierarchical organization of tau and amyloid deposits in the cerebral cortex	[93, 94]
Neuroimaging diagnosis for Alzheimer's disease and other dementias	[95]
Longitudinal positron-emission tomography (PET study showing an early and late peak in microglial activation in AD trajectory	[96]
Array tomography (AT) imaging investigating spread of tau down neural circuits precedes synapse and neuronal loss in a mouse model of early AD	[97]
Tau imaging in AD diagnosis and clinical trials	[98]
Tau imaging in staging AD revealing interactions between β-amyloid and tauopathy (http://www.alzforum.org/news/research-news/brain-imaging-suggests-av-unleashes-deadly-side-tau)	[99]
Global efforts on neuroimaging, biomarkers, and patterns for identification of AD subtypes from the Alzheimer's disease neuroimaging initiative (ADNI) (http://www.adni-info.org/)	[100]
Tau PET in vivo imaging showing tau patterns mirror clinical and neuroanatomical symptoms (cortical atrophy) in AD progression	[101]
Multimodal imaging in vivo study confirming a high regional association between tau levels, atrophy, and symptoms in early clinical stages of AD (characterized by neurodegeneration/cell death, atrophy, and cognitive symptoms) (http://www.alzforum.org/news/research-news/multimodal-imaging-ties-tau-neurodegeneration-and-symptoms)	[102, 103]
Selecting trial participants based on neurofibrillary tangle stage to improve the power of clinical trials and reduce sample sizes (http://www.alzforum.org/news/research-news/selecting-trial-participants-based-tangle-pathology-might-improve-power)	[104]

(continued)

Table 2
(continued)

Description of method/study	References
Next-generation tau PET tracers being developed. New available tau PET tracers (at early stage of development) overcoming limitations of earlier compounds: higher brain uptake, more specific binding, yielding cleaner scans with sharper distinction between positive and negative findings (http://www.alzforum.org/news/conference-coverage/next-generation-tau-pet-tracers-strut-their-stuff)	
Advances in studies of vascular impairment features in neurodegenerative diseases and AD	
Investigation of cerebrovascular disease features	[105]
Consortium to investigate biomarkers for vascular cognitive impairment (http://www.alzforum.org/news/community-news/consortium-seek-biomarkers-vascular-cognitive-impairment)	
III. Relevant methods for the study of mechanisms, pathways/networks underlying AD	
(Main bulk experimental methods. New single-cell technologies being incorporated, below)	
APP processing, including oxidative stress	[106, 107]
β-Amyloid aggregation in vitro and in vivo. Super-resolution microscopy methods	[108]
Protocols for monitoring the development of tau pathology in AD	[109]
Tau prion strains dictate patterns of cell pathology, progression rate, and regional vulnerability in vivo	[110]
Disturbance of endoplasmic reticulum (ER) proteostasis, and unfolded protein response (UPR) in NDs	[111]
Autophagic activity	[112]
Autophagy-mediated regulation of BACE1 protein trafficking and degradation	[113]
Mitochondrial dysfunction	[114]
Microglial proliferation	[115]
Disease-associated amyloid and misfolded protein aggregates activate the inflammasome	[116]
Role of infection and neuroinflammation in neurodegeneration: new insights	[117]
Neuroinflammation can both help and harm AD. Right kind of immune response? (http://www.alzforum.org/news/conference-coverage/inflammation-helps-microglia-clear-amyloid-ad-brains)	
The immune system. Balancing health and disease	
(http://www.the-scientist.com/?articles.view/articleNo/47289/title/Immune-System-Maintains-Brain-Health/)	
Aβ drainage from the brain. The glymphatic system (http://www.alzforum.org/news/research-news/dearth-water-channels-sign-glymphatic-breakdown-alzheimers)	[118, 119]
IV. Experimental systems biology. Omics levels. Interactomes and networks involved in AD. Next-generation molecular and high-throughput omics methods for the study of disease susceptibility and network dynamics in multifactorial diseases and AD	[2, 3]

(continued)

Table 2
(continued)

Description of method/study	References
Use of "omics" technologies to dissect neurologic disease	[120]
Next-generation genomics. AD genomic susceptibility. Latest methods (see Table 1)	
Transcriptomics. RNA gene expression analysis	
RNA-sequencing (RNA-Seq) to elucidate early patterns of dysregulation underlying AD	[121]
RNA-Seq advanced studies to unveil genetic disorder-causing mutations in coding and noncoding regions (http://www.the-scientist.com/?articles.view/articleNo/49236/title/RNA-Seq-Reveals-Previously-Hidden--Genetic-Disorder-Causing-Mutations/)	[73]
Experimental methods applied to the study of RNA networks in AD. The role of miRNAs	[122]
The miRNome of Alzheimer's disease	[123]
RNA-sequencing studies showing RNA splicing alterations in AD	[124]
Regulation of endogenous tau exon 10 splicing by Dyrk1A in Ts65Dn mice, a model of Down syndrome	[125]
Proteomics and methods to investigate posttranslational mechanisms/networks	
Metalloproteomics in AD research	[126]
Redox proteomics in biofluids. Posttranslational modifications analysis	[127]
Proteomics study showing Aβ amyloid impair splicing mechanisms and the spliceosome	[128]
Proteomics in systems biology. Methods and protocols	[129]
Plasma proteomics biomarkers in Alzheimer's disease	[130]
Integrated approaches analyzing RNA splicing abnormalities and impaired RNA processing in AD	[131–133]
Metabolomics	
Metabolomics to study central nervous system diseases	[134]
Alterations in metabolic pathways and networks in AD	[135]
Metabolic network studies in AD. A biochemical road map	[136]
Lipidomics. Lipid metabolites in AD	[137, 138]
Interactomes. Networks	
The architecture of the human interactome defines protein modules and disease networks	[139]
Amyloid β and tau network interplay. Tau aggregation in the presence of amyloid β	[140]
V. Computational systems biology. Network biology: Next-generation computational and integrative network biology approaches for the study of modules, network dynamics, and their interplay in multifactorial diseases and AD	[2, 3]
Computational analyses of neuroimaging patterns toward identification of AD subtypes (ADNI)	[100]

(continued)

Table 2
(continued)

Description of method/study	References
Network-based analysis for uncovering mechanisms underlying AD	[141, 142]
Computational network biology approach to uncover novel genes related to AD	[143]
Characterization of genetic networks associated with AD	[144]
Amyloid β and tau network interplay. Tau aggregation in the presence of amyloid β	[140]
Computational systems biology-network approaches to study miRNA networks in AD	[122]
Defining endoplasmic reticulum-associated degradation (ERAD) networks through a systems-level integrative mapping strategy	[145]
Progressive impairment of the ubiquitin proteasome system (UPS) during AD progression revealed by computational network biology	[146]
Methods for studying signaling and regulatory response networks and disease progression	[147]
A method to cluster longitudinal data (time series) according to their patterns	[148]
VI. Specific approaches and methods using comprehensive disease models recapitulating AD features to characterize underlying mechanisms and subtypes: From single-celled models to human	
(Yeast, *Drosophila*, mouse, human trisomy 21 iPSCs and neurons; cortical neurons after differentiation of human pluripotent cells and others)	
(Yeast) *Saccharomyces cerevisiae*	[149, 150]
(Fruit fly) *Drosophila*	[151]
(Mouse) *Mus musculus*	[97, 125, 152]
(Human cell lines, mouse, fly, rat models)	
Sustained protein folding ER stress activates the unfolded protein response (UPR) and builds up levels of death cell receptor DR5. If stress is relieved soon enough receptor levels decay back to normal and the cells stay alive (effect counteracted/reversed; homeostasis restored), otherwise induction of apoptotic cell death	[153]
Tau accumulation activates the UPR by impairing UPS/ERAD. The reversibility of the process suggests that tau-based therapeutics could delay cell death and disease progression	[154]
Tau association with synaptic vesicles causes presynaptic dysfunction	[155]
Spread of tau down neural circuits precedes synapse and neuronal loss in a mouse model of early AD	[97]
Amyloid β and tau network interplay. Tau aggregation in the presence of amyloid β	[140]
Early treatments in Ts65Dn mice, a model of Down syndrome	[125, 156]
Latest studies investigating the role of APOE isoforms (http://www.alzforum.org/news/research-news/apoe-risk-explained-isoform-dependent-boost-app-expression-uncovered)	[74, 75]

(continued)

Table 2
(continued)

Description of method/study	References
Human trisomy 21 iPSC-derived neurons; iPSC-derived cortical neurons	[157, 158]
3D culture models of AD. Recapitulating AD pathogenic cascades in 3D human neural cell culture models using AD patient-derived induced pluripotent stem cells (iPSCs) or genetically modified human stem cell lines	[159, 160]
Advances in mini-brain technology. Brain organoids. 3D cultured tissues resembling human brain structures to study neuronal development and how brain regions interact	[161]
VII. Next-generation genome editing methods. Application to AD studies	
(Clustered regularly interspaced short palindromic repeats/Cas9 (CRISPR/Cas9) and others)	
CRISPR proof-of-principle studies and methods (http://www.the-scientist.com/?articles.view/articleNo/48576/title/A-Selection-of-CRISPR-Proof-of-Principle-Studies/)	
Measuring and reducing off-target activities of programmable nucleases including CRISPR–Cas9	[162]
Genome-wide CRISPR screens identifying essential components of inflammasome activation	[163]
Generation of human induced pluripotent stem cells with heterozygous and homozygous dominant early-onset AD-causing mutations, and derived cortical neurons displaying genotype-dependent disease-associated phenotypes (CRISPR/Cas9-based scarless genome editing method)	[164]
Use of genome editing techniques to reduce genomic variability. Modeling AD with human induced pluripotent stem (iPS) cells and differentiation into different neural cell types. Generation of two- and three-dimensional iPS cell models	[165]
New CRISPR screening technique enabling high-throughput analysis of functional regulatory elements in the human genome (CRISPR-Cas9 epigenome method). Probing the regulatory roles of specific noncoding DNA sequences (http://www.the-scientist.com/?articles.view/articleNo/49055/title/CRISPR-Screen-Detects-Functional-Gene-Regulation/)	[76]
In vivo CRISPR interference (CRISPRi) study to investigate how ApoE isoforms activate a signaling cascade that enhances transcription of APP and production of Aβ (http://www.alzforum.org/news/research-news/apoe-risk-explained-isoform-dependent-boost-app-expression-uncovered)	[75]
VIII. Single-cell technologies/methods for single-cell functional analysis	
(Single-cell genomics. Single-cell genome sequencing, single-cell transcriptomics, RNA sequencing (RNA-Seq), single-cell combinatorial indexing (SCI) and others)	[166–174]
Single-cell RNA Seq: unraveling the brain one cell at a time	[175]
Optical cell positioning for long-term in vivo single-cell tracking of adult-born cells	[176]

(continued)

Table 2
(continued)

Description of method/study	References
Single-cell RNA-Seq and component analysis to unveil cellular heterogeneity in tumors and complex diseases for characterization of subtypes	[177]
Single-cell genomic techniques to study single-cell diversity in the brain. Somatic mutations and their relevance in neuropsychiatric disorders. The brain somatic mosaicism network (BSMN)	[77]
Combining CRISPR gene editing with single-cell sequencing for genotype-phenotype screenings (http://www.the-scientist.com/?articles.view/articleNo/48539/title/Massively-Parallel-Perturbations/)	
Single-cell RNA-seq identifies a novel microglia type (DAM) associated with restricting development of AD	[178]

Alzheimer's disease: toward molecular, cellular, and physiological hallmarks as standard biomarkers to characterize AD stages (preclinical (asymptomatic), mild, intermediate, and late AD) and subtypes for comprehensive stratification, and targets for mechanism-based, tailored interventions (preventive and therapeutic) and precision medicine. Next-generation genomics, neuroimaging, experimental and computational systems biology reference methods for holistic studies including latest genome analysis approaches, genome editing, molecular and high-throughput omics studies, bulk and new single-cell technologies in vitro and in vivo, from simple model organisms to human, to be applied in longitudinal cohort studies and trials. Several techniques and studies presented in refs. [2, 3, 41] and references therein

Main advances in neuroimaging methods and discoveries toward characterization of AD subtypes and stages are emerging from the progressive incorporation of next-generation amyloid-β and tau tracers for in vivo imaging, which are revealing new links between amyloid-β deposition and tauopathy and new insights into underlying mechanisms during AD progression. Most relevant are (a) tau imaging in staging AD studies revealing interactions between β-amyloid and tauopathy [99]; (b) an array tomography imaging study which has revealed that the spread of tau down neural circuits precedes synapse and neuronal loss [97]; (c) a tau positron-emission tomography (PET) in vivo imaging study showing that tau patterns mirror clinical and neuroanatomical symptoms (cortical atrophy) during AD progression [101]; (d) a multimodal imaging in vivo study which confirmed a high regional association between tau levels, atrophy, and symptoms in early clinical stages of AD [102, 103]; and (e) a longitudinal PET study which revealed an early and late peak in microglial activation in AD trajectory [96]. More recently, new multitracer technologies for in vivo imaging revealed a hierarchical organization of tau and amyloid deposits in the cerebral cortex [93, 94]. The novel neuroimaging methods and discoveries are paving the way to more comprehensive characterization of AD subtypes and stages [84, 88–92, 95, 179] and latest studies from the Alzheimer's disease neuroimaging initiative (ADNI) (http://www.adni-info.org/) [100].

2.2.2 Advanced Methods for the Study of Mechanisms, Pathways, and Networks Underlying AD

These include the most relevant techniques and protocols to investigate the essential role of, among others, APP processing pathways and tau networks, including oxidative stress and β-amyloid aggregation; the development of tau pathology; tau prion strains; disturbance of endoplasmic reticulum (ER) proteostasis and unfolded protein response (UPR); autophagic activity and interlinked networks; mitochondrial dysfunction; microglial proliferation; inflammation; role of infection and neuroinflammation in neurodegeneration; the immune system balancing health and disease; and role of Aβ clearance mechanisms and drainage from the brain (including the glymphatic system) (*see* Table 2, section III).

2.2.3 Experimental Systems Biology Approaches: Omics Levels, Interactomes, and Networks—Next-Generation Molecular and High-Throughput Omics Methods

Advanced systems biology methods, experimental and computational, include next-generation molecular, high-throughput omics approaches studying genome, transcriptome, proteome, and metabolome patterns and interactions, and integrative approaches ([1, 3] and references therein). Relevant examples of advanced studies using systems biology approaches in multifactorial diseases (cancers, neurodegenerative diseases) include (1) multi-omics studies in longitudinal studies using integrative personal omics profiling (iPOP) monitoring panels of biomarkers and patterns toward diagnosis and personalized medicine [4]; (2) integrative genomic approaches including transcriptomics (RNA-Seq) for tumor profiling toward personalized cancer therapy [180]; (3) identification of key regulators of pancreatic cancer progression through multidimensional systems-level analysis [181]; and (4) systems biology proteomics studies identifying a molecular signature, group of plasma proteins, as biomarkers and potential therapeutic targets for patients with glioblastoma [182]. More omics-driven studies and initiatives are in progress to revolutionize healthcare toward precision medicine [183].

Among most relevant systems-level approaches including the application of omics technologies to dissect neurologic disease and AD [120] are for instance:

1. Transcriptomics: RNA-Seq to elucidate early patterns of dysregulation underlying AD [121]; experimental methods applied to the study of RNA networks in AD [122, 123]; RNA-Seq studies showing RNA splicing alterations in AD [124, 131–133].

2. Proteomics studies showing Aβ amyloid impair splicing mechanisms [128]; metalloproteomics and redox proteomics studies in AD [126, 127]; plasma proteomics biomarkers in AD [130].

3. Metabolomics: Alterations in metabolic pathways and networks in AD [135, 136, 138].

4. Amyloid-β and tau network interplay: Tau aggregation in the presence of amyloid [140]. For more integrative systems-level studies applied to NDs and AD *see* Table 2, section IV ([2, 3] and references therein, [184–186]).

2.2.4 Computational Systems Biology: Network Biology—Next-Generation Computational and Integrative Network Biology Approaches

Selected systems-level computational, network biology methods and studies applied to neurodegenerative diseases and AD (*see also* Table 2, section V) are as follows: computational network biology approaches to uncover novel genes related to AD [143]; characterization of genetic networks associated with AD [144]; network-based analysis for uncovering mechanisms underlying AD [141, 142]; computational analyses of neuroimaging patterns toward identification of AD subtypes ([100] and Alzheimer's disease neuroimaging initiative (ADNI)); amyloid-β and tau networks' interplay studies [140]; computational systems biology approaches to study miRNA networks in AD [122]; progressive impairment of the ubiquitin proteasome system (UPS) during AD progression revealed by computational network biology [146]; and methods for studying signaling and regulatory response networks and disease progression [147].

2.2.5 Latest Approaches Using Comprehensive Disease Models Recapitulating AD Features to Characterize Underlying Mechanisms and Subtypes: From Single-Celled Models to Human

Comprehensive studies on multifactorial complex diseases such as AD require the construction of reliable models which recapitulate the altered mechanisms and features of the disease at the molecular and cellular level, leading to the generation of the characteristic supracellular features and hallmarks of the disease (e.g., in AD, amyloid plaques and neurofibrillary tangles). The main requirement of a disease model is "to be able to recapitulate molecular and physiological features of the disease," to advance our understanding of the real events in vivo [2]. Studies and methodologies using AD disease models (*see also* Table 2, section VI) include the following:

1. The construction of simple disease models to investigate the role of essentially conserved pathways and networks in AD (e.g., homeostatic, proteostasis networks), and transgenic humanized models to study the influence of specific mechanisms in simple models under controlled conditions, from single-celled organisms to human (e.g., yeast, worm, fly, mouse, rat models) [2, 125, 149–152]), and leading to relevant new discoveries: for example: (a) the fact that the spread of tau down neural circuits precedes synapse and neuronal loss in a mouse model of early AD [97]; (b) tau association with synaptic vesicles causing presynaptic dysfunction [155]; (c) amyloid-β and tau networks' interplay and tau aggregation in the presence of amyloid-β [140]; and (d) integrative studies combining different techniques showing ApoE2, ApoE3, and ApoE4 differentially stimulating APP transcription and Aβ secretion [74, 75].

2. The construction and development of closer-to-human AD disease models, to unveil human-specific mechanisms and networks underlying AD, including (a) human cell lines, patient-derived induced pluripotent stem cells (iPSCs), human trisomy 21 iPSC-derived neurons, and iPSC-derived cortical neurons [157, 158]; (b) 3D culture models. Recapitulating AD pathogenic cascades in 3D human neural cell culture models using AD patient-derived iPSCs or genetically modified human stem cell lines

[159, 160]; (c) advances in brain organoid technology. 3D cultured tissues resembling human brain structures to study neuronal development and how brain regions interact [161].

2.2.6 Next-Generation Genome Editing Methods: Application to Multifactorial Diseases and AD

New advances in comprehensive and reliable genome editing methods are opening the way to new discoveries in multifactorial diseases and AD. For instance: (a) New CRISPR screening techniques enabling high-throughput analysis of functional regulatory elements in the human genome (CRISPR-Cas9 epigenome method) probing the regulatory roles of specific noncoding DNA sequences [76]; (b) genome-wide CRISPR screens identifying essential components of inflammasome activation [163]; (c) generation of human iPSCs with heterozygous and homozygous dominant early-onset AD-causing mutations, and derived cortical neurons displaying genotype-dependent disease-associated phenotypes (CRISPR/Cas9-based scarless genome editing method) [164]; (d) in vivo CRISPR interference (CRISPRi) study which allows to investigate how ApoE isoforms activate a signaling cascade that enhances transcription of APP and production of Aβ [75] (Table 2, section VII).

2.2.7 Single-Cell Technologies for Single-Cell Functional Analysis: Application to Multifactorial Diseases and AD

The progressive incorporation of single-cell technologies to the repertoire of holistic, systems biology methods is allowing the analysis of complex diseases at the single-cellular level. These are revealing cellular heterogeneity in multifactorial diseases and AD, with new discoveries opening the way to more comprehensive characterization of AD subtypes and stages. The most relevant methods and discoveries (*see also* Table 2, section VIII) include the following:

(a) Single-cell genome sequencing, single-cell RNA-Seq, and single-cell combinatorial indexing (SCI) and others [166–174]; (b) single-cell genomic techniques to study single-cell diversity in the brain. Somatic mutations and their relevance in neuropsychiatric disorders [77]; (c) single-cell RNA Seq: unraveling the brain one cell at a time [175]; (d) single-cell RNA-Seq and component analysis to unveil cellular heterogeneity in tumors and complex diseases for characterization of subtypes [177]; (e) single-cell RNA-Seq recently identified a novel microglia type (disease-associated microglia, DAM) targeting neurodegeneration, associated with restricting development of AD [178].

Next-generation genomics, neuroimaging, and systems biology methods as summarized in this work will require continuous refining, validation, and update in public databases, book series, and repositories (e.g., Cold Spring Harbour protocols; Springer protocols; Springer MiMB methods series; Nature Methods; Nature Protocols; Methods in Enzymology; Methods), to be readily available to researchers and experts worldwide [41]. These will need to be progressively incorporated into new, next-generation comprehensive cohort studies and trials (*see* below), to advance in the discovery of mechanism-based molecular markers and signatures for classification and disease staging as well as candidate targets for tailored treatments and precision medicine [2, 3, 12, 13] (Fig. 1).

3   Systems Biology Methods to Be Applied in AD Cohort Studies and Trials: Strategies and Challenges—The European Prevention of Alzheimer's Dementia (EPAD) Project

If new systems biology methods should be incorporated into cohort studies and trials, what is required? We suggest that the following will be needed. First, new systems-level approaches, molecular high-throughput techniques, and computational tools will need to be continuously developed and refined, compared with previous ones and, once validated, lead to the implementation of new standards and guidelines. This is a continuous process until reliable and affordable methods and biomarkers are approved by medicine agencies (e.g., US Food and Drug Administration (FDA) clinical trial guidances, with adherence to the principles of good clinical practice (GCP): http://www.fda.gov/regulatoryinformation/guidances/ucm122046.htm;   http://clinicaltrials.gov; European Medicine Agency (EMA) and European Clinical Trials Database (EudraCT): https://eudract.ema.europa.eu/). Main advances on standardization and guidelines in AD are coming from global efforts on neuroimaging and standard biomarkers, for example, from the Alzheimer's disease neuroimaging initiative (ADNI) and the Dominantly Inherited Alzheimer Network (DIAN) (*see also* [2] and references therein, and [187, 188]).

Together with this, raw data, methods, and approaches will need to be deposited in well-curated repositories, protocol series, and databases, together with their associated metadata (e.g., conditions and methods used) to guide in the identification of truly comparable datasets for efficient *Big Data* analyses [82, 83]. Progress is being made and advances are steadily produced in both the experimental and computational systems biology areas ([1–3] and references therein, and [6, 12, 41, 184, 186, 189]) (Tables 1 and 2).

With this perspective, a selection of relevant trials (*see also* the ClinicalTrials.gov registry) which may benefit from incorporating new holistic systems biology methods can include the following:

1. The Dominantly Inherited Alzheimer Network (DIAN) trial: Assessing the safety, tolerability, and biomarker efficacy of the drugs gantenerumab and solanezumab in individuals who have a genetic mutation for autosomal dominant Alzheimer's disease (ADAD).

2. Alzheimer's disease in Down syndrome (DS-AD) trials: *See also* DS Consortium and DS-Connect resource, and London Down Syndrome Consortium (LonDownS) studies.

   (a) The Anti-Amyloid Treatment in Asymptomatic Alzheimer's study (the A4 study): Testing whether solanezumab can slow the progression of memory problems associated with amyloid.

3. Prevention trial: Lifestyle (FINGER) trial: A 2-year multidomain intervention of diet, exercise, cognitive training, and vascular risk monitoring versus control to prevent cognitive decline in at-risk elderly people: a randomized controlled trial. Extended for 7 years [190].

4. The European Prevention of Alzheimer's Dementia (EPAD) project: A major component of a global approach to improve trial design and delivery for the secondary prevention of Alzheimer's dementia (*see* below).

Most relevant systems biology methods which may be incorporated into these and new next-generation cohort studies and trials, to provide essential information for proper classification/stratification and to improve new trial design, are the following:

1. Latest amyloid-β, tau, and microglia tracers for in vivo imaging and new advanced neuroimaging methods (Table 2, section II).

2. High-throughput expression studies to characterize and dissect early altered molecular signatures such as transcriptome patterns and splicing (e.g., using RNA-Seq and proteomics techniques), and to monitor impaired and homeostatic networks and their interplay in different subtypes and stages (Table 2, section IV).

3. Single-cell technologies such as single-cell RNA-Seq, to dissect the role of different cellular entities, their activities and interplay, including a novel disease-associated microglia (DAM) restricting development of AD [178] (Table 2, section VIII).

The incorporation of these and new, progressively more affordable, systems biology methods is expected to allow the discovery of basic mechanisms, pathways, and regulatory networks in different subtypes and stages, molecular signatures, and markers for improved classification, better trial design, and earlier diagnostics (preferably at the earliest preclinical stage), toward timely tailored interventions (precision medicine) [2, 12, 13].

3.1 The European Prevention of Alzheimer's Dementia (EPAD) Project: A Comprehensive and Integrated Clinical Research Platform for the Secondary Prevention of Alzheimer's Dementia

The European Prevention of Alzheimer's Dementia (EPAD) Project was initiated in January 2015 [191]. It will provide a pan-European platform and environment for the effective and efficient undertaking of Phase2 Proof of Concept (PoC) Bayesian Adaptive Clinical Trials of purported disease-modifying interventions (pharmacological and non-pharmacological) for the secondary prevention of Alzheimer's dementia (http://ep-ad.org/).

Since the turn of the century and despite massive drug discovery efforts, there have been no significant therapeutic breakthroughs in the management of AD (Fig. 2). The key mediator to this is the fact that disease-modifying interventions were being used too late in the disease course to have any realistic expectation (in retrospect)

3.1.1 Background

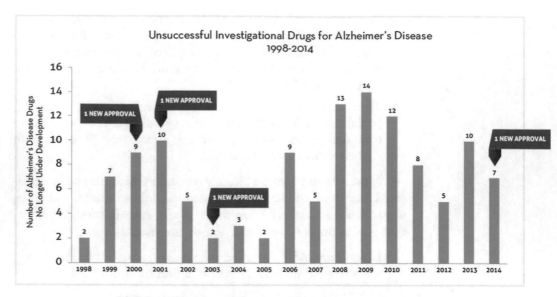

Fig. 2 Unsuccessful investigational drugs for Alzheimer's disease (1998–2014)

of success. It is accepted now by most that AD is a disease of midlife that may present with Alzheimer's dementia as a late-stage manifestation [192]. Going too late in the disease course was compounded by the lack of homogeneity that can only come from empirically based stratification of the trial populations. While success 20 years ago was manifest with drugs specifically affecting the cholinergic deficits seen in Alzheimer's dementia [193] (and other prevalent dementias, e.g., Lewy body dementia and vascular dementia)—their perturbation of the "cholinergic hypothesis" was measurable given the tight tethering of cholinergic manipulation to clinical (primarily amnestic) symptoms. In the later stage of AD observed in Alzheimer's dementia, the correlation between amyloid pathology and clinical symptoms is not high. It is hypothesized therefore that earlier and perhaps multimodal interventions will have a greater chance of success, i.e., in a preclinical population when disease is at its genesis but clinical symptoms many decades away.

The targeting of preclinical populations for disease modification though requires several hurdles to be overcome:

1. A critical requirement for biologically based stratification

2. An understanding of the trajectories of decline in biological and clinical outcomes in these strata

3. Data sharing between research programs that are independent but dedicated to the same objectives

4. The need to develop cognitive outcome measures with the necessary psychometric properties that also reflect underlying core Alzheimer's disease pathologies

5. Recruitment of preclinical populations who (by definition) do not present in large numbers to clinical centers

6. Ethical and societal aspects of testing for biomarker and cognitive abnormalities in asymptomatic individuals [194]

In addition to these challenges, a review of pharmacological failures to date has highlighted that these exceptionally expensive studies will have continued to recruit and follow up research participants at a point after the futility of the drug could (and perhaps should) have been known. There is also a strong sense that major Phase 3 programs were embarked upon with insufficient knowledge gained on the drug, ideal population, and optimal outcome measures in Phase 2.

To address all of these issues concurrently, the EPAD project was established in 2015 with €64,000,000 of funding from the Innovative Medicines Initiative (IMI) (http://www.imi.europa.eu/) to establish the platform. Additional funding will be forthcoming for the running of the actual adaptive trial by the intervention owners.

3.1.2 The EPAD Structure

EPAD is divided in several ways; there are eight work packages across two primary domains (Fig. 3). There are also four major component parts to the participant and associated data flow; these are as follows: the EPAD Virtual Register, PrePAD, the EPAD Longitudinal Cohort Study (EPAD-LCS), and the EPAD PoC Trial (EPAD-PoC).

The recruitment of research participants into EPAD is exclusively from preexisting parent cohorts and registers that are both clinically and population based. The data already held in those data environments is considered as the *EPAD Virtual Register* and is viewed by the PrePAD solution that can identify individuals who fulfil certain risk algorithms, e.g., ApoEe4+, evidence of hippocampal atrophy, and cognitive impairment. On the basis of these searches participants are invited to attend an EPAD Trial Delivery Centre (TDC) where they may consent for inclusion in the *EPAD Longitudinal Cohort Study (LCS)*. The EPAD LCS is a cohort with two primary objectives—firstly to act as a readiness cohort for the *EPAD PoC Trial*. The second objective is to be the largest and most deeply phenotyped cohort for disease modeling in preclinical and prodromal AD ever assembled. This second objective will inform stratification and illness trajectories as data accumulates both in volume and length of follow-up. These models will then be translated to determine the "readiness strata" that will push the adaptation of the inclusion criteria (strata) that are approached for the EPAD PoC Trial.

The EPAD PoC Trial is a Bayesian adaptive trial with evolutionary analysis on the basis of safety as well as success/futility against prespecified criteria on trajectories of change in intermediary biomarker phenotypes and then the primary cognitive outcome. The choice of primary outcome as the RBANS (Repeatable

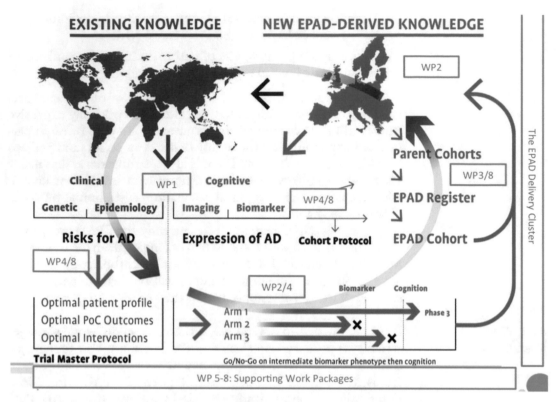

Fig. 3 Summary of EPAD structure. WP = Work Package. WP1 = Scientific Advisory Groups, WP2 = PoC and Disease Modeling Statistics, WP3 = PrePAD and EPAD Virtual Register, WP4 = EPAD LCS, PoC and TDC Establishment and Management, WP5 = Project Management, WP6 = Communication and Public Engagement, WP7 = Sustainability and WP8 = Ethics, Legal, and Social Implications

Battery for the Assessment of Neuropsychological Status) total score was based on the output of the Cognitive Scientific Advisory Group [195, 196].

The trial is a single project with multiple appendices. The majority of the trial procedures are articulated in the master protocol. Appendix-specific adaptations may add safety, cognitive, or biomarker outcomes but cannot take away from the master protocol. This has the key advantages of being able to build significant efficiencies in terms of trial delivery and secondly in terms of the capacity to share placebo between appendices.

The EPAD LCS started recruitment in 2016 and is on target to reach over 1000 participants by late 2017. The EPAD Virtual Register, PrePAD, and recruitment into EPAD LCS have all proved both feasible and efficient.

In summary, the EPAD Project is a major component of a global approach to improve trial design and delivery for the secondary prevention of Alzheimer's dementia. It works in tandem with other contributing projects to this goal namely the Global Alzheimer's Platform (GAP) (http://globalalzplatform.org/),

DIAN-TU (https://dian-tu.wustl.edu/en/home/), and initiating aligned initiatives in Canada, Australia, and Japan. The fundamental objective of EPAD is to understand disease mechanisms and their associated clinical phenotype in a preclinical Alzheimer's disease population agnostic to currently preeminent hypothesis. In doing so the within platform PoC will be designed and adapted on empirical, unbiased cohort data emerging from the same individuals and TDCs that enter the trial.

4   Conclusions: Future Perspectives—From Systems Biology Methods to Underlying Mechanisms, AD Subtypes and Staging, Timely Tailored Interventions, and Precision Medicine

Alzheimer's disease (AD) is a complex multifactorial disease starting decades before the appearance of first cognitive symptoms [197, 198]. This evidence emphasizes the urgent need to study the pathophysiological mechanisms underlying impairments and the interplay of networks at the molecular and cellular levels. Experimental approaches targeting small sets of genes and proteins may overlook key elements of pathways and regulatory networks, ultimately limiting the opportunity to develop early diagnostic tools and multitarget therapeutics. A more comprehensive insight into potential treatment options for AD can be achieved only through the integrative and holistic approaches offered by systems biology. "For mechanisms-based Precision Medicine strategies of multifactorial diseases to succeed, holistic systems-level methods are necessary" [2, 3, 12, 41].

Systems biology methods, experimental and computational, offer the potential to unveil new fundamental insights, basic mechanisms, and networks and their interplay. These may lead to the characterization of mechanism-based molecular signatures and AD hallmarks at the earliest molecular and cellular levels (and beyond) for comprehensive classification/stratification and the development of rational targeted interventions in the framework of precision medicine (Fig. 1). "The notion that we will find one single treatment that cures all patients with AD is quickly losing ground. Far more likely is the idea that in the future, specific subtypes of AD could benefit from specific treatments." Efforts are being directed toward timely targeted treatments ("right treatment at the right time"), preferably at the earliest asymptomatic stage, well before irreversible cell damage [2, 12, 78].

In this chapter, an update on advanced systems biology methods, including next-generation genomics, neuroimaging, and multiomics methods, experimental and computational, relevant disease models, latest genome editing, and single-cell technologies applicable to AD and other multifactorial diseases, is presented (Tables 1 and 2). The progressive incorporation of these methods into new studies and trials is expected to follow the path previously observed in other more advanced fields of medicine (e.g., oncology), with findings from basic research (including genomic and molecular signatures), helping to identify reliable markers for classification and targeted therapies. Such a strategy is already delivering relevant insights and major translational benefits [180–182, 199–201]. In this context, the recent first FDA approval of a cancer treatment for any solid tumor with a specific molecular signature (molecular marker) regardless of the tumor's location represents a major milestone. This first success in targeting a molecular signature will pave the way to the investigation of new marker-based approaches using latest systems biology methods and molecular profiling approaches such as those presented in this chapter. These are expected to unveil new molecular markers for proper classification and staging, improved trial design, and mechanism-based, timely tailored interventions [2, 3, 12] (Fig. 1).

The systems biology methods and approaches presented here can be incorporated into several studies and trials, with the European Prevention of Alzheimer's Dementia (EPAD) project being a relevant reference example (*see* Subheading 3). Furthermore, they can also be applied to studies and trials investigating benefits of protective, modifiable risk factors (e.g., diet, exercise, enriched environment, active lifestyle) [190, 202, 203], to provide additional mechanism-based evidence to support Health Public initiatives and incentives, and expedite their implementation [2, 3, 12]. In all, only multidisciplinary worldwide collaborations will allow us to progress from systems biology approaches to precision medicine and public health. For a solid, coordinated progress, most relevant national and multinational projects may benefit from adhering to the guidelines of the recently approved Global Plan on Dementia 2017–2025 (29 May 2017; WHO adopts Global Plan of Action on the Public Health Response to Dementia 2017-2025).

Acknowledgments

This work was supported by Genetadi Biotech SL (Bizkaia, Spain). J.I.C. is the beneficiary of a senior prossgram (mode A) of Bizkaia:Xede Foundation. H.H. is supported by the AXA Research Fund, the Fondation Université Pierre et Marie Curie, and the Fondation pour la Recherche sur Alzheimer, Paris, France. Ce travail a bénéficié d'une aide de l'Etat "Investissements d'avenir" ANR-10-IAIHU-06 (H.H.). The research leading to these results has received funding from the program "Investissements d'avenir" ANR-10-IAIHU-06 (Agence Nationale de la Recherche-10-IA Agence Institut Hospitalo-Universitaire-6) (H.H.).

References

1. Castrillo JI, Oliver SG (2011) Yeast systems biology. Methods and protocols. Methods in molecular biology 759 (MiMB series. Editor-in-chief. Prof. John M. Walker). Humana Press/Springer, New York

2. Castrillo JI, Oliver SG (2016a) Alzheimer's as a systems-level disease involving the interplay of multiple cellular networks. Methods Mol Biol 1303:3–48

3. Castrillo JI, Oliver SG (2016b) Systems biology of Alzheimer's disease. Methods in molecular biology (MiMB) series. Humana Press/Springer, New York

4. Chen R, Mias GI, Li-Pook-Than J et al (2012) Personal omics profiling reveals dynamic molecular and medical phenotypes. Cell 148:1293–1307

5. Castrillo JI, Pir P, Oliver SG (2013) Yeast systems biology: towards a systems understanding of regulation of eukaryotic networks in complex diseases and biotechnology. In: Walhout M, Vidal M, Dekker J (eds) Handbook of systems biology. Elsevier, New York, pp 343–365

6. Walhout M, Vidal M, Dekker J (2013) Handbook of systems biology. Elsevier, New York

7. Kosik KS (2015) Personalized medicine for effective Alzheimer disease treatment. JAMA Neurol 72:497–498

8. Montine TJ, Montine KS (2015) Precision medicine: clarity for the clinical and biological complexity of Alzheimer's and Parkinson's diseases. J Exp Med 212:601–605

9. Kovacs GG (2016) Molecular pathological classification of neurodegenerative diseases: turning towards precision medicine. Int J Mol Sci 17:pii: E189

10. Reitz C (2016) Toward precision medicine in Alzheimer's disease. Ann Transl Med 4:107

11. Swanton C, Soria JC, Bardelli A et al (2016) Consensus on precision medicine for metastatic cancers: a report from the MAP conference. Ann Oncol 27:1443–1448

12. Hampel H, O'Bryant SE, Castrillo JI et al (2016) Precision medicine - the golden gate to detect, prevent and cure Alzheimer's disease. J Prev Alz Dis 3:243–259

13. Hampel H, O'Bryant SE, Durrleman S, Alzheimer Precision Medicine Initiative et al (2017) A precision medicine initiative for Alzheimer's disease: the road ahead to biomarker-guided integrative disease modeling. Climacteric 20:107–118

14. Collins FS, Varmus H (2015) A new initiative on precision medicine. N Engl J Med 372:793–795

15. Goodwin S, McPherson JD, McCombie WR (2016) Coming of age: ten years of next-generation sequencing technologies. Nat Rev Genet 17:333–351

16. Berg J (2016) Gene-environment interplay. Science 354:15

17. Kitano H (2002) Systems biology: a brief overview. Science 295:1662–1664

18. Castrillo JI, Oliver SG (2006) Metabolomics and systems biology in *Saccharomyces cerevisiae*. In: Karl Esser K (ed) The mycota. A comprehensive treatise on fungi as experimental systems for basic and applied research, Fungal genomics, vol XIII. Springer, New York, pp 3–18

19. Castrillo JI, Oliver SG (2014) Yeast as a model for systems Biology studies on complex Diseases. In: Nowrousian M (ed) The mycota. A comprehensive treatise on fungi as experimental systems for basic and applied research. Fungal genomics, 2nd edn (Karl Esser, Series Editor). Springer, Berlin, pp 3–30

20. Hampel H, Frank R, Broich K et al (2010) Biomarkers for Alzheimer's disease: academic, industry and regulatory perspectives. Nat Rev Drug Discov 9:560–574

21. Hampel H, Lista S, Khachaturian ZS (2012) Development of biomarkers to chart all Alzheimer's disease stages: the royal road to cutting the therapeutic Gordian Knot. Alzheimers Dement 8:312–336

22. Hampel H, Lista S (2013) Use of biomarkers and imaging to assess pathophysiology, mechanisms of action and target engagement. J Nutr Health Aging 17:54–63

23. Hampel H, Lista S, Teipel SJ et al (2014) Perspective on future role of biological markers in clinical therapy trials of Alzheimer's disease: a long-range point of view beyond 2020. Biochem Pharmacol 88:426–449

24. Lista S, Emanuele E (2011) Role of amyloid β1-42 and neuroimaging biomarkers in Alzheimer's disease. Biomark Med 5:411–413

25. Lista S, Garaci FG, Ewers M et al (2014) CSF Aβ1-42 combined with neuroimaging biomarkers in the early detection, diagnosis and prediction of Alzheimer's disease. Alzheimers Dement 10:381–392

26. Zetzsche T, Rujescu D, Hardy J, Hampel H (2010) Advances and perspectives from genetic research: development of biological

markers in Alzheimer's disease. Expert Rev Mol Diagn 10:667–690

27. Bertram L, Hampel H (2011) The role of genetics for biomarker development in neurodegeneration. Prog Neurobiol 95:501–504

28. Hampel H, Lista S (2012) Alzheimer disease: from inherited to sporadic AD-crossing the biomarker bridge. Nat Rev Neurol 8:598–600

29. Lista S, O'Bryant SE, Blennow K et al (2015) Biomarkers in sporadic and familial Alzheimer's disease. J Alzheimers Dis 47:291–317

30. Blennow K, Hampel H, Weiner M, Zetterberg H (2010) Cerebrospinal fluid and plasma biomarkers in Alzheimer disease. Nat Rev Neurol 6:131–144

31. Blennow K, Dubois B, Fagan AM et al (2015) Clinical utility of cerebrospinal fluid biomarkers in the diagnosis of early Alzheimer's disease. Alzheimers Dement 11:58–69

32. Ghidoni R, Benussi L, Paterlini A et al (2011) Cerebrospinal fluid biomarkers for Alzheimer's disease: the present and the future. Neurodegener Dis 8:413–420

33. Ewers M, Mattsson N, Minthon L et al (2015) CSF biomarkers for the differential diagnosis of Alzheimer's disease: a large-scale international multicenter study. Alzheimers Dement 11:1306–1315

34. Lista S, Faltraco F, Prvulovic D, Hampel H (2013) Blood and plasma-based proteomic biomarker research in Alzheimer's disease. Prog Neurobiol 101–102:1–17

35. Lista S, Faltraco F, Hampel H (2013) Biological and methodical challenges of blood-based proteomics in the field of neurological research. Prog Neurobiol 101–102:18–34

36. O'Bryant SE, Lista S, Rissman RA et al (2015) Comparing biological markers of Alzheimer's disease across blood fraction and platforms: comparing apples to oranges. Alzheimers Dement (Amst) 3:27–34

37. O'Bryant SE, Gupta V, Henriksen K, STAR-B and BBBIG Working Groups et al (2015) Guidelines for the standardization of preanalytic variables for blood-based biomarker studies in Alzheimer's disease research. Alzheimers Dement 11:549–560

38. O'Bryant SE, Mielke MM, Rissman RA et al (2017) Biofluid based biomarker professional interest area. Blood-based biomarkers in Alzheimer disease: current state of the science and a novel collaborative paradigm for advancing from discovery to clinic. Alzheimers Dement 13:45–58

39. Ewers M, Sperling RA, Klunk WE et al (2011) Neuroimaging markers for the prediction and early diagnosis of Alzheimer's disease dementia. Trends Neurosci 34:430–442

40. Teipel SJ, Grothe M, Lista S et al (2013) Relevance of magnetic resonance imaging for early detection and diagnosis of Alzheimer disease. Med Clin North Am 97:399–424

41. Villa A (2016) Book review (Systems biology of Alzheimer's disease. Castrillo JI, Oliver SG (eds). Humana, Springer, New York, 2016). J Alzheimers Dis 50(4):1255–1256

42. Braak H, Braak E, Bohl J, Bratzke H (1998) Evolution of Alzheimer's disease related cortical lesions. J Neural Transm Suppl 54:97–106

43. Yankner BA, Lu T, Loerch P (2008) The aging brain. Annu Rev Pathol 3:41–66

44. Wood H (2014) Alzheimer disease: functional connectivity changes show similar trajectories in autosomal dominant and sporadic Alzheimer disease. Nat Rev Neurol 10:483

45. Blennow K, de Leon MJ, Zetterberg H (2006) Alzheimer's disease. Lancet 368:387–403

46. Acosta-Baena N, Sepulveda-Falla D, Lopera-Gómez CM et al (2011) Pre-dementia clinical stages in presenilin 1 E280A familial early-onset Alzheimer's disease: a retrospective cohort study. Lancet Neurol 10:213–220

47. Waring SC, Rosenberg RN (2008) Genome-wide association studies in Alzheimer disease. Arch Neurol 65:329–334

48. Alzheimer's Society UK (2014) What is Alzheimer's disease? Alzheimers.org.uk. https://www.alzheimers.org.uk/download/downloads/id/3379/what_is_alzheimers_disease.pdf

49. Strittmatter WJ, Saunders AM, Schmechel D et al (1993) Apolipoprotein E: high-avidity binding to beta-amyloid and increased frequency of type 4 allele in late-onset familial Alzheimer disease. Proc Natl Acad Sci U S A 90:1977–1981

50. Guerreiro R, Brás J, Hardy J (2013) SnapShot: genetics of Alzheimer's disease. Cell 155:968–968.e1

51. Budson AE, Kowall NW (2011) The handbook of Alzheimer's disease and other dementias. Willey-Blackwell, New York

52. Eisenstein M (2011) Genetics: finding risk factors. Nature 475:S20–S22. http://www.nature.com/nature/journal/v475/n7355_supp/full/475S20a.html

53. Benitez BA, Jin SC, Guerreiro R et al (2014) Missense variant in TREML2 protects against Alzheimer's disease. Neurobiol Aging 35:1510.e19–1510.e26

54. St George-Hyslop PH, Petit A (2005) Molecular biology and genetics of Alzheimer's disease. C R Biol 328:119–130

55. Morgan K, Carrasquillo MM (2013) Genetic variants in Alzheimer's disease. Springer, New York

56. Karch CM, Cruchaga C, Goate AM (2014) Alzheimer's disease genetics: from the bench to the clinic. Neuron 83:11–26

57. Novarino G, Fenstermaker AG, Zaki MS et al (2014) Exome sequencing links corticospinal motor neuron disease to common neurodegenerative disorders. Science 343:506–511

58. Tanzi RE (2014) Decoding Alzheimer's in the age of genome-wide analyses. Mol Neurodeg 8(Suppl 1):O1

59. Bertram L (2016) Next generation sequencing in Alzheimer's disease. Methods Mol Biol 1303:281–297

60. Jin SC, Benitez BA, Deming Y, Cruchaga C (2016) Pooled-DNA sequencing for elucidating new genomic risk factors, rare variants underlying Alzheimer's disease. Methods Mol Biol 1303:299–314

61. Szigeti K (2016) New genome-wide methods for elucidation of candidate copy number variations (CNVs) contributing to Alzheimer's disease heritability. Methods Mol Biol 1303:315–326

62. Rader DJ, Damrauer SM (2016) "Pheno"menal value for human health. Science 354:1534–1536

63. Huddleston J, Chaisson MJ, Meltz Steinberg K et al (2017) Discovery and genotyping of structural variation from long-read haploid genome sequence data. Genome Res 27:677–685

64. Seo JS, Rhie A, Kim J et al (2016) De novo assembly and phasing of a Korean human genome. Nature 538:243–247

65. Chiang C, Scott AJ, Davis JR et al (2017) The impact of structural variation on human gene expression. Nat Genet 49(5):692–699. https://doi.org/10.1038/ng.3834

66. Weisenfeld NI, Kumar V, Shah P et al (2017) Direct determination of diploid genome sequences. Genome Res 27(5):757–767. https://doi.org/10.1101/gr.214874.116

67. Bickhart DM, Rosen BD, Koren S et al (2017) Single-molecule sequencing and chromatin conformation capture enable de novo reference assembly of the domestic goat genome. Nat Genet 49:643–650

68. Worley KC (2017) A golden goat genome. Nat Genet 49:485–486

69. Dudchenko O, Batra SS, Omer AD et al (2017) De novo assembly of the Aedes aegypti genome using Hi-C yields chromosome-length scaffolds. Science 356(6333):92–95. https://doi.org/10.1126/science.aal3327

70. Check Hayden E (2016) A radical revision of human genetics. Nature 53:154–157

71. Patra B, Kon Y, Yadav G et al (2017) A genome wide dosage suppressor network reveals genomic robustness. Nucleic Acids Res 45:255–270

72. Lek M, Karczewski KJ, Minikel EV, Exome Aggregation Consortium et al (2016) Analysis of protein-coding genetic variation in 60,706 humans. Nature 536:285–291

73. Cummings BB, Marshall JL, Tukiainen T et al (2017) Improving genetic diagnosis in Mendelian disease with transcriptome sequencing. Sci Transl Med 9(386). https://doi.org/10.1126/scitranslmed.aal5209

74. Baker-Nigh AT, Mawuenyega KG, Bollinger JG et al (2016) Human central nervous system (CNS) ApoE isoforms are increased by age, differentially altered by amyloidosis, and relative amounts reversed in the CNS compared with plasma. J Biol Chem 291:27204–27218

75. Huang YA, Zhou B, Wernig M, Südhof TC (2017) ApoE2, ApoE3, and ApoE4 differentially stimulate APP transcription and Aβ secretion. Cell 168:427–441.e21

76. Klann TS, Black JB, Chellappan M et al (2017) CRISPR-Cas9 epigenome editing enables high-throughput screening for functional regulatory elements in the human genome. Nat Biotechnol 35:561–568. https://doi.org/10.1038/nbt.3853

77. McConnell MJ, Moran JV, Abyzov A, The Brain Somatic Mosaicism Network et al (2017) Intersection of diverse neuronal genomes and neuropsychiatric disease: The Brain Somatic Mosaicism Network. Science 356(6336). https://doi.org/10.1126/science.aal1641

78. Van der Flier WM (2016) Clinical heterogeneity in familial Alzheimer's disease. Lancet Neurol 15:1296–1298

79. Hatami A, Monjazeb S, Milton S, Glabe CG (2017) Familial Alzheimer's disease mutations within the amyloid precursor protein alter the aggregation and conformation of the amyloid-β peptide. J Biol Chem 292:3172–3185

80. Senthil G, Dutka T, Bingaman L, Lehner T (2017) Genomic resources for the study of neuropsychiatric disorders. Mol Psychiatry 22:1659–1663. https://doi.org/10.1038/mp.2017.29

81. Litton JE (2017) We must urgently clarify data-sharing rules. Nature 541:437

82. Editorial (2016) The power of big data must be harnessed for medical progress. Nature 539:467–468

83. Auffray C, Balling R, Barroso I et al (2016) Making sense of big data in health research: towards an EU action plan. Genome Med 8:71

84. Dubois B, Feldman HH, Jacova C et al (2014) Advancing research diagnostic criteria for Alzheimer's disease: the IWG-2 criteria. Lancet Neurol 13:614–629

85. Mar J, Soto-Gordoa M, Arrospide A, Moreno-Izco F, Martínez-Lage P (2015) Fitting the epidemiology and neuropathology of the early stages of Alzheimer's disease to prevent dementia. Alzheimers Res Ther 7(1):2. https://doi.org/10.1186/s13195-014-0079-9

86. Jack CR Jr, Bennett DA, Blennow K et al (2016) A/T/N: an unbiased descriptive classification scheme for Alzheimer disease biomarkers. Neurology 87:539–547

87. Jack CR Jr, Wiste HJ, Weigand SD et al (2017) Age-specific and sex-specific prevalence of cerebral β-amyloidosis, tauopathy, and neurodegeneration in cognitively unimpaired individuals aged 50–95 years: a cross-sectional study. Lancet Neurol 16:435–444. https://doi.org/10.1016/S1474-4422(17)30077-7

88. Johnson KA, Minoshima S, Bohnen NI et al (2013) Appropriate use criteria for amyloid PET: a report of the amyloid imaging task force, the Society of Nuclear Medicine and Molecular Imaging, and the Alzheimer's Association. Alzheimers Dement 9 :e-1–e16

89. Mak E, Gabel S, Mirette H et al (2016) Structural neuroimaging in preclinical dementia: from microstructural deficits and grey matter atrophy to macroscale connectomic changes. Ageing Res Rev 35:250–264. https://doi.org/10.1016/j.arr.2016.10.001

90. Nichols TE, Das S, Eickhoff SB et al (2017) Best practices in data analysis and sharing in neuroimaging using MRI. Nat Neurosci 20:299–303

91. Sepulcre J, Masdeu JC (2016) Advanced neuroimaging methods towards characterization of early stages of Alzheimer's disease. Methods Mol Biol 1303:509–519

92. Masdeu JC (2017) Future directions in imaging neurodegeneration. Curr Neurol Neurosci Rep 17:9

93. Sepulcre J, Grothe MJ, Sabuncu M et al (2017) Hierarchical organization of tau and amyloid deposits in the cerebral cortex. JAMA Neurol 74:813–820. https://doi.org/10.1001/jamaneurol.2017.0263

94. Vemuri P, Schöll M (2017) Linking amyloid-β and tau deposition in Alzheimer disease. JAMA Neurol 74:766–768. https://doi.org/10.1001/jamaneurol.2017.0323

95. Matsuda H, Asada T, Tokumaru AM (2017) Neuroimaging diagnosis for Alzheimer's disease and other dementias. Springer, Tokyo

96. Fan Z, Brooks DJ, Okello A, Edison P (2017) An early and late peak in microglial activation in Alzheimer's disease trajectory. Brain 140:792–803. https://doi.org/10.1093/brain/aww349

97. Pickett EK, Henstridge CM, Allison E et al (2017) Spread of tau down neural circuits precedes synapse and neuronal loss in the rTgTauEC mouse model of early Alzheimer's disease. Synapse. https://doi.org/10.1002/syn.21965

98. Brosch JR, Farlow MR, Risacher SL, Apostolova LG (2017) Tau imaging in Alzheimer's disease diagnosis and clinical trials. Neurotherapeutics 14:62–68

99. Wang L, Benzinger TL, Su Y et al (2016) Evaluation of tau imaging in staging Alzheimer disease and revealing interactions between β-amyloid and tauopathy. JAMA Neurol 73:1070–1077

100. Park JY, Na HK, Kim S, The Alzheimer's Disease Neuroimaging Initiative et al (2017) Robust identification of Alzheimer's disease subtypes based on cortical atrophy patterns. Sci Rep 7:43270

101. Ossenkoppele R, Schonhaut DR, Schöll M et al (2016) Tau PET patterns mirror clinical and neuroanatomical variability in Alzheimer's disease. Brain 139:1551–1567

102. Xia C, Makaretz SJ, Caso C et al (2017) Association of in vivo [18F]AV-1451 tau PET imaging results with cortical atrophy and symptoms in typical and atypical Alzheimer disease. JAMA Neurol 74:427–436. https://doi.org/10.1001/jamaneurol.2016.5755

103. Masdeu JC (2017b) Tau and cortical thickness in Alzheimer disease. JAMA Neurol 74:390–392. https://doi.org/10.1001/jamaneurol.2016.5701

104. Qian J, Hyman BT, Betensky RA (2017) Neurofibrillary tangle stage and the rate of progression of Alzheimer symptoms: Modeling using an autopsy cohort and application to clinical trial design. JAMA Neurol 74:540–548. https://doi.org/10.1001/jamaneurol.2016.5953

105. Perneczky R, Tene O, Attems J et al (2016) Is the time ripe for new diagnostic criteria of cognitive impairment due to cerebrovascular disease? Consensus report of the international congress on vascular dementia working group. BMC Med 14:162

106. Tan J, Li QX, Evin G (2016) Effects of mild and severe oxidative stress on BACE1 expression and APP amyloidogenic processing. Methods Mol Biol 1303:101–116

107. García-Osta A, Cuadrado-Tejedor M (2016) Advanced assay monitoring APP-carboxyl-terminal fragments as markers of APP processing in Alzheimer disease mouse models. Methods Mol Biol 1303:117–123

108. Pinotsi D, Kaminski Schierle GS, Kaminski CF (2016) Optical super-resolution imaging of β-amyloid aggregation in vitro and in vivo: method and techniques. Methods Mol Biol 1303:125–141

109. Rábano A, Cuadros R, Merino-Serráis P et al (2016) Protocols for monitoring the development of tau pathology in Alzheimer's disease. Methods Mol Biol 1303:143–160

110. Kaufman SK, Sanders DW, Thomas TL et al (2016) Tau prion strains dictate patterns of cell pathology, progression rate, and regional vulnerability in vivo. Neuron 92:796–812

111. Hetz C, Mollereau B (2014) Disturbance of endoplasmic reticulum proteostasis in neurodegenerative diseases. Nat Rev Neurosci 15:233–249

112. Streeter A, Menzies FM, Rubinsztein DC (2016) LC3-II tagging and western blotting for monitoring autophagic activity in mammalian cells. Methods Mol Biol 1303:161–170

113. Feng T, Tammineni P, Agrawal C et al (2017) Autophagy-mediated regulation of BACE1 protein trafficking and degradation. J Biol Chem 292:1679–1690

114. Grimm A, Schmitt K, Eckert A (2016) Advanced mitochondrial respiration assay for evaluation of mitochondrial dysfunction in Alzheimer's disease. Methods Mol Biol 1303:171–183

115. Gomez-Nicola D, Perry VH (2016) Analysis of microglial proliferation in Alzheimer's disease. Methods Mol Biol 1303:185–193

116. Masters SL, O'Neill LA (2011) Disease-associated amyloid and misfolded protein aggregates activate the inflammasome. Trends Mol Med 17:276–282

117. McManus RM, Heneka MT (2017) Role of neuroinflammation in neurodegeneration: new insights. Alzheimers Res Ther 9:14

118. Jessen NA, Munk AS, Lundgaard I, Nedergaard M (2015) The glymphatic system: a beginner's guide. Neurochem Res 40:2583–2599

119. Zeppenfeld DM, Simon M, Haswell JD et al (2017) Association of perivascular localization of aquaporin-4 with cognition and Alzheimer disease in aging brains. JAMA Neurol 74:91–99

120. Tosto G, Reitz C (2016) Use of "omics" technologies to dissect neurologic disease. Handb Clin Neurol 138:91–106

121. Chen BJ, Mills JD, Janitz C, Janitz M (2016) RNA-sequencing to elucidate early patterns of dysregulation underlying the onset of Alzheimer's disease. Methods Mol Biol 1303:327–347

122. Roth W, Hecker D, Fava E (2016) Systems biology approaches to the study of biological networks underlying Alzheimer's disease: role of miRNAs. Methods Mol Biol 1303:349–377

123. Pichler S, Gu W, Hartl D et al (2017) The miRNome of Alzheimer's disease: consistent downregulation of the miR-132/212 cluster. Neurobiol Aging 50:167.e1–167.e10

124. Bai B, Hales CM, Chen PC et al (2013) U1 small nuclear ribonucleoprotein complex and RNA splicing alterations in Alzheimer's disease. Proc Natl Acad Sci U S A 110:16562–16567

125. Yin X, Jin N, Shi J et al (2017) Dyrk1A overexpression leads to increase of 3R-tau expression and cognitive deficits in Ts65Dn Down syndrome mice. Sci Rep 7(1):619. https://doi.org/10.1038/s41598-017-00682-y

126. Hare DJ, Rembach A, Roberts BR (2016) The emerging role of metalloproteomics in Alzheimer's disease research. Methods Mol Biol 1303:379–389

127. Di Domenico F, Perluigi M, Butterfield DA (2016) Redox proteomics in human biofluids: sample preparation, separation and immunochemical tagging for analysis of protein oxidation. Methods Mol Biol 1303:391–403

128. Nuzzo D, Inguglia L, Walters J et al (2017) A shotgun proteomics approach reveals a new toxic role for Alzheimer's disease Aβ peptide: Spliceosome impairment. J Proteome Res 16:1526–1541. https://doi.org/10.1021/acs.jproteome.6b00925

129. Reinders J (2016) Proteomics in systems biology. Methods and protocols, Methods in molecular biology (MIMB) series. Humana Press/Springer, New York

130. Perneczky R, Guo LH (2016) Plasma proteomics biomarkers in Alzheimer's disease: latest advances and challenges. Methods Mol Biol 1303:521–529

131. Bai B, Chen PC, Hales CM et al (2014) Integrated approaches for analyzing U1-70K cleavage in Alzheimer's disease. J Proteome Res 13:4526–4534

132. Hales CM, Seyfried NT, Dammer EB et al (2014a) U1 small nuclear ribonucleoproteins (snRNPs) aggregate in Alzheimer's disease due to autosomal dominant genetic mutations and trisomy 21. Mol Neurodegener 9:15

133. Hales CM, Dammer EB, Diner I et al (2014b) Aggregates of small nuclear ribonucleic acids (snRNAs) in Alzheimer's disease. Brain Pathol 24:344–351

134. Kaddurah-Daouk R, Krishnan KR (2009) Metabolomics: a global biochemical approach to the study of central nervous system diseases. Neuropsychopharmacology 34:173–186

135. Kaddurah-Daouk R, Zhu H, Sharma S, Pharmacometabolomics Research Network et al (2013) Alterations in metabolic pathways and networks in Alzheimer's disease. Transl Psychiatry 3:e244

136. Toledo JB, Arnold M, Kastenmüller G, The Alzheimer's Disease Neuroimaging Initiative and the Alzheimer Disease Metabolomics Consortium et al (2017) Metabolic network failures in Alzheimer's disease-A biochemical road map. Alzheimers Dement 13:965–984. https://doi.org/10.1016/j.jalz.2017.01.020

137. Wang M, Han X (2016) Advanced shotgun lipidomics for characterization of altered lipid patterns in neurodegenerative diseases and brain injury. Methods Mol Biol 1303:405–422

138. Proitsi P, Kim M, Whiley L et al (2017) Association of blood lipids with Alzheimer's disease: a comprehensive lipidomics analysis. Alzheimers Dement 13:140–151

139. Huttlin EL, Bruckner RJ, Paulo JA et al (2017) Architecture of the human interactome defines protein communities and disease networks. Nature 545:505–509. https://doi.org/10.1038/nature22366

140. Bennett RE, DeVos SL, Dujardin S et al (2017) Enhanced tau aggregation in the presence of amyloid β. Am J Pathol 187:1601–1612. https://doi.org/10.1016/j.ajpath.2017.03.011

141. Kikuchi M, Ogishima S, Mizuno S et al (2016) Network-based analysis for uncovering mechanisms underlying Alzheimer's disease. Methods Mol Biol 1303:479–491

142. Yerbury J, Bean D, Favrin G (2016) Network approaches to the understanding of Alzheimer's disease: from model organisms to humans. Methods Mol Biol 1303:447–458

143. Zanzoni A (2016) A computational network biology approach to uncover novel genes related to Alzheimer's disease. Methods Mol Biol 1303:435–446

144. Zhang B, Tran L, Emilsson V, Zhu J (2016) Characterization of genetic networks associated with Alzheimer's disease. Methods Mol Biol 1303:459–477

145. Christianson JC, Olzmann JA, Shaler TA et al (2011) Defining human ERAD networks through an integrative mapping strategy. Nat Cell Biol 14:93–105

146. Kikuchi M, Ogishima S, Miyamoto T et al (2013) Identification of unstable network modules reveals disease modules associated with the progression of Alzheimer's disease. PLoS One 8:e76162

147. Gitter A, Bar-Joseph Z (2016) The SDREM method for reconstructing signaling and regulatory response networks: applications for studying disease progression. Methods Mol Biol 1303:493–506

148. Genolini C, Ecochard R, Benghezal M et al (2016) kmlShape: an efficient method to cluster longitudinal data (time-series) according to their shapes. PLoS One 11:e0150738

149. Verduyckt M, Vignaud H, Bynens T et al (2016) Yeast as a model for Alzheimer's disease: latest studies and advanced strategies. Methods Mol Biol 1303:197–215

150. Porzoor A, Macreadie I (2016) Yeast as a model for studies on Aβ aggregation toxicity in Alzheimer's disease, autophagic responses, and drug screening. Methods Mol Biol 1303:217–226

151. Lim JY, Ott S, Crowther DC (2016) Drosophila melanogaster as a model for studies on the early stages of Alzheimer's disease. Methods Mol Biol 1303:227–239

152. Cuadrado-Tejedor M, García-Osta A (2016) Chronic mild stress assay leading to early onset and propagation of Alzheimer's disease phenotype in mouse models. Methods Mol Biol 1303:241–246

153. Lu M, Lawrence DA, Marsters S (2014b) Cell death. Opposing unfolded-protein-response signals converge on death receptor 5 to control apoptosis. Science 345:98–101

154. Abisambra JF, Jinwal UK, Blair LJ et al (2013) Tau accumulation activates the unfolded protein response by impairing endoplasmic reticulum-associated degradation. J Neurosci 33:9498–9507

155. Zhou L, McInnes J, Wierda K et al (2017) Tau association with synaptic vesicles causes presynaptic dysfunction. Nat Commun

8:15295. https://doi.org/10.1038/ncomms15295

156. Kazim SF, Blanchard J, Bianchi R, Iqbal K (2017) Early neurotrophic pharmacotherapy rescues developmental delay and Alzheimer's-like memory deficits in the Ts65Dn mouse model of Down syndrome. Sci Rep 7:45561. https://doi.org/10.1038/srep45561

157. Weick JP, Kang H, Bonadurer GF 3rd, Bhattacharyya A (2016) Gene expression studies on human Trisomy 21 iPSCs and neurons: towards mechanisms underlying Down's syndrome and early Alzheimer's disease-like pathologies. Methods Mol Biol 1303:247–265

158. Saurat NG, Livesey FJ, Moore S (2016) Cortical differentiation of human pluripotent cells for in vitro modeling of Alzheimer's disease. Methods Mol Biol 1303:267–278

159. Choi SH, Kim YH, Hebisch M et al (2014) A three-dimensional human neural cell culture model of Alzheimer's disease. Nature 515:274–278

160. Choi SH, Kim YH, Quinti L et al (2016) 3D culture models of Alzheimer's disease: a road map to a "cure-in-a-dish". Mol Neurodegener 11:75

161. Camp JG, Treutlein B (2017) Human development: advances in mini-brain technology. Nature 545:39–40. https://doi.org/10.1038/545039a

162. Koo T, Lee J, Kim JS (2015) Measuring and reducing off-target activities of programmable nucleases including CRISPR-Cas9. Mol Cells 38:475–481

163. Schmid-Burgk JL, Chauhan D, Schmidt T et al (2016) A genome-wide CRISPR (clustered regularly interspaced short palindromic repeats) screen identifies NEK7 as an essential component of NLRP3 inflammasome activation. J Biol Chem 291:103–109

164. Paquet D, Kwart D, Chen A et al (2016) Efficient introduction of specific homozygous and heterozygous mutations using CRISPR/Cas9. Nature 533:125–129

165. Mungenast AE, Siegert S, Tsai LH (2016) Modeling Alzheimer's disease with human induced pluripotent stem (iPS) cells. Mol Cell Neurosci 73:13–31

166. Owens B (2012) Genomics: the single life. Nature 491:27–29

167. Single-cell technology Focus Issue (2016) In this issue. Nat Biotechnol 34:vii. doi: https://doi.org/10.1038/nbt.3732

168. De Strooper B, Karran E (2016) The cellular phase of Alzheimer's disease. Cell 164:603–615

169. Ledford H (2017) The race to map the human body - one cell at a time. Nature 542:404–405

170. Xu Y, Mizuno T, Sridharan A et al (2016) Single-cell RNA sequencing identifies diverse roles of epithelial cells in idiopathic pulmonary fibrosis. JCI Insight 1:e90558

171. Frazer S, Prados J, Niquille M et al (2017) Transcriptomic and anatomic parcellation of 5-HT(3A)R expressing cortical interneuron subtypes revealed by single-cell RNA sequencing. Nat Commun 8:14219. https://doi.org/10.1038/ncomms14219

172. Pavličev M, Wagner GP, Chavan AR et al (2017) Single-cell transcriptomics of the human placenta: inferring the cell communication network of the maternal-fetal interface. Genome Res 27:349–361

173. Zenobi R (2013) Single-cell metabolomics: analytical and biological perspectives. Science 342:1243259

174. Clyde D (2017) Technique: barcoding the nucleus. Nat Rev Genet 18:4–211. https://doi.org/10.1038/nrg.2017.11

175. Ofengeim D, Giagtzoglou N, Huh D et al (2017) Single-cell RNA sequencing: unraveling the brain one cell at a time. Trends Mol Med 23:563–576. https://doi.org/10.1016/j.molmed.2017.04.006

176. Liang Y, Li K, Riecken K et al (2016) Long-term in vivo single-cell tracking reveals the switch of migration patterns in adult-born juxtaglomerular cells of the mouse olfactory bulb. Cell Res 26:805–821

177. Li H, Courtois ET, Sengupta D et al (2017) Reference component analysis of single-cell transcriptomes elucidates cellular heterogeneity in human colorectal tumors. Nat Genet 49:708–718. https://doi.org/10.1038/ng.3818

178. Keren-Shaul H, Spinrad A, Weiner A et al (2017) A unique microglia type associated with restricting development of Alzheimer's disease. Cell 169:1276–1290.e17. https://doi.org/10.1016/j.cell.2017.05.018

179. Dubois B, Hampel H, Feldman HH et al (2016) Preclinical Alzheimer's disease: definition, natural history, and diagnostic criteria. Alzheimers Dement 12:292–323

180. Uzilov AV, Ding W, Fink MY et al (2016) Development and clinical application of an integrative genomic approach to personalized cancer therapy. Genome Med 8:62

181. Rajamani D, Bhasin MK (2016) Identification of key regulators of pancreatic cancer progression through multidimensional systems-level analysis. Genome Med 8:38

182. Ghosh D, Funk CC, Caballero J et al (2017) A cell-surface membrane protein signature for glioblastoma. Cell Syst 4:516–529

183. Sheridan C (2015) Omics-driven startups challenge healthcare model. Nat Biotechnol 33:887–889

184. Lausted C, Lee I, Zhou Y et al (2014) Systems approach to neurodegenerative disease biomarker discovery. Annu Rev Pharmacol Toxicol 54:457–481

185. Lista S, Khachaturian ZS, Rujescu D et al (2016) Application of systems theory in longitudinal studies on the origin and progression of Alzheimer's disease. Methods Mol Biol 1303:49–67

186. Rollo JL, Banihashemi N, Vafaee F et al (2016) Unraveling the mechanistic complexity of Alzheimer's disease through systems biology. Alzheimers Dement 12:708–718

187. Burton A (2016) Kaj Blennow: the route to biomarkers and the Söderberg prize. Lancet Neurol 15(9):906. https://doi.org/10.1016/S1474-4422(16)30097-7

188. Zwan MD, Rinne JO, Hasselbalch SG et al (2016) Use of amyloid-PET to determine cutpoints for CSF markers: a multicenter study. Neurology 86:50–58

189. FitzGerald GA (2016) Measure for measure: biomarker standards and transparency. Sci Transl Med 8:343fs10

190. Kivipelto M, Håkansson K (2017) A rare success against Alzheimer's. Sci Am 316:32–37

191. Ritchie CW, Molinuevo JL, Satlin A et al (2016) The European Prevention of Alzheimer's Dementia (EPAD) Consortium: a platform to enable the secondary prevention of Alzheimer's dementia through improved Proof of Concept Trials. Lancet Psychiatry 3:179–186

192. Ritchie K, Ritchie CW, Yaffe K et al (2015) Is late-onset Alzheimer's disease really a disease of midlife? Alzheimers Dement 1(2):122–130

193. Ritchie CW, Ames D, Clayton T, Lai R (2004) A meta-analysis of randomised trials for the efficacy and safety of donepezil, galantamine and rivastigmine for the treatment of Alzheimer's disease. Am J Geriatr Psychiatry 12:358–369

194. Molinuevo JL, Jordi C, Came X et al (2016) Ethical challenges in preclinical Alzheimer's disease observational studies and trials: results of the Barcelona Summit. Alzheimers Dement 12:614–622

195. Ritchie K, Ropacki M, Albala B et al (2017) Recommended cognitive outcomes in preclinical Alzheimer's disease: consensus statement from the European Prevention of Alzheimer's Dementia project. Alzheimers Dement 13:186–195

196. Mortamais M, Ash JA, Harrison J et al (2017) Detecting cognitive changes in preclinical Alzheimer's disease: a review of its feasibility. Alzheimers Dement 13:468–492

197. Bateman RJ, Xiong C, Benzinger TL, Dominantly Inherited Alzheimer Network et al (2012) Clinical and biomarker changes in dominantly inherited Alzheimer's disease. N Engl J Med 367:795–804

198. Fagan AM, Xiong C, Jasielec MS, Dominantly Inherited Alzheimer Network et al (2014) Longitudinal change in CSF biomarkers in autosomal-dominant Alzheimer's disease. Sci Transl Med 6:226ra30

199. Imamura K, Izumi Y, Watanabe A et al (2017) The Src/c-Abl pathway is a potential therapeutic target in amyotrophic lateral sclerosis. Sci Transl Med 9. https://doi.org/10.1126/scitranslmed.aaf3962

200. Sun C, Fang Y, Yin J et al (2017) Rational combination therapy with PARP and MEK inhibitors capitalizes on therapeutic liabilities in RAS mutant cancers. Sci Transl Med 9. https://doi.org/10.1126/scitranslmed.aal5148

201. Cancer Genome Atlas Research Network (2017) Comprehensive and integrative genomic characterization of hepatocellular carcinoma. Cell 169:1327–1341.e23

202. Norton S, Matthews FE, Barnes DE et al (2014) Potential for primary prevention of Alzheimer's disease: an analysis of population-based data. Lancet Neurol 13:788–794

203. World Alzheimer Report (2014) Dementia and risk reduction: an analysis of protective and modifiable factors. ADI (http://www.alz.co.uk/research/world-report-2014)

204. Sperling RA, Karlawish J, Johnson KA (2013) Preclinical Alzheimer disease-the challenges ahead. Nat Rev Neurol 9:54–58

205. Epelbaum S, Genthon R, Cavedo E et al (2017) Preclinical Alzheimer's disease: a systematic review of the cohorts underlying the concept. Alzheimers Dement 13:454–467

Part II

Innovative Approaches to Cerebrospinal Fluid
Biomarker Discovery

Chapter 4

CSF Lipidomics Analysis: High-Resolution Mass Spectrometry Analytical Platform

Paul L. Wood and Randall L. Woltjer

Abstract

High-resolution mass spectrometry provides the resolution required for direct infusion allowing detection and characterization of a vast array of lipids with a single injection. This chapter presents the methodology utilized for both unbiased and targeted lipidomics of cerebrospinal fluid.

Key words High-resolution mass spectrometry, Lipidomics, CSF

1 Introduction

Cerebrospinal fluid (CSF) offers a unique biofluid for bioanalysis of neuronal function in diverse clinical conditions [1–3], including Alzheimer's disease (AD) [4–8]. However, as aqueous solution, CSF is not as lipid rich as plasma, necessitating the utilization of highly sensitive and specific methods for monitoring specific CSF lipids.

2 Materials and Methods

2.1 Lipidomics Standards

1. Internal standards are made up as 1 mM solutions in methanol and are stored at −20 °C. Chloroform and/or water are utilized with lipids insoluble in methanol alone.

2. All standard solutions should be warmed to room temperature before removing aliquots for the internal standard cocktail, since some lipids precipitate at −20 °C.

3. Bromocriptine is included as an internal standard to monitor for potential mass axis drift and to evaluate isotopic resolution (Br^{81} = 49.3%). Bromocriptine can be monitored both in positive electrospray ionization (ESI) and negative ESI.

Robert Perneczky (ed.), *Biomarkers for Alzheimer's Disease Drug Development*, Methods in Molecular Biology, vol. 1750, https://doi.org/10.1007/978-1-4939-7704-8_4, © Springer Science+Business Media, LLC 2018

2.2 High-Resolution Mass Spectrometry

An orbitrap mass spectrometer is utilized for direct infusion analyses (Q Exactive; Thermo Fischer). This is a benchtop quadrupole orbitrap mass spectrometer with high mass resolution (140,000), high mass accuracy (0.4–3 ppm), high analytical sensitivity, excellent mass axis stability, and a maintenance-free analyzer [9, 10].

2.3 CSF Extraction (See Notes 1 and 2)

1. 500 μL of CSF is vortexed with 1 mL of methanol containing the internal standards in 7 mL polypropylene tubes (Table 1).

2. Next 1 mL of water and 2 mL of t-butyl methyl ether are added.

3. The tubes are capped and shaken vigorously at *room temp* for 30 min using a vortexer.

4. Centrifuge the tubes at 4000 × *g* for 15 min at *room temperature*.

5. 1 mL of the upper organic lipid layer is transferred to a screw-top 1.5 mL microfuge tube and the samples are dried for 4 h in an Eppendorf Vacufuge.

6. Dissolve the dried samples in 150 μL of the infusion solvent.

7. Centrifuge at 30,000 × *g* for 5 min in an Eppendorf microfuge to precipitate any particulates.

2.4 Lipidomics Mass Spectrometer Platform (See Note 3)

1. The dried sample is dissolved in the infusion solvent (80 mL 2 propanol + 40 mL methanol + 20 mL chloroform + 0.5 mL water containing 164 mg ammonium acetate).

2. The sample is infused into the ESI source at a flow rate of 10 μL/min.

3. Scan in Pos-ESI (200–1400 amu) mode for 0.5 min, followed by Neg-ESI (180–1400 amu) mode for 0.5 min with a resolution of 140,000.

4. Minimize memory effects by washing the syringe and infusion line with a large excess of solvent between sample infusions. Wash first with 1 mL of methanol followed by 1 mL of hexane: ethyl acetate: chloroform (3:2:1).

2.5 Mass Spectrometric Data Reduction

From the high-resolution mass spectrometric data, the top 1000 masses, for successive 250 amu bins, and their associated ion intensities are transferred to an Excel spreadsheet. Within the spreadsheet is a list of lipids along with their exact masses (5 decimals), and the scanned ions for the biomolecules which are searched within the data table. If the calculated ppm mass error is determined to be ≤3 for the extracted ion, then the ratio of the ion intensity to the ion intensity of an appropriate internal standard (R) is calculated and added to the spreadsheet. The major lipids monitored in human CSF are tabulated in Table 2.

Table 1
Internal standards to analyze 500 μL CSF samples

Int. std.	nmoles	Exact mass	[M + H]$^+$
PtdC 28:0 [D54]	1	729.8257	730.8330
PtdC 32:0 [D62]	0.5	793.9337	794.9410
PtdC 34:1 [D31]	4	790.7720	791.7793
MAG 18:1 [D5]	1	361.3240	362.3313
Cer [D31]	1	568.7070	569.7143
Bromocriptine	0.5	653.2213	654.2285
Bromocriptine-81		655.2192	656.2265

Int. std.	nmoles	Exact mass	[M + NH$_4$]$^+$
DAG 36:2 [C3]	1	623.5480	641.5824
TAG 48:0 [D5]	3	811.7677	829.8021

Int. std.	nmoles	Exact mass	[M–H]$^-$
PtdE 34:1 [D31]	1.2	747.7191	746.7119
PtdC 28:0 [D54]	0.5	687.7783	686.7710
PtdS 34:1 [D31]	4	791.0837	790.7011
PG 32:0 [D62]	0.25	784.8990	883.8917
PG 34:1 [D31]	0.5	779.7200	778.7127
Arachidonic acid [D7]	0.1	312.2905	311.2832
DHA [D5]	0.5	333.2716	332.2643
VLCFA 26:0 [D4]	1.25	400.4218	399.4146
DC 16:0 [D28]	1.5	314.3902	313.3829
Cholesterol sulfate [D7]	1	473.3556	472.3483
PA 34:1 [D31]	1	704.6763	703.6690
Bromocriptine	0.5	653.2213	652.21398
Bromocriptine-81		655.2192	654.2119

nmoles = nanomoles of internal standard per 500 μL CSF

Table 2
Major CSF lipids (0.5 mL)

Lipid	Int. std.	Exact mass	ppm	R	AD %C
Fatty acids [M–H]⁻	AA-D8				
Arachidonic		304.24023	0.48	7.69	90
Docosahexaenoic (DHA)		328.2403	1.14	1.98	75
Phosphatidylglycerols [M–H]⁻	PG 32:0-D62				
PG 34:0		750.5410	0.27	0.56	70
Very-long-chain fatty acids [M–H]⁻	VLCFA 26:0-D28				
VLCFA 26:0		396.3967	0.49	0.025	49
Phosphatidylinositols [M–H]⁻	PE 34:1-D31				
PI 38:4		886.5571	2.5	0.72	95
Phosphatidylserines[M–H]⁻	PE 34:1-D31				
PS 38:0		819.5989	0.92	0.35	97
Phosphatidylethanolamines [M–H]⁻	PE 34:1-D31				
PE 38:4		767.5465	2.4	0.92	79
Phosphatidylcholines [M + H]⁺	PC 32:0-D62				
PC 32:0		733.5622	0.30	2.5	100
PC 34:1		759.5778	0.5	5.8	110
PC 36:4		781.5621	2.0	34.0	105
PC 38:4		809.5935	2.2	6.5	120
Ethanolamine Plasmalogens [M–H]⁻	PE 28:0-D54				
PlsE 36:4		723.5203	2.1	1.45	80
PlsE 38:4		751.5516	2.7	1.62	75
Choline plasmalogens [M + H]⁺	PC 28:0-D54				100
PlsC 34:0		745.5985	2.2	0.33	100
PlsC 36:4		765.5673	1.3	0.64	100
PlsC 40:6		817.5985	0.36	0.76	100
Sphingomyelins [M + H]⁺	PC 32:0-D62				
SM d18:1/18:0		730.5989	1.3	3.7	100
SM d18:1/24:1		814.6928	0.58	0.7	100
Sulfatides [M–H]⁻	AA-D8				
Sulf d18:1/24:1		889.6313	2.3	0.50	100

(continued)

Table 2
(continued)

Lipid	Int. std.	Exact mass	ppm	R	AD %C
Ceramides [M + H]⁺	PC 34:0-D31				
Cer d18:1/16:0		537.5121	0.41	0.46	100
Cer d18:1/18:0		565.5434	0.21	0.61	100
Diacylglycerols [M + NH₄]⁺	DAG-C3				
DAG 36:1		622.5536	0.11	2.5	100
DAG 38:1		650.5849	0.48	2.2	100
DAG 38:4		644.5379	0.04	3.8	100
Lysophosphatidylcholines [M + H]⁺	PC 34:0-D31				
LPC 16:0		495.3325	0.33	1.3	266
Acylcarnitines [M + H]⁺	MAG-D5				
AC 16:0		399.3349	0.88	0.19	100
AC 18:0		427.3662	0.17	0.28	100
AC 18:1		425.3505	0.76	0.38	100

AD%C, AD ($N = 3$) CSF value as a percent of that observed with control ($N = 3$) CSF; ppm, parts per million mass error; R, ratio of the ion intensity of the biological molecule to the ion intensity of the internal standard

3   Notes

1. It is critical to perform the lipid extractions at room temperature to maximize extraction efficiency.

2. This extraction method is not optimal for the extraction of gangliosidcs.

3. Calibration of the mass axis is best performed with the Thermo-Fisher PESI and NESI calibration solutions. In the case of the NESI calibrant it is best diluted 1:1 with the infusion solvent (2.4) for stable scanning.

Acknowledgments

This work was supported by Lincoln Memorial University.

References

1. Kantae V, Ogino S, Noga M, Harms AC, van Dongen RM, Onderwater GL, van den Maagdenberg AM, Terwindt GM, van der Stelt M, Ferrari MD, Hankemeier T (2017) Quantitative profiling of endocannabinoids and related N-acylethanolamines in human CSF using nano LC-MS/MS. J Lipid Res 58:615–624

2. Seyer A, Boudah S, Broudin S, Junot C, Colsch B (2016) Annotation of the human cerebrospinal fluid lipidome using high resolution mass spectrometry and a dedicated data processing workflow. Metabolomics 12:91

3. Gonzalo H, Brieva L, Tatzber F, Jové M, Cacabelos D, Cassanyé A, Lanau-Angulo L, Boada J, Serrano JC, González C, Hernández L, Peralta S, Pamplona R, Portero-Otin M (2012) Lipidome analysis in multiple sclerosis reveals protein lipoxidative damage as a potential pathogenic mechanism. J Neurochem 123:622–634

4. Koal T, Klavins K, Seppi D, Kemmler G, Humpel C (2015) Sphingomyelin SM(d18:1/18:0) is significantly enhanced in cerebrospinal fluid samples dichotomized by pathological amyloid-β42, tau, and phospho-tau-181 levels. J Alzheimers Dis 44:1193–1201

5. Trushina E, Dutta T, Persson XM, Mielke MM, Petersen RC (2013) Identification of altered metabolic pathways in plasma and CSF in mild cognitive impairment and Alzheimer's disease using metabolomics. PLoS One 8:e63644

6. Kaddurah-Daouk R, Zhu H, Sharma S, Bogdanov M, Rozen SG, Matson W, Oki NO, Motsinger-Reif AA, Churchill E, Lei Z, Appleby D, Kling MA, Trojanowski JQ, Doraiswamy PM, Arnold SE, Pharmacometabolomics Research Network (2013) Alterations in metabolic pathways and networks in Alzheimer's disease. Transl Psychiatry 3:e244

7. Ibáñez C, Simó C, Martín-Álvarez PJ, Kivipelto M, Winblad B, Cedazo-Mínguez A, Cifuentes A (2012) Toward a predictive model of Alzheimer's disease progression using capillary electrophoresis-mass spectrometry metabolomics. Anal Chem 84:8532–8540

8. Wood PL, Barnette BL, Kaye JA, Quinn JF, Woltjer RL (2015) Non-targeted lipidomics of CSF and frontal cortex gray and white matter in control, mild cognitive impairment, and Alzheimer's disease subjects. Acta Neuropsychiatrica 27:270–278

9. Wood PL (2017) Non-targeted lipidomics utilizing constant infusion high resolution ESI mass spectrometry. In Springer Protocols. Meuromethods. Lipidomics 125:13–19 (PL Wood, Ed)

10. Wood PL (2017) High-resolution mass spectrometry of glycerophospholipid oxidation products. In Springer Protocols Neuromethods. Lipidomics 125:237–241 (PL Wood, Ed)

Chapter 5

CSF N-Glycomics Using MALDI MS Techniques in Alzheimer's Disease

Angelo Palmigiano, Angela Messina, Rosaria Ornella Bua, Rita Barone, Luisa Sturiale, Mario Zappia, and Domenico Garozzo

Abstract

In this chapter, we present the methodology currently applied in our laboratory for the structural elucidation of the cerebrospinal fluid (CSF) N-glycome. N-glycans are released from denatured carboxymethylated glycoproteins by digestion with peptide-N-glycosidase F (PNGase F) and purified using both C18 Sep-Pak® and porous graphitized carbon (PGC) HyperSep™ Hypercarb™ solid-phase extraction (SPE) cartridges. The glycan pool is subsequently permethylated to increase mass spectrometry sensitivity. Molecular assignments are performed through matrix-assisted laser desorption/ionization time-of-flight mass spectrometry (MALDI TOF MS) analysis considering either the protein N-linked glycosylation pathway or MALDI TOF MS/MS data. Each stage has been optimized to obtain high-quality mass spectra in reflector mode with an optimal signal-to-noise ratio up to m/z 4800. This method has been successfully adopted to associate specific N-glycome profiles to the early and the advanced phases of Alzheimer's disease.

Key words AD, CSF, N-glycans, MALDI MS, MCI

1 Introduction

Although the role of N-glycosylation in the development and progression of AD is still to elucidate [1], several findings show that it has a considerable impact on central nervous system (CNS) neurodegeneration processes [2–6]. Among all posttranslational modifications that regulate protein processing, glycosylation is a common and versatile form that is vital for proper brain function. Glycans regulate how the proteins are processed and sorted inside the cells and play a role in cell adhesion, recognition, and signaling. Protein N-glycosylation is a highly ordered, sequential process that encompasses different cellular compartments. The nascent protein is glycosylated in the endoplasmic reticulum, where the precursor oligosaccharide Glc3Man9GlcNAc2 is first transferred *en bloc* to the polypeptide chain, and then processed in the Golgi [7]. Based on the last process, N-glycan structures are distinguished in

Robert Perneczky (ed.), *Biomarkers for Alzheimer's Disease Drug Development*, Methods in Molecular Biology, vol. 1750, https://doi.org/10.1007/978-1-4939-7704-8_5, © Springer Science+Business Media, LLC 2018

complex, hybrid, and high-mannose types [7]. The huge variability of N-glycan structures basically relies on the type and position of attached sugars and branching.

CSF N-glycomics using MALDI MS techniques represents a reliable and a feasible approach for the characterization of brain glycoproteome enabling to identify possible alterations on different pathological processes affecting the CNS. Here we report the N-glycan CSF profile of a 79-year-old man with absence of neurological and cognitive concerns (obtained with the procedure briefly outlined in the summary), considered as a representative spectrum of a healthy reference control (*see* Fig. 1a). The developed protocol allowed us to pinpoint in human CSF a relevant incidence of biantennary N-glycans with bisecting GlcNAc and proximal fucosylation ($\alpha1, 6$ fucosylation at the chitobiosyl core), the so-called brain-type N-glycosylation (Fig. 2a), whereas representative serum N-glycans are complex glycans with almost absent bisecting GlcNAc (Fig. 2b) [3, 8].

Our strategy led to a full identification of brain-type and serum-type glycoforms by MALDI TOF MS/MS analyses on representative (not-derivatized) model compounds, as the biantennary, bisected, fucosylated species FA2B and the isobaric triantennary fucosylated analogue FA3 (letter code described by Royle et al. [9]). The typical MS/MS fragmentation patterns of FA2B and FA3 glycoforms (precursor ion at m/z 1688.6, as sodium adduct) considered as model compounds for bisected and triantennary fucosylated N-glycoforms, respectively (*see* Figs. 3a, b), show B-type and Y-type ions due to glycoside bond cleavages (Domon and Costello nomenclature [10]). In addition, FA3 spectrum (Fig. 3b) is characterized by intense Z-type (m/z 1524.6) and C-type (m/z 1339.7) ion fragments, not present in the MS/MS spectrum of the bisected FA2B species (Fig. 2a). The fragmentation spectrum associated to FA2B, matched with those from the same precursor ion belonging to CSF profiles from healthy individuals and AD patients (Fig. 3c, d), thus suggesting that the CSF glycoform at m/z 1688.6 and, consequently, the corresponding permethylated derivative at m/z 2080.9 (*see* Fig. 1a) are both associated to a bisected, core fucosylated structure [2].

N-glycans with bisecting GlcNAc, referred as bisected N-glycans, are synthesized by $\beta1,4$-N-acetylglucosaminyltransferase III enzyme (GnT-III; EC 2.4.1.144) (encoded by *MGAT3*) that catalyzes GlcNAc attachment to the core β-mannose residue of N-glycans with $\beta1,4$ linkage [11]. GnT-III is overexpressed in the brain of AD patients [12] and it has been found to modulate the innate immune response of blood monocytes to Aβ [12, 13]. GnT-III plays moreover a regulatory role of N-glycan biosynthesis, as bisecting GlcNAc, preventing the action of further GlcNAc-transferases, leads to an overall reduction of the N-glycan branching [7, 14]. We have compared, in a recent study [2], the N-glycosylation profile of CSF samples from patients with AD, mild cognitive impairment (MCI) and from healthy controls. Principal compo-

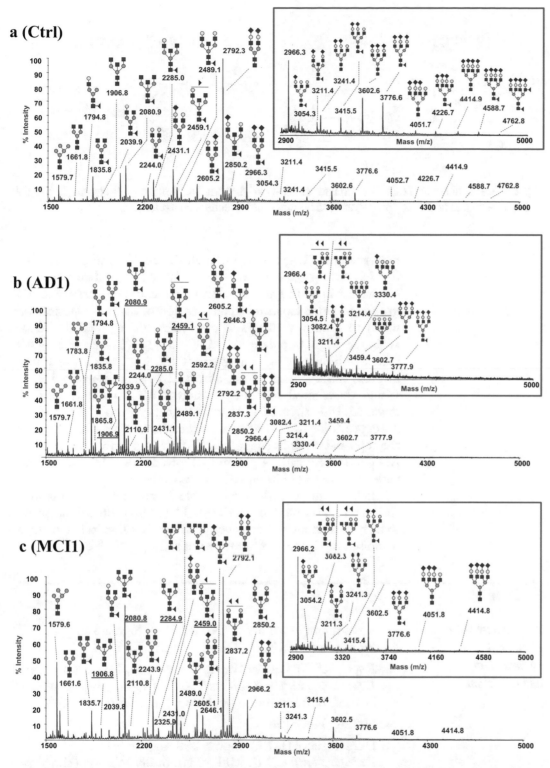

Fig. 1 MALDI-TOF spectra of permethylated CSF N-glycans from (**a**) healthy control (age 79 years), (**b**) AD1 patient (age 76 years), (**c**) MCI1 patient (age 75 years). Each figure inset highlights differences and/or similarities at high mass range between control, AD1, and MC1 profiles. N-acetylglucosamine (GlcNAc): blue square; mannose (Man): green circle; galactose (Gal): yellow circle; sialic acid (NeuAc): purple lozenge; fucose (Fuc): red triangle

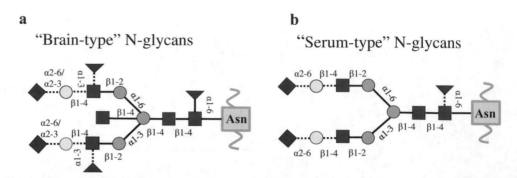

Fig. 2 Typical features of "brain-type" (**a**) and "serum-type" (**b**) complex biantennary N-glycans. Dotted linkages are related to additional "brain-type" and "serum-type" structural characteristics

nent analysis (PCA) showed that all the 24 AD patients are classified into two groups, namely AD1 (10 patients) characterized by an increase in brain-type glycoforms (bisected N-glycans) and AD2 group (14 patients) showing a reduction of the same species compared to healthy controlrs. Noteworthy, PCA revealed also two analogue MCI populations: MCI1 group (5 out of 11) with increased bisected N-glycans and MCI2, showing a lower amount of these species. Surprisingly, all MCI1 patients converted to AD within the clinical follow-up, whereas MC2 patients remained unvaried, thus suggesting that CSF changes proceed the clinical onset providing useful biomarker for early AD diagnosis. Moreover, the reported findings suggest GnT-III as a possible target for the AD pharmaceuticals. N-glycan CSF profiles of a AD1 and a MC1 patient are reported in Fig. 2b, c, respectively.

Below, our procedure to profile N-glycans from 200 μL of CSF samples is described in detail. The same protocol has proved to be robust enough to achieve spectra with still satisfactory signal-to-noise ratio by employing up to only 20 μL of CSF.

2 Materials

2.1 Denaturation of Proteins by Reduction and Alkylation

1. Ammonium bicarbonate (NH_4HCO_3), Sigma-500 g.
   Buffer solution. NH_4HCO_3 50 mM pH 7.8 in MilliQ water.

2. *Rapi*Gest™ SF Powder Waters Corporation, 1 pack of 1 mg vials.
   *Denaturing buffer. Rapi*Gest™ 0.1% (w/v). 1 mg *Rapi*Gest™ in 1 mL buffer solution (stable several months at −20 °C).

3. Heating block (56 °C).

4. Dithiothreitol (DTT), Sigma-250 mg.
   Reducing buffer. DTT 100 mM in buffer solution (always prepare fresh).

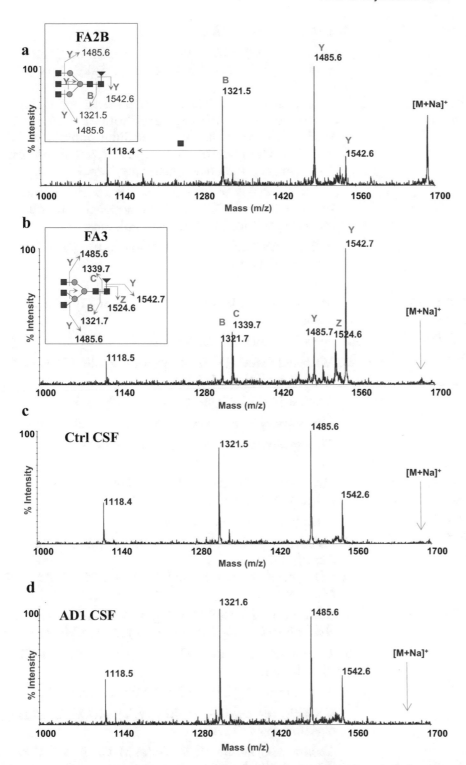

Fig. 3 MALDI-TOF/TOF fragmentation analysis of the parent ion at *m/z* 1688.6 from (**a**) FA2B model compound, (**b**) FA3 model compound, (**c**) healthy control CSF profile, and (**d**) AD1 CSF profile. N-acetylglucosamine (GlcNAc): blue square; mannose (Man): green circle; galactose (Gal): yellow circle; sialic acid (NeuAc): purple lozenge; fucose (Fuc): red triangle

5. Iodoacetamide (IAA), Sigma-5 g.

    Alkylating buffer. IAA 100 mM in buffer solution (always prepare fresh; light sensitive, keep in the dark).

2.2 PNGase F digestion

1. N-glycosidase F (PNGase F, EC 3.5.1.52) of *Flavobacterium meningosepticum*, recombinant from *E. coli*, 250 units, 0.25 mL, solution in 50 mM sodium phosphate, 12.5 mM EDTA, 50% glycerol (v/v), pH 7.2 (Roche Molecular Biochemicals, Mannheim, Germany) (*see* **Note 1**).

    PNGase F is an amidase that cleaves the linkage between the innermost GlcNAc and the asparagine residues of high mannose, hybrid, and complex N-glycans.

2. 500 mM Hydrochloric acid (HCl) reagent grade 37%, Aldrich, 5 L, in MilliQ water.

2.3 C$_{18}$ Sep-Pak Purification of the Released N-Glycans

1. Sep-Pak® Vac tC18 1cc, part # WAT036820 (Waters, Milford, MA).

2. SpeedVac™ vacuum concentrator.

3. Methanol (MeOH) HPLC gradient grade, J.T. Baker®, 2.5 L.
    Cleaning solution: MeOH.

4. Acetic acid (HAc) ≥99.9%, Sigma Aldrich-1 L.
    Conditioning solution: 5% (v/v) HAc in MilliQ water.
    Eluting solution: 5% (v/v) HAc in MilliQ water.

2.4 Solid-Phase Extraction of the Released N-Glycans

1. HyperSep™ Hypercarb™ SPE Cartridges 50 mg/1 mL (Thermo Scientific™, Bellefonte, PA USA).

2. SpeedVac™ vacuum concentrator.

3. NaOH, beads/pellets, 99.99% (metal basis), Alfa Aesar®-100 g.
    Basic priming solution: Sodium hydroxide (NaOH) 1 M in MilliQ water.

4. Acetic acid (HAc) ≥99.9%, Sigma Aldrich-1 L.
    Acidic priming solution: 30% (v/v) HAc in MilliQ water.

5. Trifluoroacetic acid (TFA) ≥99.9% Purified B, Sigma Aldrich-25 g.

6. Acetonitrile (MeCN) UHPLC-MS, Scharlau-1 L.

    Conditioning solution 1: 50% (v/v) MeCN in MilliQ water plus 0.1% (v/v) TFA.

    Conditioning solution 2: 5% (v/v) MeCN in MilliQ water plus 0.1% (v/v) TFA.

    Washing solution: 5% (v/v) MeCN, in MilliQ water plus 0.1% (v/v) TFA.

    Eluting solution: 50% (v/v), MeCN, in MilliQ water plus 0.1% (v/v) TFA.

2.5 Glycan Permethylation	1. Permethylation is performed in PYREX screw-cap culture tubes (13 × 100 mm, Corning™) with phenolic PTFE-lined caps (Corning™).
	2. Syringe Driven Filter Unit Millex®-HV 0.45 μm, PVDF.
	3. Freeze dryer.
	4. NaOH, beads/pellets, 99.99% (metal basis), Alfa Aesar®-100 g.
	5. Methyl sulfoxide (DMSO) 99.7 + % extra dry over molecular sieves, AcroSeal™, ACROS Organics™-100 mL.
	6. Iodomethane (ICH_3), contains copper as stabilizer, ReagentPlus®, 99.5%, Sigma Aldrich-100 g (*see* **Note 2**).
	7. Chloroform ($CHCl_3$) HPLC grade, ≥ 99.9%, Sigma Aldrich-2 5 L.
2.6 MALDI MS Analysis of Permethylated Glycans	1. *MALDI TOF instrument.* 4800 Proteomic Analyzer (Applied Biosystems) equipped with a Nd:YAG laser operating at a wavelength of 355 nm with <500-ps pulse and 200-Hz firing rate.
	2. *Calibration mixture.* The instrument is calibrated externally using the AB SCIEX TOF/TOF™ 4700 Peptide Calibration Standard Mixture (TOF/TOF Calibration Mixture), containing des-Arg1-bradykinin ($[MH]^+$ *m/z* 904.4681), angiotensin I ($[MH]^+$ *m/z* 1296.6853), human [Glu1] fibrinopeptide B ($[MH]^+$ *m/z* 1570.6774), ACTH (adrenocorticotropic hormone)-(1–17) ($[MH]^+$ *m/z* 2093.0867), ACTH-(18–39) ($[MH]^+$ *m/z* 2465.1989) and ACTH-(7–38) ($[MH]^+$ *m/z* 3657.9294).
	3. MeOH, HPLC gradient grade, J.T. Baker®-2.5 L.
	4. 5-Chloro-2-mercaptobenzothiazole (CMBT) technical grade, ≥90%, Aldrich-5 g.
	CMBT matrix solution: 10 mg/mL CMBT in 80/20 (v/v) MeOH/MilliQ water.
	5. TFA ≥99.9% Purified B, Sigma Aldrich-25 g.
	6. MeCN, UHPLC-MS, Scharlau-1 L.
	7. 5α-Cyano-4-hydroxycinnamic acid (CHCA) purum ≥99.0%, Fluka-10 g.
	CHCA matrix solution: 10 mg/mL solution of CHCA in 60/40 (v/v) 0.1% TFA/MeCN.
2.7 MALDI TOF/TOF MS/MS Differential Analysis of Bisected/ Triantennary Glycans	1. FA2B model compound oligosaccharide, asialo, agalacto, bisected, fucosylated, bi-antennary N-linked glycan from Dextra Laboratories Ltd-20 μg.
	2. Citric acid ($C_6H_8O_7$) 99 + %, Aldrich-100 g.

3. Sodium phosphate dibasic heptahydrate (Na$_2$HPO$_4$·7H$_2$O) Sigma-250 g.

4. *Exoglycosidase digestion buffer.* Citrate/phosphate buffer 50 mM, pH 5. A 0.1 M citric acid solution is adjusted to pH 5 with 0.2 M Na$_2$HPO$_4$·7H$_2$O solution and diluted 1:1 (v/v) with MilliQ water.

5. Neuraminidase (Sialidase, EC 3.2.1.18) from *Arthrobacter ureafaciens* 1 U (100 μL) in 10 mM sodium phosphate, 0.1% Micr-O-Protect (w/v), 0.25 mg/mL bovine serum albumin, pH 7 (Roche Molecular Biochemicals, Mannheim, Germany).

    Neuraminidase is an exosialidase which cleaves the α-ketosidic linkage between sialic acid and an adjacent sugar residue.

6. β-Galactosidase from bovine testes (EC 3.2.1.23): Ammonium sulfate suspension, 1.0–3.0 units/mg protein (modified Warburg-Christian), 0.26 mL, 0.4 mg protein/mL (WC), 1.9 units/mg protein.

    β-Galactosidase is a hydrolase enzyme that catalyzes the hydrolysis of β-galactosides into monosaccharides.

7. 2,5-Dihydroxybenzoic acid (DHB) Sigma-10 g.

8. TFA ≥99.9% Purified B, Sigma Aldrich-25 g.

9. MeCN, UHPLC-MS, Scharlau-1 L.

10. MeOH, HPLC gradient grade, J.T. Baker®-2.5 L.

    DHB matrix solution: 50 mg/mL in 80/20 (v/v) 0.1% TFA/MeCN.

3   Methods

3.1   Denaturation of Proteins by Reduction and Alkylation

Denaturation of glycoproteins by reduction of disulfide bridges with DTT and subsequent alkylation of the free thiol groups with IAA is a crucial step to ensure a better availability of the glycosylation sites throughout PNGase F digestion. The use of *Rapi*Gest™ surfactant as denaturing agent provides a rapid and efficient sample deglycosylation.

1. 200 μL of CSF sample is freeze-dried and dissolved in 50 μL of denaturing buffer, *Rapi*Gest™ 0.1% (w/v) in NH$_4$HCO$_3$ 50 mM (*see* **Note 3**).

2. Add reducing buffer to the protein sample to obtain a final 5 mM DTT solution.

3. Incubate at 56 °C for 30 min.

4. Let the sample cool at room temperature.

5. Add alkylating buffer to the protein sample to obtain a final 15 mM IAA solution.

6. Let it react at room temperature in the dark for 40 min.

3.2 PNGase F Digestion

1. This step is carried out by adding 2 μL PNGase F (2 U) (*see* **Note 4**).

2. Incubate at 37 °C overnight.

3. PNGase digestion is terminated by adding HCl 500 mM to a final concentration between 30 and 50 mM, pH ≤2 (*see* **Note 5**).

4. Incubate at 37 °C for 45 min.

5. Dilute the sample with MilliQ water to a final volume of 500 μL.

3.3 C₁₈ Sep-Pak Purification of the Released N-Glycans

N-glycans are separated from hydrophobic contaminants using a Sep-Pak® C18 cartridge. Impurities are adsorbed by the C18 stationary phase whereas N-glycans elute with HAc 5%.

A vacuum manifold is employed to speed up this cleaning stage.

1. Clean the Sep-Pak® C18 cartridges with 3 mL of MeOH.

2. Condition the cartridge with 9 mL of HAc 5%.

3. Load the sample (500 μL).

4. Elute with 3 mL HAc 5% and recover the sample.

5. Remove sample solvent in a SpeedVac™ vacuum concentrator.

3.4 Solid-Phase Extraction of the Released N-Glycans

A further cleanup step using graphite cartridges is performed to remove salts and hydrophilic species. N-glycans are adsorbed by the hydrophilic graphite-based stationary phase, while impurities are discarded by washing solutions.

A vacuum manifold is employed to speed up this cleaning stage.

1. Wash the SPE cartridge with 1 mL of NaOH 1 M (basic priming solution), followed by 2 mL of MilliQ water, 1 mL of HAc 30% (acidic priming solution), and finally 1 mL of MilliQ water.

2. Condition the cartridge with 1 mL of 50% ACN in 0.1% TFA (conditioning solution 1) followed by 2 mL of 5% MeCN in 0.1% TFA (conditioning solution 2).

3. Load the sample (redissolved in 500 μL of MilliQ water).

4. Wash with 1 mL of MilliQ water followed by 1 mL of 5% MeCN in 0.1% TFA (washing solution).

5. Elute the sample with 4 × 0.25 mL of 50% MeCN in 0.1% TFA (eluting solution) and collect in a unique Eppendorf™ tube.

6. Remove solvent in a SpeedVac™ vacuum concentrator.

3.5 Glycan Permethylation

Glycans are permethylated prior to MALDI mass spectrometry analysis. This derivatization method aims at reducing the high hydrophilic nature of the oligosaccharide sample, decreasing sample-to-sample and sample-to-matrix aggregation and enhancing about two orders of magnitude signal sensitivity upon MALDI MS. Our permethylation protocol is performed according to

Ciucanu and Kerek procedure [15]. All the reaction steps are accomplished in a fume hood because of the presence of iodomethane. The use of anhydrous DMSO and dry glassware is strictly recommended to reduce moisture absorption before permethylation.

1. Redissolve glycan sample in 400 μL of MilliQ water.

2. Clarify sample solution by a 0.45 μm filter unit. Put the filtered sample in a PYREX screw-cap culture tube and add a magnetic stir bar (*see* **Note 6**).

3. Freeze-dry overnight.

4. About five pellets of NaOH are quickly crushed in a dry agate mortar, after the addition of 3 mL of anhydrous DMSO by a glass syringe, to obtain a NaOH slurry in DMSO.

5. With an end-broken Pasteur pipette, add 1 mL of the slurry solution into the glass tube containing the freeze-dried N-glycan pool.

6. Add about 400 μL of ICH_3 with a Pasteur pipette, vortex, and let it react in a magnetic stirrer at room temperature for 20 min.

7. Stop permethylation by adding, dropwise, 1 mL of MilliQ cold water (*see* **Note 7**).

8. Add 2 mL of chloroform.

9. Vortex and centrifuge at $300 \times g$ for 2 min. Sample centrifugation allows the mixture to settle into two layers. Remove the upper water phase containing impurities and reagent excess.

10. Add 1 mL of MilliQ water and repeat **step 9**.

11. Transfer the chloroform phase into a clean screw-capped glass tube.

12. Wash the sample chloroform solution with 1 mL of MilliQ water at least seven times or until the water phase has a neutral pH.

13. Transfer the final sample solution into another clean screw-capped glass tube and let it dry at room temperature under a gentle stream of nitrogen.

3.6 MALDI MS Analysis of Permethylated Glycans

1. Permethylated glycans are dissolved in MeOH to obtain a concentration of about 10 pmol/μL.

2. Prepare matrix solution by dissolving CMBT at a concentration of 10 mg/mL matrix in 80% MeOH (*see* **Note 8**). Help CMBT dissolution by sonicating and then mild heating until matrix solution is clarified.

3. Mix 2–3 μL of sample solution with the same quantity of matrix solution.

4. Put 1 μL of the sample-matrix mixture on the cleaned stainless steel MALDI target allowing solvent evaporation and sample/matrix co-crystallization at room temperature and atmospheric pressure (dried drop method).

Spectra are acquired in positive ion reflectron mode allowing detection of monoisotopic masses. Each sample spot is submitted to multiple laser shots (1000–3000) and the extracted ions are detected by a TOF analyzer over a mass range of 1000–5000. Laser radiance is set slightly above the ion detection threshold. Typical voltages on the Sciex 4800 TOF/TOF mass spectrometer are source voltage 20 kV, delayed extraction time 500 ns, grid voltage 16 kV, source 1 lens voltage 10 kV, lens 1 voltage 4.2 kV, and mirror 2 voltage 20.494 kV.

External calibration is performed using 1 μL of TOF/TOF Calibration Mixture in 24 μL of CHCA matrix solution and putting 1 μL of calibration mix/matrix on the MALDI target, thus allowing co-crystallization with the dried drop method (*see* **Note 9**). Mass accuracy resulted better than 50 ppm. Data are processed using DataExplorer™ 4.9 software.

3.7 MALDI TOF/TOF MS/MS Differential Analysis of Bisected/ Triantennary Glycans

To confirm the presence of bisected N-glycans in human CSF, we performed the differential MALDI TO/TOF MS/MS analysis on two isobaric compounds: FA2B as a representative model compound of bisected N-glycans ("brain-type" structures) and F3A as a representative model of complex triantennary glycoform ("serum-type" structures); then we compared the MS/MS spectrum of the same precursor ion in the human CSF N-glycan profile(s) to those obtained from the models (*see* Fig. 2a–d).

FA2B glycan is a commercial compound purchased from Dextra Laboratories Ltd., whereas FA3 is obtained by serum treatment with neuraminidase and subsequently with β-galactosidase by the following method (*see* **Note 10**).

1. N-glycans are released and purified from 10 μL of control human serum as described for CSF samples (Subheadings 3.1–3.4.).

2. The obtained glycan pool is dissolved in 200 μL of citrate/ phosphate buffer 50 mM, pH 5.

3. Add 4 μL of neuraminidase (50 mU).

4. Incubate at 37 °C overnight.

5. Stop the reaction by deactivating the enzyme at 100 °C for 10 min.

6. Let the sample cool at room temperature.

7. Add 13 μL of β-galactosidase (10 mU).

8. Incubate at 37 °C overnight.

9. Stop the reaction by deactivating the enzyme at 100 °C for 10 min.

10. Let the sample cool at room temperature.

11. Desalt glycan sample by SPE cartridge as described in Subheading 3.4.

MS analysis is finally performed on the obtained sample to confirm the presence of FA3 compound in the glycan mixture.

12. Prepare sample solution by adding 15 μL di TFA 0.1% to the dried glycan pool.

13. Prepare matrix solution by dissolving DHB at a concentration of 50 mg/mL in 80/20 (v/v) 0.1% TFA/MeCN.

14. Mix 2 μL of sample solution with the same quantity of matrix solution.

15. Put 1 μL of the sample-matrix mixture on the cleaned stainless steel MALDI target allowing solvent evaporation and sample/matrix co-crystallization at room temperature and atmospheric pressure (dried drop method).

16. Once the spot is dried, recrystallize the sample by adding 0.3 μL of MeOH (*see* **Note 11**).

17. Spectra are acquired in positive reflector mode.

MS/MS analysis is performed on this same FA3 solution, on FA2B model compound and on not-derivatized CSF samples (obtained as described from Subheadings 3.1–3.4.). Sample preparation for MS/MS analysis is the same as described for MS (from **steps 12** to **16**).

Typical voltages on the Sciex 4800 TOF/TOF mass spectrometer for MS/MS acquisitions are source 1 voltage 4.2 kV, source 2 voltage 15.0 kV, delayed extraction time 1330 ns, delayed extraction time 2 40,841 ns, source 1 lens voltage 3.2 kV, lens 1 voltage 2.525 kV, lens 2 voltage 4.00 kV, lens 3 voltage 2.1 kV, mirror 1 voltage 10.256 kV, mirror 2 voltage 17.4785 kV, metastable suppressor 1.0 kV, time ion selector enabled, precursor mass window resolution 400 (FWHM), and CID gas off.

Laser radiance is set higher (25–35%) above the threshold of ion detection.

External calibration is performed by using, as the precursor ion, the protonated molecular ion of the human [Glu1]-fibrinopeptide B at m/z 1570.6774 present in the Sciex TOF/TOF standard calibration mixture. The calibrant/matrix solution is loaded as for MALDI TOF MS.

3.8 Assignments of Molecular Ions of Native and Permethylated Glycans

Glycans are detected in positive polarity by MALDI MS as sodiated ions $[M+ Na]^+$. Structural assignments were primarily based on the knowledge of the accurate molecular weight and the N-glycan biosynthetic pathway. N-glycan species were also identified with the help of bioinformatics tools as those provided by the Consortium for Functional Glycomics (CFG; http://www.functionalglycomics.org/) and Glycoworkbench v2.1 [16]. For practical reasons Fig. 1a–c shows only major CSF permethylated N-glycans. The complete peak assign-

Table 1
Structures of permethylated *N*-glycans from control CSF identified by MALDI-TOF MS

STRUCTURE	*m/z*	STRUCTURE	*m/z*	STRUCTURE	*m/z*
	1579.7		1999.0		2244.0
	1590.8		2010.0		2285.0
	1620.8		2029.0		2315.1
	1661.6		2039.9		2326.1
	1753.8		2069.9		2360.1
	1783.8		2081.0		2390.1
	1794.8		2110.9		2396.1
	1835.8		2152.0		2401.1
	1865.9		2156.0		2418.1
	1906.8		2192.0		2431.1
	1981.9		2214.0		2459.1
	1987.9		2227.0		2472.2

(continued)

**Table 1
(continued)**

STRUCTURE	m/z	STRUCTURE	m/z	STRUCTURE	m/z
	2489.1		2704.2		2908.4
	2519.1		2717.2		2921.4
	2530.1		2734.3		2966.3
	2560.2		2749.3		3024.4
	2564.2		2764.2		3037.4
	2592.2		2792.2		3054.4
	2605.1		2820.3		3082.4
	2646.2		2837.3		3140.5
	2663.2		2850.3		3198.4
	2676.2		2880.4		3211.4
	2693.2		2891.4		3241.4

(continued)

Table 1
(continued)

STRUCTURE	m/z	STRUCTURE	m/z	STRUCTURE	m/z
	3269.5		3503.5		3864.7
	3282.5		3602.5		4051.7
	3299.5		3647.6		4226.7
	3415.5		3660.6		4414.8
	3443.5		3690.6		4588.8
	3456.6		3776.6		4762.8
	3473.5		3834.7		

Linkages are not indicated on the cartoons; thus most structures may refer to two or more isomers as, for example, those due to different branching elongation or fucosylation at the 3-linked or 6-linked mannosyl residue of the core

ments (a total of about 90 species for control CSF, ranging from *m/z* 1579.7 to *m/z* 4762.8) are reported in Table 1.

4　Notes

1. Some authors recommend the use of PNGase F in water (storage at 4 °C) because glycerol could inhibit matrix crystallization prior to MS. In our experience PNGase F storage in glycerol is preferable as it ensures a perfect enzyme stability for a longer period at −20 °C. Sample will be separated from the digestion buffer including glycerol through the subsequent cleanup steps.

2. All operations with ICH_3 should be performed in a fume hood.

3. All reagent amounts used for reduction and alkylation are calculated for 200 μL of CSF.

4. Proteolytic digestion before PNGase F addition is not necessary when utilizing *Rapi*Gest™ as denaturing agent.

5. Lowering the pH serves either to stop the reaction or to hydrolyze *Rapi*Gest™ whose by-products are easily removed from the sample by the subsequent cleanup steps.

6. Permethylation requires perfectly dry conditions; for this reason magnetic stir bar is added to sample before freeze-drying and is mandatory using anhydrous reagents and dry glasses.

7. As water addition has an exothermic effect, it should be accomplished by placing the reaction tube in an ice-cold bath and shaking frequently.

8. The most used matrix for permethylated glycans is DHB. We tested a number of matrices and found that CMBT gives much better results with remarkable increased sensitivity and resolution.

9. In general, it is a good practice to use the same matrix solution for the sample and the calibration mixture (in this case CMBT solution used as matrix for permethylated oligosaccharides). In our experience no improvement on accuracy of MS measurements was observed by performing calibration with the standard SCIEX peptide mixture in CHCA, probably because the laser irradiation threshold is very similar for the two matrices.

10. This comparison can be performed by MS/MS analysis either on native or on permethylated glycans. The first choice is preferable as native (not-derivatized) glycans give a set of intense and well-defined ion fragments providing a clear-cut fingerprint identification.

11. Sample recrystallization with methanol or ethanol is sometimes useful, when using DHB as matrix, to redistribute sample and matrix crystals in a more homogeneous thin layer.

Acknowledgements

Generous donation from Stellalucente Trust is gratefully acknowledged. This chapter is dedicated to our dear friend and colleague Francesco Le Pira, University of Catania, who too early passed away.

References

1. Schedin-Weiss S, Winblad B, Tjernberg LO (2014) The role of protein glycosylation in Alzheimer disease. FEBS J 281:46–62

2. Palmigiano A, Barone R, Sturiale L et al (2016) CSF N-glycoproteomics for early diagnosis in Alzheimer's disease. J Proteome 131:29–37

3. Barone R, Sturiale L, Palmigiano A et al (2012) Glycomics of pediatric and adulthood diseases of the central nervous system. J Proteome 75:5123–5139

4. Kizuka Y, Kitazume S, Fujinawa R, Saito T, Iwata N, Saito T et al (2015) An aberrant sugar modification of BACE1 blocks its lysosomal targeting in Alzheimer's disease. EMBO Mol Med 7:175–189

5. Kizuka Y, Nakano M, Kitazume S, Saito T et al (2016) Bisecting GlcNAc modification stabilizes BACE1 protein under oxidative stress conditions. Biochem J 473(1):21–30

6. Kizuka Y, Kitazume S, Taniguchi N (2017) N-glycan and Alzheimer's disease. Biochim Biophys Acta 1861(10):2447–2454. https://doi.org/10.1016/j.bbagen.2017.04.012

7. Stanley P, Schachter H, Taniguchi N (2009) N-glycans. In: Varki A, Cummings R, Esko J, Freeze H, Stanley P, Bertozzi CR, Hart GW, Etzler ME (eds) Essentials of glycobiology, 2nd edn. Cold Spring Harbor Laboratory Press, Cold Spring Harbor, NY

8. Hoffmann A, Nimtz M, Getzlaff R, Conradt HS (1995) 'Brain-type' N-glycosylation of asialo-transferrin from human cerebrospinal fluid. FEBS Lett 359(2–3):164–168

9. Royle LI, Campbell MP, Radcliffe CM, White DM, Harvey DJ et al (2008) HPLC-based analysis of serum N-glycans on a 96-well plate platform with dedicated database software. Anal Biochem 376:1–12

10. Domon B, Costello CE (1988) A systematic nomenclature for carbohydrate fragmentations in FAB-MS/MS spectra of glycoconjugates. Glycoconj J 5:397–409

11. Schachter H (1986) Biosynthetic controls that determine the branching and microheterogeneity of protein-bound oligosaccharides. Biochem Cell Biol 64(3):163–181

12. Akasaka-Manya K, Manya H, Sakurai Y et al (2010) Protective effect of N-glycan bisecting GlcNAc residues on β-amyloid production in Alzheimer's disease. Glycobiology 20(1):99–106

13. Avagyan H, Goldenson B, Tse E, Masoumi A et al (2009) Immune blood biomarkers of Alzheimer disease patients. J Neuroimmunol 210:67–72

14. Ikeda Y, Ihara H, Tsukamoto H et al (2014) Mannosyl (beta-1,4-)-glycoprotein beta-1,4-N-acetylglucosaminyltransferase (MGAT3); β1,4-N-acetylglucosaminyltransferase III (GnT-III, GlcNAcT-III). In: Taniguchi N et al (eds) Handbook of glycosyltransferase and related genes, 2nd edn. Springer, Tokyo

15. Ciucanu I, Kerek F (1984) A simple and rapid method for the permethylation of carbohydrates. Carbohydr Res 131:209–217

16. Ceroni A, Maass K, Geyer H, Geyer R, Dell A, Haslam SM (2008) GlycoWorkbench: a tool for the computer-assisted annotation of mass spectra of glycans. J Proteome Res 7:1650–1659

Chapter 6

MicroRNA Profiling of Alzheimer's Disease Cerebrospinal Fluid

Johannes Denk and Holger Jahn

Abstract

MicroRNAs (miRNAs) are a class of small, highly conserved, and noncoding RNAs that modulate gene expression by regulating the activity and stability of target mRNAs. MiRNAs play significant roles by controlling fundamental cellular processes and its deregulation is associated with various diseases. Ubiquitous expression and its release into circulation make them interesting biomarkers, which can be measured by different platforms. In this book chapter, we provide a specific protocol that describes the detection of circulating miRNAs in CSF by using RT-qPCR.

Key words RT-qPCR, CSF, MicroRNA, MIQE, Biomarker, SYBR-green, CNS disorders

1 Introduction

What was once called Junk-DNA now serves at least in parts as a mirror of a cornucopia of so-called noncoding RNA species present in every cell and tissue. There is evidence that these RNA types, e.g., circular RNAs and especially the large number of different miRNAs, have an important role in cell differentiation and regulation of cell biochemistry in general. The investigation of miRNAs may help us to understand the pathology of psychiatric diseases, e.g., neurodegenerative diseases, as these small molecules interact with mRNAs. By controlling epigenetically the translation of mRNA into proteins, miRNAs may offer an explanation for the often milieu-dependent incomplete penetrance and multigenetic character of many psychiatric disorders. MiRNAs are ubiquitously expressed and can be found in all cell types and body fluids including serum, cerebrospinal fluid (CSF), saliva, urine, and breast milk [1]. They are stable at room temperature for longer periods of time, resistant to RNase activity [2], and easier to detect and quantify compared to other protein-based biomarkers. Hence miRNAs fulfil key requirements toward an ideal biomarker. So far, despite considerable efforts, no CSF miRNA has been firmly established as a

Robert Perneczky (ed.), *Biomarkers for Alzheimer's Disease Drug Development*, Methods in Molecular Biology, vol. 1750, https://doi.org/10.1007/978-1-4939-7704-8_6, © Springer Science+Business Media, LLC 2018

clinically relevant biomarker for any psychiatric condition. Many basic questions are still unanswered, e.g., the source of miRNAs in the CSF and a secured function for free and exosomal miRNA drifting in CSF. A recent paper points at the plexus choroideus as a major provider of miRNAs in CSF and suggests that miRNA released in extracellular vesicles from the choroid plexus may enter brain parenchyma to activate astrocytes and microglia as a mechanism to regulate inflammation processes [3]. RNA content in CSF is very low and reproducible results remain a challenge mainly due to different protocols and methods in the field. Pre-analytical and analytical factors such as sampling, RNA isolation, and detection methods as well as different normalization strategies contribute to conflicting results. In addition, many studies do not adhere to established guidelines (e.g., MIQE), which complicates interpretability, comparability, and thus reproducibility. In the following sections we describe a protocol that allows the accurate detection of circulating miRNAs in CSF by using RT-qPCR. Our protocol includes the following main steps: (1) general considerations, (2) sampling, (3) preparation of spike-in mixes, (4) RNA isolation, (5) reverse transcription, (6) quantitative PCR, (7) absolute quantification, and (8) recommendations for data analysis.

2   Material

2.1 Preparation of Spike-In Mixes

1. miRCURY LNA™ Universal RT microRNA PCR, RNA Spike-in kit, Exiqon (see Note 1).

   (a) Synthetic UniSp2 RNA (22 nt), 160 fmole, 2 fmole/µL (resuspended).
   Synthetic UniSp4 RNA (22 nt), 1.6 fmole, 0.02 fmole/µL (resuspended).
   Synthetic UniSp5 RNA (22 nt), 0.016 fmole, 0.0002 fmole/µL (resuspended).
   MS2 total RNA, 50 ng, 0.625 ng/µL (resuspended).

   (b) Synthetic cel-miR-39-3p RNA, 0.16 fmole, 0.002 fmole/µL (resuspended).

2.2 RNA Isolation

1. miRNeasy Serum/Plasma Kit (50), Qiagen (see Note 2).

   (a) 50 RNeasy® MinElute® Spin Columns (each packaged with a 2 mL collection tube) (store at 2–8 °C).

   (b) 50 Collection tubes (1.5 mL).

   (c) 50 mL QIAzol® Lysis Reagent (store at 15–25 °C).

   (d) 15 mL Buffer RWT (store at 15–25 °C) (see Note 3).

   (e) 11 mL Buffer RPE (store at 15–25 °C) (see Note 4).

   (f) Ce_miR-39_1 miScript® Primer Assay (see Note 5).

   (g) 10 mL RNase-free water (store at 15–25 °C).

2. Chloroform (without added isoamyl alcohol).

3. Ethanol (80 and 100%) (*see* **Note 6**).

4. MS2 RNA, Roche.

5. Microcentrifuge (with rotor for 2 mL tubes).

6. Phase Lock GeI™ (PLG) tubes, heavy 2 mL, 200 tubes, 5Prime (*see* **Note 7**).

2.3 Reverse Transcription

1. Eppendorf® PCR Cooler, 0.1 mL tubes, Eppendorf.

2. Multiply®-Pro 0.2 mL Biosphere®, Sarstedt.

3. Universal cDNA synthesis kit II, 8-64 rxns, Exiqon (*see* **Note 8**).

   (a) 5× Reaction buffer, 128 μL, 5× concentrated.

   (b) Enzyme mix, 64 μL, 10× concentrated.

   (c) Nuclease-free water, 1 mL.

   (d) UniSp6, RNA spike-in template, 12 fmol, dried down.

2.4 Quantitative PCR

1. Eppendorf® PCR Cooler, 0.1 mL tubes, Eppendorf.

2. CoolRack XT PCR384, Biocision.

3. qPCR Seal, sheets (140 × 77 mm), 4titude (*see* **Note 9**).

4. Q-Stick™ qPCR Seal, sheets (133 × 76 mm), 4ti-0565, 4titude (*see* **Note 9**).

5. ExiLENT SYBR® Green master mix, 20 mL, Exiqon (*see* **Note 10**).

6. Multipette® E3, Eppendorf (*see* **Note 25**).

7. Individual microRNA primer set(s) or ready-to-use panels ordered from Exiqon (www.exiqon.com) (*see* **Note 11**).

8. Any thermal cycler that is compatible with Exiqons microRNA primer system (e.g., LC480 from Roche).

2.5 Absolute Quantification Using Standard Curve Method

1. Synthetic RNA oligos, RNase-free HPLC purity, 5′ phosphorylated, IDT (*see* **Note 12**).

2. MS2 RNA, Roche.

3 Methods

Carry out all procedures at room temperature and vortex all reagents and spin them down before use unless otherwise specified. Make sure to work with calibrated pipettes.

3.1 General Considerations

This protocol provides a means to accurately detect circulating miRNAs isolated from human antemortem CSF by using RT-qPCR. However, many different protocols and methods exist and conflicting results are still a problem in this field of research.

Certain key aspects should be taken into account to increase the generation of more reliable and reproducible results. Providing detail would go beyond the scope of this chapter but we would like to draw the attention to the following key points: (a) miRNA profiling (*see* Refs [4–6]), (b) standardization (*see* Refs [7–11]), and (c) normalization (*see* Refs [12–14]). These references will provide profound knowledge to support the reader in carefully planning and evaluating miRNA profiling studies.

3.2 Sampling

We adhere to a CSF sampling procedure, which was developed as a SOP in the German Research Consortium of frontotemporal lobar degeneration:

1. The lumbar puncture should be performed ideally between 8 am and 11 am.

2. Follow local guidelines/routines for antiseptic cleansing and anesthesia.

3. Position the patient in a reclining or sitting position with back arched.

4. Use whenever possible an atraumatic lumbar puncture system (spinal needle (20–22 gauge) for the LP.

5. Insert the needle through the L3/L4 or L4/L5 interspace.

6. Collect 10 mL of CSF from the subject. Use a POLYPROPYLENE TUBE ONLY for CSF collection. Cell count and Reiber schema done on an aliquot.

7. Mix the CSF gently by turning the tube upside down three to four times (cap on).

8. Within 15 min centrifuge the CSF in the polypropylene tube at $1600 \times g$ for 10 min at +4 °C, to eliminate cells and debris.

9. Aliquot CSF in 0.25–1 mL aliquots, into sterile PRELABELED POLYPROPYLENE CRYOVIALS with a screw cap.

10. Store aliquots of CSF at −80 °C until use. Do not snap freeze, e.g., in liquid nitrogen.

3.3 RNA Isolation Spike-In Mix

1. Spin down vial including UniSp2, UniSp4, and UniSp5 (*see* Subheading 2.2, **item 1a**) before opening and resuspend the spike-in mix by adding 80 µL nuclease-free water to the vial. Leave for 20 min on ice to properly dissolve the RNA pellet. Then mix again by vortexing and shortly spin down. Store in aliquots at −20 °C to avoid freeze-thaw cycles.

3.4 cDNA Synthesis RNA Spike-In Mix

1. Spin down UniSp6 RNA spike-in (*see* Subheading 2.3, **item 3d**) before opening and resuspend by adding 80 µL nuclease-free water to the vial and mix by vortexing and spin down. Leave for 20–30 min on ice to properly dissolve the RNA spike-in. Then mix again by vortexing and spin down.

2. Resuspend the cel-miR-39-3p RNA spike-in (*see* Subheading 2.2, **item 1b**) by adding the 80 µL resuspended UniSp6 RNA spike-in to the vial and mix by vortexing and spin down. Leave for 20–30 min on ice to properly dissolve the RNA spike-in. Then mix again by vortexing and spin down. Store in aliquots at −20 °C.

3.5 RNA Isolation

1. Thaw CSF samples on ice (*see* **Note 13**).

2. Centrifuge 2 mL Phase Lock Gel (PLG) tubes at $12,000 \times g$ for 20 s to pellet the gel.

3. Centrifuge CSF samples at $3000 \times g$ for 5 min and store on ice (*see* **Note 14**).

4. Pipette 1000 µL QIAzol Lysis Reagent in a sterile 2 mL microcentrifuge tube.

5. (Optional) Add 1.25 µL MS2 RNA (0.8 µg/µL) (*see* **Note 15**).

6. Add 1 µL RNA isolation spike-in mix (*see* Subheading 3.2 and **Note 16**).

7. Add 200 µL CSF (*see* **Note 17**) to the QIAzol spike-in mix and mix by vortexing. Leave at room temperature for 5 min.

8. Add 200 µL chloroform and mix by vortexing for 15 s.

9. Pipette the QIAzol-chloroform-CSF mix (appr. 1400 µL) into the PLG tube, carefully mix by inverting, and leave at room temperature for 3 min.

10. Centrifuge the QIAzol-chloroform-CSF mix at $12,000 \times g$ for 15 min (*see* **Note 18**).

11. Pipette 1170 µL 100% ethanol (*see* **Note 19**) in sterile 2 mL microcentrifuge tubes.

12. Pipette 780 µL aqueous phase from the PLG tubes to the ethanol and mix by pipetting up and down (*see* **Note 20**).

13. Pipette 650 µL of your mixture on the MinElute® Spin Column, centrifuge at $8000 \times g$ for 15 s at room temperature, and discard the flow-through (*see* **Note 21**).

14. Repeat **step 13** until the complete mixture is filtered.

15. Pipette 700 µL buffer RWT on the spin column, centrifuge at $8000 \times g$ for 15 s at room temperature, and discard the flow-through.

16. Pipette 500 µL buffer RPE on the spin column, centrifuge at $8000 \times g$ for 15 s at room temperature, and discard the flow-through.

17. Pipette 500 µL buffer 80% ethanol on the spin column, centrifuge at $8000 \times g$ for 2 min at room temperature, and discard the flow-through.

18. Place the spin column into a new 2 mL collection tube, open the spin column, and centrifuge at full speed for 5 min to dry the membrane.

19. Place the spin column into a new, sterile 1.5 mL collection tube and add 14 μL RNase-free water (*see* **Note 22**) directly to the center of the spin column membrane. Close the lid and centrifuge for 1 min at full speed to elute the RNA.

3.6 Reverse Transcription

Keep reagents and reactions on ice (or at 4 °C) at all times.

1. Gently thaw the 5× reaction buffer and nuclease-free water, and immediately place on ice. Mix by vortexing. Immediately before use, remove the enzyme mix from the freezer, mix by flicking the tubes, and place on ice. Spin down all reagents.

2. Prepare the required amount of RT working solution (*see* **Note 23**) according to Table 1 in a sterile microcentrifuge tube, mix by flicking, and spin down.

3. Pipette 12 μL RT working solution into sterile 0.2 mL nuclease-free tubes cooled on ice.

4. Pipette 8 μL isolated total RNA into each tube. Mix by flicking and spin down (*see* **Note 24**).

5. Use the following thermal cycling protocol to synthesize cDNA:

Incubate for 60 min at 42 °C. Heat-inactivate the reverse transcriptase for 5 min at 95 °C. Immediately cool to 4 °C. Store at 4 °C or freeze (*see* **Note 25**).

Table 1
Reverse transcription (RT) reaction setup

RT working solution (*see* Note 23)	μL	10% PL (for one sample)	10 samples
5× Reaction buffer	4	4.4	44.0
Nuclease-free water	5	5.5	55.0
Enzyme mix	2	2.2	22.0
cDNA synthesis RNA spike-in mix, optional replace with H₂O if omitted	1	1.1	11.0
RT working solution	12	13.2	132.0
(Total) RNA (*see* Note 23)	8	–	–
Total reaction	20	–	–

PL pipette loss

3.7   Quantitative PCR

1. Place cDNA (*see* Subheading 3.5, **step 5**), nuclease-free water, and 2× PCR master mix (*see* Subheading 2.4, **item 5**) on ice and thaw for 15–20 min. Protect the 2× PCR master mix vial from light. Immediately before use, mix the 2× PCR master mix by pipetting up and down. The rest of the reagents are mixed by vortexing and spun down.

2. Dilute the cDNA with nuclease-free water to give a final 50× dilution (*see* Table 2, column 3). Do not freeze or store the diluted cDNA.

3. Before removing the seal from the ready-to-use plate, briefly spin down the plate in a plate centrifuge and place it on a cooled PCR rack (96- or 384-well).

4. Combine 2× PCR master mix (*see* Subheading 2.4, **item 5**) and 50× diluted cDNA (*see* Subheading 3.6, **step 2**) 1:1, mix gently by inverting the tube, and spin down (*see* Table 2, column 5, and **Note 26**).

5. Pipette 10 µL 2× PCR master mix:cDNA mix to each well (*see* **Note 27**).

6. Seal the plate with optical sealing as recommended by the instrument manufacturer (*see* **Notes 9** and **28**).

Table 2
Different pick-and-mix configurations and the resulting cDNA and master mix dilution procedures

Pick-and-mix plate configuration[a]	Plate format	cDNA dilution procedure[b] (µL) (RNA + H$_2$O)	Diluted cDNA (µL) needed for each sample[c]	Composition (µL) of final PCR master mix (diluted cDNA +H$_2$O)	Number of required PCR master mixes
8 × 12	96 well	4 + 196 (1:50)	66 (10% PL)	66 + 66 (1:1)	8×
4 × 24	96-well	4 + 196 (1:50)	132 (10% PL)	132 + 132 (1:1)	4×
1 × 96	96-well	10 + 490 (1:50)	500 (4% PL)	500 + 500 (1:1)	1×
16 × 24	384-well	4 + 196 (1:50)	132 (10% PL)	132 + 132 (1:1)	16×
8 × 48	384-well	6 + 294 (1:50)	264 (10% PL)	264 + 264 (1:1)	8×
4 × 96	384-well	10 + 490 (1:50)	500 (4% PL)	500 + 500 (1:1)	4×
2 × 192	384-well	20 + 980 (1:50)	1000 (4% PL)	1000 + 1000 (1:1)	2×

[a]Samples × number of miRNA assays per sample
[b]*See* Subheading 3.6, **step 2**
[c]*See* Subheading 3.6, **step 4**; *PL* pipette loss

Table 3
Thermal cycling protocol for amplification and fluorescent real-time detection of miRNA transcripts

Process step	Settings, LC480 instrument	Settings, other instruments
Polymerase activation/ denaturation	95 °C, 10 min	95 °C, 10 min
Amplification	45 amplification cycles at 95 °C, 10 s 60 °C, 1 min, ramp-rate 1.6 °C/s[a] optical read	40 amplification cycles at 95 °C, 10 s 60 °C, 1 min, ramp-rate 1.6 °C/s[a] Optical read
Melting curve analysis	Yes	Yes

[a]The ramp rate of cooling from 95 °C to 60 °C should be set to 1.6 °C/s

7. Spin plate briefly in a plate centrifuge at $1500 \times g$ for 1 min to remove air bubbles.

8. Perform real-time PCR amplification followed by melting curve analysis according to Table 3.

9. Perform initial data analysis using the software supplied with the real-time PCR instrument to obtain raw Cq values. Check each assay for a clear, single peak and remove values that display more than one peak.

3.8 Absolute Quantification Using Standard Curve Method

The standard curve method provides a means to assess the absolute copy number and the efficiency of a particular miRNA assay by using synthetic RNA oligonucleotides. The following protocol allows the detection of $n = 8$ different miRNAs on a 384-well plate including technical replicates on the cDNA ($n = 2$) and PCR ($n = 3$) level (*see* **Note 29**, Fig. 1).

1. Resuspend each synthetic RNA oligo ($n = 8$) to give a stock concentration of 100 µM resulting in ~6.02×10^{13} copies/µL.

2. Pool each miRNA oligo to generate a miRNA oligo pool of 10 µM. Combine 80 µL of each oligo stock (100 µM) with 160 µL nuclease-free water.

3. Serially dilute oligo pool down to 0.001 µM using 1:10 dilution steps. For example dilute 100 µL oligo pool in 900 µL nuclease-free water and transfer 100 µL from this dilution to another 900 µL nuclease-free water. Proceed until a concentration of 0.001 µM is achieved.

4. Serially dilute the oligo pool (0.001 µM) in 1:4 dilution steps. Start by diluting 4 µL oligo pool in 118.1 µL nuclease-free water (1:30.5) containing 10 ng/µL MS2 carrier RNA resulting in 1.97×10^7 copies/µL (Standard 0).

	1	2	3	4	5	6	7	8	9	10	11	12	13	14	15	16	17	18	19	20	21	22	23	24	PCR MM	Replicate
A	STD 1 primer 1	STD 1 primer 1	STD 1 primer 1	STD 1 primer 2	STD 1 primer 2	STD 1 primer 2	STD 1 primer 3	STD 1 primer 3	STD 1 primer 3	STD 1 primer 4	STD 1 primer 4	STD 1 primer 4	STD 1 primer 5	STD 1 primer 5	STD 1 primer 5	STD 1 primer 6	STD 1 primer 6	STD 1 primer 6	STD 1 primer 7	STD 1 primer 7	STD 1 primer 7	STD 1 primer 8	STD 1 primer 8	STD 1 primer 8	STD 1	cDNA 1
B	STD 2 primer 1	STD 2 primer 1	STD 2 primer 1	STD 2 primer 2	STD 2 primer 2	STD 2 primer 2	STD 2 primer 3	STD 2 primer 3	STD 2 primer 3	STD 2 primer 4	STD 2 primer 4	STD 2 primer 4	STD 2 primer 5	STD 2 primer 5	STD 2 primer 5	STD 2 primer 6	STD 2 primer 6	STD 2 primer 6	STD 2 primer 7	STD 2 primer 7	STD 2 primer 7	STD 2 primer 8	STD 2 primer 8	STD 2 primer 8	STD 2	
C	STD 3 primer 1	STD 3 primer 1	STD 3 primer 1	STD 3 primer 2	STD 3 primer 2	STD 3 primer 2	STD 3 primer 3	STD 3 primer 3	STD 3 primer 3	STD 3 primer 4	STD 3 primer 4	STD 3 primer 4	STD 3 primer 5	STD 3 primer 5	STD 3 primer 5	STD 3 primer 6	STD 3 primer 6	STD 3 primer 6	STD 3 primer 7	STD 3 primer 7	STD 3 primer 7	STD 3 primer 8	STD 3 primer 8	STD 3 primer 8	STD 3	
D	STD 4 primer 1	STD 4 primer 1	STD 4 primer 1	STD 4 primer 2	STD 4 primer 2	STD 4 primer 2	STD 4 primer 3	STD 4 primer 3	STD 4 primer 3	STD 4 primer 4	STD 4 primer 4	STD 4 primer 4	STD 4 primer 5	STD 4 primer 5	STD 4 primer 5	STD 4 primer 6	STD 4 primer 6	STD 4 primer 6	STD 4 primer 7	STD 4 primer 7	STD 4 primer 7	STD 4 primer 8	STD 4 primer 8	STD 4 primer 8	STD 4	
E	STD 5 primer 1	STD 5 primer 1	STD 5 primer 1	STD 5 primer 2	STD 5 primer 2	STD 5 primer 2	STD 5 primer 3	STD 5 primer 3	STD 5 primer 3	STD 5 primer 4	STD 5 primer 4	STD 5 primer 4	STD 5 primer 5	STD 5 primer 5	STD 5 primer 5	STD 5 primer 6	STD 5 primer 6	STD 5 primer 6	STD 5 primer 7	STD 5 primer 7	STD 5 primer 7	STD 5 primer 8	STD 5 primer 8	STD 5 primer 8	STD 5	
F	STD 6 primer 1	STD 6 primer 1	STD 6 primer 1	STD 6 primer 2	STD 6 primer 2	STD 6 primer 2	STD 6 primer 3	STD 6 primer 3	STD 6 primer 3	STD 6 primer 4	STD 6 primer 4	STD 6 primer 4	STD 6 primer 5	STD 6 primer 5	STD 6 primer 5	STD 6 primer 6	STD 6 primer 6	STD 6 primer 6	STD 6 primer 7	STD 6 primer 7	STD 6 primer 7	STD 6 primer 8	STD 6 primer 8	STD 6 primer 8	STD 6	
G	STD 7 primer 1	STD 7 primer 1	STD 7 primer 1	STD 7 primer 2	STD 7 primer 2	STD 7 primer 2	STD 7 primer 3	STD 7 primer 3	STD 7 primer 3	STD 7 primer 4	STD 7 primer 4	STD 7 primer 4	STD 7 primer 5	STD 7 primer 5	STD 7 primer 5	STD 7 primer 6	STD 7 primer 6	STD 7 primer 6	STD 7 primer 7	STD 7 primer 7	STD 7 primer 7	STD 7 primer 8	STD 7 primer 8	STD 7 primer 8	STD 7	
H	STD 8 primer 1	STD 8 primer 1	STD 8 primer 1	STD 8 primer 2	STD 8 primer 2	STD 8 primer 2	STD 8 primer 3	STD 8 primer 3	STD 8 primer 3	STD 8 primer 4	STD 8 primer 4	STD 8 primer 4	STD 8 primer 5	STD 8 primer 5	STD 8 primer 5	STD 8 primer 6	STD 8 primer 6	STD 8 primer 6	STD 8 primer 7	STD 8 primer 7	STD 8 primer 7	STD 8 primer 8	STD 8 primer 8	STD 8 primer 8	STD 8	
I	STD 1 primer 1	STD 1 primer 1	STD 1 primer 1	STD 1 primer 2	STD 1 primer 2	STD 1 primer 2	STD 1 primer 3	STD 1 primer 3	STD 1 primer 3	STD 1 primer 4	STD 1 primer 4	STD 1 primer 4	STD 1 primer 5	STD 1 primer 5	STD 1 primer 5	STD 1 primer 6	STD 1 primer 6	STD 1 primer 6	STD 1 primer 7	STD 1 primer 7	STD 1 primer 7	STD 1 primer 8	STD 1 primer 8	STD 1 primer 8	STD 1	cDNA 2
J	STD 2 primer 1	STD 2 primer 1	STD 2 primer 1	STD 2 primer 2	STD 2 primer 2	STD 2 primer 2	STD 2 primer 3	STD 2 primer 3	STD 2 primer 3	STD 2 primer 4	STD 2 primer 4	STD 2 primer 4	STD 2 primer 5	STD 2 primer 5	STD 2 primer 5	STD 2 primer 6	STD 2 primer 6	STD 2 primer 6	STD 2 primer 7	STD 2 primer 7	STD 2 primer 7	STD 2 primer 8	STD 2 primer 8	STD 2 primer 8	STD 2	
K	STD 3 primer 1	STD 3 primer 1	STD 3 primer 1	STD 3 primer 2	STD 3 primer 2	STD 3 primer 2	STD 3 primer 3	STD 3 primer 3	STD 3 primer 3	STD 3 primer 4	STD 3 primer 4	STD 3 primer 4	STD 3 primer 5	STD 3 primer 5	STD 3 primer 5	STD 3 primer 6	STD 3 primer 6	STD 3 primer 6	STD 3 primer 7	STD 3 primer 7	STD 3 primer 7	STD 3 primer 8	STD 3 primer 8	STD 3 primer 8	STD 3	
L	STD 4 primer 1	STD 4 primer 1	STD 4 primer 1	STD 4 primer 2	STD 4 primer 2	STD 4 primer 2	STD 4 primer 3	STD 4 primer 3	STD 4 primer 3	STD 4 primer 4	STD 4 primer 4	STD 4 primer 4	STD 4 primer 5	STD 4 primer 5	STD 4 primer 5	STD 4 primer 6	STD 4 primer 6	STD 4 primer 6	STD 4 primer 7	STD 4 primer 7	STD 4 primer 7	STD 4 primer 8	STD 4 primer 8	STD 4 primer 8	STD 4	
M	STD 5 primer 1	STD 5 primer 1	STD 5 primer 1	STD 5 primer 2	STD 5 primer 2	STD 5 primer 2	STD 5 primer 3	STD 5 primer 3	STD 5 primer 3	STD 5 primer 4	STD 5 primer 4	STD 5 primer 4	STD 5 primer 5	STD 5 primer 5	STD 5 primer 5	STD 5 primer 6	STD 5 primer 6	STD 5 primer 6	STD 5 primer 7	STD 5 primer 7	STD 5 primer 7	STD 5 primer 8	STD 5 primer 8	STD 5 primer 8	STD 5	
N	STD 6 primer 1	STD 6 primer 1	STD 6 primer 1	STD 6 primer 2	STD 6 primer 2	STD 6 primer 2	STD 6 primer 3	STD 6 primer 3	STD 6 primer 3	STD 6 primer 4	STD 6 primer 4	STD 6 primer 4	STD 6 primer 5	STD 6 primer 5	STD 6 primer 5	STD 6 primer 6	STD 6 primer 6	STD 6 primer 6	STD 6 primer 7	STD 6 primer 7	STD 6 primer 7	STD 6 primer 8	STD 6 primer 8	STD 6 primer 8	STD 6	
O	STD 7 primer 1	STD 7 primer 1	STD 7 primer 1	STD 7 primer 2	STD 7 primer 2	STD 7 primer 2	STD 7 primer 3	STD 7 primer 3	STD 7 primer 3	STD 7 primer 4	STD 7 primer 4	STD 7 primer 4	STD 7 primer 5	STD 7 primer 5	STD 7 primer 5	STD 7 primer 6	STD 7 primer 6	STD 7 primer 6	STD 7 primer 7	STD 7 primer 7	STD 7 primer 7	STD 7 primer 8	STD 7 primer 8	STD 7 primer 8	STD 7	
P	STD 8 primer 1	STD 8 primer 1	STD 8 primer 1	STD 8 primer 2	STD 8 primer 2	STD 8 primer 2	STD 8 primer 3	STD 8 primer 3	STD 8 primer 3	STD 8 primer 4	STD 8 primer 4	STD 8 primer 4	STD 8 primer 5	STD 8 primer 5	STD 8 primer 5	STD 8 primer 6	STD 8 primer 6	STD 8 primer 6	STD 8 primer 7	STD 8 primer 7	STD 8 primer 7	STD 8 primer 8	STD 8 primer 8	STD 8 primer 8	STD 8	
Replicate	PCR 1	PCR 2	PCR 3	PCR 1	PCR 2	PCR 3	PCR 1	PCR 2	PCR 3	PCR 1	PCR 2	PCR 3	PCR 1	PCR 2	PCR 3	PCR 1	PCR 2	PCR 3	PCR 1	PCR 2	PCR 3	PCR 1	PCR 2	PCR 3		

Fig. 1 Detection of $n = 8$ different miRNAs on a 334-well plate including technical replicates on the cDNA ($n = 2$) and PCR ($n = 3$) level

5. Dilute 20 μL Standard 0 in 60 μL nuclease-free water containing 10 ng/μL MS2 carrier RNA resulting in 4.93×10^6 copies/μL (Standard 1).

6. Continue dilution series by following the procedure in **step 5** to generate Standard 1–8. Standard 8 will contain 3.01×10^2 copies/μL.

7. Considering subsequent dilution factors from the cDNA reaction (1:2.5), cDNA dilution (1:50), and PCR master mix (1:1), Standard 8 will result in 1.2 copies/μL or 12 copies in the final PCR reaction. Standards 1–8 will cover a range of $12–1.97 \times 10^5$ copies.

8. Use the protocol described in Subheadings 3.6 and 3.7 to quantify the copy number of Standards 1–8 (*see* **Note 27**).

9. Plot the obtained Ct values against the log copy number of the synthetic oligos. The standard curve is the regression line through these points, which allows to determine the number of copies in your biological sample and gives you a good estimate about the efficiency (E) of your assay by using the following equation: $E = 10^{-1/\text{slope}}$.

3.9 Recommendations for Data Analysis

We advise to consider the following aspects when evaluating miRNA expression data:

1. We used a Cq > 37 as a general cutoff. However, we recommend to test the sensitivity, also referred to the limit of detection (LOD), of a representative set of assays to determine a protocol-specific cutoff. This can be achieved by using at least six replicate standard curves. The last dilution where all six replicates give a positive and specific amplification (Cq and Tm) can be considered as the LOD with a 95% confidence level (*see* Refs [15, 16]).

2. No-template controls (NTC) are used to measure the background of your protocol. This can be achieved by isolating and measuring an aliquot of nuclease-free water like the biological CSF samples. We recommend to consider a $dCq = Cq_{\text{NTC}} - Cq_{\text{miRNA}} < 5$ as background.

3. Check the expression levels of the spike-ins to evaluate the efficiency of the RNA isolation and cDNA synthesis reaction. UniSp2 is present at a concentration 100-fold higher than UniSp4, and UniSp4 is present at a concentration 100-fold higher than UniSp5. Therefore UniSp2 should amplify at the level of very abundant miRNAs, UniSp4 should amplify ~6.6 cycles later than UniSp2, and UniSp5 ~6.6 cycles later than UniSp4. Cel-miR-39-3p also amplifies ~6.6 cycles later than UniSp6. Exclude samples from further analysis, if expression is inconsistent or the variation too large.

4. We recommend to analyze the expression data with GeNorm (*see* Ref. [17]) and NormFinder (*see* Ref. [18]). These approaches are based on comparing variances and are able to identify reference miRNAs expressed at consistent levels. NormFinder also allows to include several experimental groups and considers the variance in between. We recommend to use at least three stable reference miRNAs for normalization. The data are then normalized by using the average of the identified reference miRNAs. The global mean method can be used as an alternative or when analyzing >100 miRNAs per sample. Here, the average of all expressed miRNAs per sample is used (*see* Ref. [13]).

4   Notes

1. Quality control based on OD measurements such as NanoDrop or Bioanalyzer is not suitable for miRNA detection in CSF since RNA content is very low and other classes of small RNA molecules and degradation products may be co-purified. The primary purpose of the RNA spike-in kit is to provide a control for the quality of the RNA isolation, cDNA synthesis, and PCR amplification based on synthetic miRNA standards.

2. This kit is usually designed for purification of cell-free total RNA—primarily miRNA and other small RNA—from small volumes of serum and plasma. However, we adapted the protocol to isolate total RNA from CSF. The kit works also for other body fluids (*see* Ref. [1]) and scored significantly better compared to other kits in this area (*see* Ref. [19]).

3. Buffer RWT is supplied as a concentrate. Before using for the first time, add 30 mL ethanol (96–100%) as indicated on the bottle to obtain a working solution.

4. Buffer RPE is supplied as a concentrate. Before using for the first time, add 24 mL ethanol (96–100%) as indicated on the bottle to obtain a working solution.

5. Not used in this protocol.

6. Do not use denatured alcohol, which contains other substances such as methanol and methyl ethyl ketone.

7. miRNeasy Serum/Plasma Kit applies organic extraction combined with phase separation using phenol and chloroform. Using CSF, there is no visible interphase compared to serum and pipetting the upper aqueous phase (containing RNA) can be challenging. PLG tubes act as a barrier between the organic and aqueous phases, allowing the RNA-containing phase to be easily decanted or pipetted off—saving time while optimizing the recovery of nucleic acids and minimizing the contamination of DNA that partitions to the interphase.

8. The miRCURY LNA™ Universal RT microRNA PCR system is a microRNA-specific, LNA™-based system designed for sensitive and accurate detection of microRNA by quantitative real-time PCR using SYBR® Green (*see* Ref. [5]). The method is based on universal reverse transcription (RT) followed by real-time PCR amplification with LNA™ enhanced primers. This kit also contains the UniSp6 RNA spike-in template for the preparation of the cDNA synthesis RNA spike-in mix to control for variations in the cDNA reaction.

9. We recommend the sealing foil P/N 4ti-560 for 384-well plates and P/N 4ti-0565 for 96-well plates. These fit all standard SBS footprint PCR and qPCR plates, microplates, assay, and storage plates.

10. The ExiLENT SYBR® Green master mix does not include the ROX passive reference dye. Please follow instrument manufacturer's recommendations.

11. For biomarker screening in CSF, we recommend human miR-Nome or focus panels for a preliminary pilot profiling and customized panels for downstream validation studies including more technical replicates on the RNA, cDNA, and PCR level.

12. The RNA oligonucleotides should match the sequences of the mature miRNAs of your interest.

13. We recommend isolating no more than four to six CSF samples simultaneously to avoid long waiting periods due to pipetting.

14. CSF samples should already be centrifuged after lumbar puncture at this stage. This is just an additional control centrifugation step to ensure the removal of cellular debris and red blood cells.

15. The idea behind MS2 RNA is that other (total) RNA is able to bind to carrier RNA potentially increasing RNA yield. However, opinions tend to differ at this step while some report increased and others unchanged RNA recovery (*see* Ref. [20]). Own data show slightly increased RNA recovery with MS2 RNA as compared without.

16. The RNA isolation spike-in RNA template must be mixed with the lysis buffer before mixing with the sample—if added directly to the sample it may be rapidly degraded.

17. The kit is intended to process a maximum of 200 μL input volume. However, one can upscale the CSF volume by simply adjusting the volumes of QIAzol lysis reagent, chloroform, and ethanol likewise (*see* Ref. [20]). An additional sterile tube >2 mL is needed to compensate the increased volume of the CSF-QIAzol-chloroform-ethanol mix as a result. However, higher sample volumes may result in co-purification of inhibi-

tors for downstream qPCR, which should be considered by using increased reaction volumes for cDNA synthesis (e.g., 40 μL instead of 20 μL). We recommend testing this in a separate experiment.

18. After centrifugation, the sample separates into three phases: an upper, colorless, aqueous phase containing RNA, which is separated by the phase-lock gel from a white interphase (hardly visible) and a lower, red, organic phase. The aqueous phase yields approximately 780–800 μL.

19. This amount of ethanol equals 1.5 volumes of the aqueous phase (*see* **Note 18**). If your aqueous phase may contain less/more volume, simply adjust the amount of ethanol by multiplying the aqueous phase times 1.5 volumes.

20. Make sure not to touch the phase-lock gel when pipetting the 780 μL aqueous phase.

21. Make sure that the bottom of the spin column does not contact the flow-through and if necessary clean the outer surface of the spin column with a clean towel to avoid contamination and carryover.

22. The dead volume of the RNeasy MinElute spin column is 2 μL: elution with 14 μL RNase-free water results in a 12 μL eluate. The amount of elution volume may be variable and eluting with only 10 μL is possible. However, yield will be reduced by approximately 20%. The more elution volume the less concentrated your total RNA and vice versa. Depending on the input CSF volume, eluting in higher volumes may further dilute co-purified inhibitors, which may increase the performance of your downstream RT-qPCR. Also consider how many total RNA you may need for other applications, technical replicates, and reference samples. We usually use 22 μL RNase-free water to elute ~20 μL total RNA.

23. CSF contains low amounts of total RNA and potential PCR inhibitors. Using 8 μL RNA input in a total cDNA reaction volume of 20 μL results in an acceptable combination of lower Cq values, saving reagents and sufficient cDNA volume to use different plate layouts and/or replicate measurements.

24. For absolute standard curve method, use Standards 1–8 (*see* Subheading 3.8), respectively.

25. The protocol can be interrupted at this stage. The undiluted cDNA may be kept at −20 °C for up to 5 weeks (optional store at 4 °C for up to 4 days). It is recommended that synthesized cDNA is stored in "low-nucleic acid-binding" tubes or plates.

26. For each CSF sample and its synthesized cDNA, a separate PCR master mix has to be prepared. When analyzing for example 4 CSF samples on a 384-well plate without any technical replicates on the RNA, cDNA, or PCR level, 96 miRNAs can be analyzed per sample, which would result in the preparation of 4 separate PCR master mixes. Fully customized layouts may include technical replicates. The dilutions for these layouts may be adjusted to the specific replicate scheme. Remember that the cDNA of each sample always has to be diluted with nuclease water 1:50 first and then diluted 1:1 with 2× PCR master mix.

27. Primers are pre-spotted at the bottom of each ready-to-use plate ordered from Exiqon. This allows to use the same pipette tip for each PCR master mix and its corresponding wells. Carryover of lyophilized primers can be avoided by holding the pipette tip in a 45° angle while slightly touching the inner surface at the top of the well. This greatly facilitates pipetting and consumes less time and material. We recommend an electronic dispenser able to dispense liquid in equal partial volumes down to 10 μL (*see* Subheading 2.4, **item 6**).

28. The experiment can be paused at this point. Store the reactions protected from light at 4 °C for up to 24 h.

29. If required, the number of miRNAs and technical replicates can be adjusted individually.

References

1. Weber JA, Baxter DH, Zhang S et al (2010) The microRNA spectrum in 12 body fluids. Clin Chem 56(11):1733–1741. https://doi.org/10.1373/clinchem.2010.147405

2. Mitchell PS, Parkin RK, Kroh EM et al (2008) Circulating microRNAs as stable blood-based markers for cancer detection. Proc Natl Acad Sci U S A 105(30):10513–10518. https://doi.org/10.1073/pnas.0804549105

3. Balusu S, Van Wonterghem E, De Rycke R et al (2016) Identification of a novel mechanism of blood-brain communication during peripheral inflammation via choroid plexus-derived extracellular vesicles. EMBO Mol Med 8(10):1162–1183. https://doi.org/10.15252/emmm.201606271

4. Pritchard CC, Cheng HH, Tewari M (2012) MicroRNA profiling: approaches and considerations. Nat Rev Genet 13(5):358–369. https://doi.org/10.1038/nrg3198

5. Mestdagh P, Hartmann N, Baeriswyl L et al (2014) Evaluation of quantitative miRNA expression platforms in the microRNA quality control (miRQC) study. Nat Methods 11(8):809–815. https://doi.org/10.1038/nmeth.3014

6. Witwer KW, Halushka MK (2016) Toward the promise of microRNAs—enhancing reproducibility and rigor in microRNA research. RNA Biol 13(11):1103–1116. https://doi.org/10.1080/15476286.2016.1236172

7. Bustin SA, Benes V, Garson JA et al (2009) The MIQE guidelines: minimum information for publication of quantitative real-time PCR experiments. Clin Chem 55(4):611–622. https://doi.org/10.1373/clinchem.2008.112797

8. Bustin SA (2010) Why the need for qPCR publication guidelines? The case for MIQE. Methods 50(4):217–226. https://doi.org/10.1016/j.ymeth.2009.12.006

9. Bustin SA, Beaulieu JF, Huggett J et al (2010) MIQE précis: practical implementation of minimum standard guidelines for fluorescence-

based quantitative real-time PCR experiments. BMC Mol Biol 11:74. https://doi.org/10.1186/1471-2199-11-74

10. Kirschner MB, van Zandwijk N, Reid G (2013) Cell-free microRNAs: potential biomarkers in need of standardized reporting. Front Genet 4:56. https://doi.org/10.3389/fgene.2013.00056

11. Kirschner MB, Edelman JJB, Kao SCH et al (2013) The impact of hemolysis on cell-free microRNA biomarkers. Front Genet 4:94. https://doi.org/10.3389/fgene.2013.00094, Article No.: 94

12. Mestdagh P, Van Vlierberghe P, De Weer A et al (2009) A novel and universal method for microRNA RT-qPCR data normalization. Genome Biol 10(6):R64. https://doi.org/10.1186/gb-2009-10-6-r64

13. D'Haene B, Mestdagh P, Hellemans J et al (2012) miRNA expression profiling: from reference genes to global mean normalization. Methods Mol Biol 822:261–272. https://doi.org/10.1007/978-1-61779-427-8_18

14. Schwarzenbach H, da Silva AM, Calin G et al (2015) Data normalization strategies for MicroRNA quantification. Clin Chem 61(11):1333–1342. https://doi.org/10.1373/clinchem.2015.239459

15. Broeders S, Huber I, Grohmann L et al (2014) Guidelines for validation of qualitative real-time PCR methods. Trends Food Sci Tech 37(2):115–126. https://doi.org/10.1016/j.tifs.2014.03.008

16. Kralik P, Ricchi M (2017) A basic guide to real time PCR in microbial diagnostics: definitions, parameters, and everything. Front Microbiol 8:108. https://doi.org/10.3389/fmicb.2017.00108

17. Vandesompele J, De Preter K, Pattyn F et al (2002) Accurate normalization of real-time quantitative RT-PCR data by geometric averaging of multiple internal control genes. Genome Biol 3(7):Research0034

18. Andersen CL, Jensen JL, Orntoft TF (2004) Normalization of real-time quantitative reverse transcription-PCR data: a model-based variance estimation approach to identify genes suited for normalization, applied to bladder and colon cancer data sets. Cancer Res 64(15):5245–5250. https://doi.org/10.1158/0008-5472.CAN-04-0496

19. El-Khoury V, Pierson S, Kaoma T et al (2016) Assessing cellular and circulating miRNA recovery: the impact of the RNA isolation method and the quantity of input material. Sci Rep 6:19529. https://doi.org/10.1038/srep19529

20. McAlexander MA, Phillips MJ, Witwer KW (2013) Comparison of methods for miRNA extraction from plasma and quantitative recovery of RNA from cerebrospinal fluid. Front Genet 4:83. https://doi.org/10.3389/fgene.2013.00083

Part III

Novel Blood-Based Biomarkers

Validation of a Chemiluminescence Immunoassay for Measuring Amyloid-β in Human Blood Plasma

Jonathan Vogelgsang, Jens Wiltfang, and Hans W. Klafki

Abstract

The technical performance of immunological assays and their suitability for the intended use should be carefully validated before implementation in research, clinical studies or routine. We describe here the evaluation of a sandwich electrochemiluminescence immunoassay for measuring total Amyloid-β levels in human blood plasma as an example of a laboratory protocol for a partial "fit for purpose" assay performance validation. We tested two different assay protocols and addressed impact of sample dilution, parallelism, intra- and inter-assay variance, lower limit of quantification, lower limit of detection, and analytical spike recoveries.

Key words Amyloid-β peptide, Immunoassay, Alzheimer's disease, Biomarker, Assay validation

1 Introduction

A low concentration of amyloid-β 42 peptide ($A\beta_{42}$) in cerebrospinal fluid (CSF) is a biomarker of Alzheimer's disease (AD) neuropathology, which has been confirmed in numerous studies [1]. The measurement of CSF $A\beta_{42}$ and of the $A\beta_{42}/A\beta_{40}$ concentration ratio, which can outperform $A\beta_{42}$ as a diagnostic AD biomarker [2–5], is usually done with immunological assays, such as enzyme linked immunosorbent assay (ELISAs) or related assay formats. Currently, there is no compelling evidence that Aβ-peptides in blood plasma can qualify as useful diagnostic biomarkers, as well [1]. Nevertheless, there is need for reliable and reproducible assays for the measurement of Aβ peptides in blood. For example, plasma $A\beta_{40}$ has been proposed to represent a "moderate risk marker" of AD [6], and total Aβ plasma levels were reported to be associated with cognitive decline in chronic kidney disease [7]. Furthermore, reliable measurements of total Aβ and/or specific variants of Aβ peptides in blood plasma may serve as theragnostic biomarkers for monitoring drug effects in the context of clinical trials of novel therapeutics targeting Aβ [8, 9]. Before implementation in

Robert Perneczky (ed.), *Biomarkers for Alzheimer's Disease Drug Development*, Methods in Molecular Biology, vol. 1750, https://doi.org/10.1007/978-1-4939-7704-8_7, © Springer Science+Business Media, LLC 2018

research, clinical studies, or clinical routine, immunological and other assays should be carefully validated.

In 2015, Andreasson et al. published "a practical guide to immunoassay method validation" [10]. For a full assay validation, the authors recommended to evaluate the following ten different parameters: robustness, precision, trueness, uncertainty, limits of quantification, dilutional linearity, parallelism, recovery, selectivity, and sample stability. Partial assay validation campaigns addressing only a subset of the recommended quality parameters may be eligible, depending on the specific assay and the particular purpose it is intended to be used for.

We present here a laboratory protocol for a partial "fit-for-purpose" validation campaign, which we have applied to evaluate the suitability of a commercially available custom immunoassay with chemiluminescence readout for measuring total Aβ in human EDTA blood plasma. The selected performance parameters that were addressed included the impact of sample dilution, parallelism, intra- and inter-assay variance, lower limit of quantification, lower limit of detection, and analytical spike recoveries. The sandwich immunoassay was initially performed essentially according to the manufacturer's recommendations (protocol A). In view of poor analytical spike recoveries we observed under these conditions, we elaborated a modified assay procedure (protocol B), which was subjected to a slightly more thorough assay performance evaluation.

2   Materials

2.1   For Sample Collection, Preparation, and Storage

1. Material for blood sampling: tourniquet, needle, disinfectant, swab.
2. EDTA monovettes (e.g., 9 mL) (Sarstedt, Nuembrecht, Germany).
3. Centrifuge.
4. Tubes for plasma storage (e.g., matrix tubes 0.5 mL, Thermo Fischer Scientific, Waltham, MA, USA).
5. Boxes for storage at −80 ° C (e.g., matrix boxes, Thermo Fischer Scientific, Waltham, MA, USA).

2.2   For Immunoassay

1. MSD human (6E10) Aβ40 ultra-sensitive immunoassay kit (Mesoscale Discovery, Rockville, MA, USA), which includes assay plates coated with monoclonal anti-Aβ antibody mAb6E10 for capture.
2. Sulfo-tag-labeled human mAb4G8 anti-Aβ-antibody (Mesoscale, Rockville, MA, USA) to replace the Aβ40-specific detection antibody supplied with the original Aβ40 assay kit.
3. Aβ40 blocker (Mesoscale Discovery, Rockville, MA, USA).

4. MESO QuickPlex SQ 120 reader (Mesoscale, Rockville, MA, USA) or another suitable MSD instrument.

5. Discovery Workbench 4.0 software for acquiring and analyzing data using the Quickplex SQ 120 instrument (Mesoscale, Rockville, MA, USA).

6. Centrifuge.

7. Vortex.

2.3 For Data Analysis

1. Discovery Workbench 4.0 (Mesoscale Discovery).

2. Microsoft Excel.

3 Methods

3.1 Blood Sampling, Preparation, and Storage

This study was performed with blood samples from the biobank of the Department of Psychiatry and Psychotherapy of the University Medical Centre Goettingen (ethical vote 2/5/09 and 9/2/16). All samples were collected and processed according to the Declaration of Helsinki in the current version.

1. Collect human blood samples in EDTA monovettes in an appropriate way (*see* **Note 1**). Mix the ETDA anticoagulant with the blood samples immediately by gently inverting the monovettes eight to ten times.

2. Centrifuge the monovettes at $2000 \times g$ for 10 min in a swing-out rotor at room temperature to separate plasma from cellular blood components (*see* **Note 2**).

3. Aliquot the EDTA-plasma (supernatant) in storage tubes (*see* **Note 3**).

4. Place the sample tubes in appropriate storage boxes and store the biomaterial at $-80\ ^\circ C$ until use.

3.2 Total Aβ Immunoassay Protocol (Protocol A)

All procedures should be carried out at room temperature.

1. Block each well of the MSD assay plate with 150 μL blocking buffer (delivered within the kit).

2. Cover the plate with an adhesive seal and incubate for 60 min while gently shaking.

3. Wash the plate three times with 150 μL Tris washing solution (delivered within the kit) (*see* **Note 4**).

4. Add 25 μL of Aβ1-40 standard or sample to each well, cover the plate with a seal, and incubate for 60 min while gently shaking (*see* **Notes 5** and **6**).

5. Wash the plate three times with 150 μL Tris washing solution.

6. Add 25 μL of 4G8 detection antibody solution per well (sulfo-tag-labeled anti-Aβ antibody 4G8 diluted 1:50 in dilution buffer), cover the plate with a seal, and incubate for 60 min while gently shaking.

7. Wash the plate three times with 150 μL Tris washing solution.

8. Add 150 μL reading buffer (delivered within the kit) (*see* **Note 7**) and measure immediately.

9. Read the plate using the MESO QuickPlex SQ 120 reader or another suitable MSD instrument.

3.3 Modified Assay Protocol (Protocol B)

All procedures should be carried out at room temperature.

1. Block each well of the MSD assay plate with 150 μL blocking buffer (delivered within the kit), cover the plate with a seal, and incubate for 60 min while gently shaking.

2. Wash the plate three times with 150 μL Tris washing solution (delivered within the kit) (*see* **Note 4**).

3. Add 25 μL of a modified mAb4G8 detection antibody solution (sulfo-tag-labeled anti-Aβ antibody mAb4G8 diluted 1:50 in dilution buffer containing 1% (v/v) of Aβ40 blocker) in each well.

4. Add 25 μL of Aβ standard or sample to each well, cover the plate with a seal, and incubate for 120 min while gently shaking (*see* **Note 6**).

5. Wash the plate three times with 150 μL Tris washing solution.

6. Add 150 μL reading buffer (delivered within the kit) (*see* **Note 7**) and measure immediately.

7. Read the plate using the MESO QuickPlex SQ 120 reader or another suitable MSD instrument.

3.4 Partial Assay Validation

Here we present different steps which we have performed for a partial assay validation. For that purpose, the samples are diluted, spiked, or distributed on an assay plate in a specific way and analyzed with the same assay protocol. At least three different assay plates are required to investigate all of the proposed validation parameters. Each experiment should be carried out with EDTA-plasma samples from at least three different donors.

3.4.1 Impact of Sample Dilution/Determination of a Suitable Dilution Factor for Further Analyses

1. Prepare serial dilutions in sample diluent of each sample (*see* **Note 8**).

2. Analyze each dilution in duplicates, at least.

3. Include at least four zero calibrators (blanks) per assay plate to calculate the lower limit of detection (LLOD) and lower limit of quantification (LLOQ).

4. Calculate LLOD and LLOQ (*see analysis of assay parameters*) and continue with a suitable sample dilution to minimize interference effects and, at the same time, generating signals above the LLOQ (*see* **Note 9**).

3.4.2 Spike Recoveries

1. Prepare four different tubes for each sample ("neat" and three different spike levels).

2. Calculate three different spike levels, low, medium, and high (*see* **Note 10**).

3. Pipette a defined volume of plasma into each tube, add the calculated volume of spike (Aβ calibrator), and finally fill up with the needed amount of dilution buffer (*see* **Note 10**).

4. Calculate the analytical spike recoveries (*see analysis of assay parameters*).

3.4.3 Intra-Assay Variance

1. Prepare sufficient volumes of the samples at the required dilution for multiple replicates. Andreasson and colleagues recommended to measure at least five technical replicates [10] (*see* **Note 11**). Dispense the samples on different wells spread all over the plate. Note that the different samples are equally distributed on the brink and corners.

2. Calculate the intra-assay variance (*see analysis of assay parameters*).

3.4.4 Inter-Assay Variance

1. At least two to three samples should be measured on all different plates as quality controls (QC samples).

2. Inter-assay variance can be calculated on the basis of the mean Aβ concentrations of the QC samples determined for each of the different assay plates (*see analysis of assay parameters*).

3.5 Analysis of Assay Parameters

3.5.1 Calculation of LLOD and LLOQ (LLOD and LLOQ Are Calculated for each Assay Plate)

1. Calculate the standard curve for each assay plate with the Discovery Workbench 4.0 software using the weighted four-parameter logistic fit (default setting).

2. Calculate the LLOD for each assay plate (again using the Discovery Workbench 4.0 software) as the lowest concentration generating a signal 3 × standard deviation above mean blank (or lowest standard) [11].

3. Calculate the LLOQ for each assay plate (again using the Discovery Workbench 4.0 software) as the lowest concentration generating a signal 10 × standard deviation above mean blank (or lowest standard) [12].

4. Average the LLODs and LLOQs of all assay plates investigated to obtain mean LLOD and mean LLOQ, respectively.

3.5.2 Impact of Sample Dilution (from Experiment 1 "Sample Dilution")

1. Back-calculate the total Aβ concentration in undiluted plasma ("back-calculated concentration"/"dilution corrected concentration") for each dilution and each sample by multiplying the measured concentration in the diluted sample with the corresponding dilution factor.

2. Plot the back-calculated concentrations against the respective dilution factors on a scatter diagram (*x*-axis: dilution factor; *y*-axis: back-calculated concentration). Visually evaluate the impact of sample dilution on back-calculated total Aβ concentrations to detect interference effects and estimate the minimum required dilution (MRD) at which the dilution-corrected concentrations remain essentially stable (*see* Fig. 1).

3.5.3 Parallelism (from Experiment 1 "Sample Dilution")

1. Parallelism is investigated to compare the immunological detection of endogenous human Aβ with that of the synthetic Aβ calibrator peptide.

2. Linearize the relations between measured signals and the respective dilution factors using a Logit-log model [13]: For each tested dilution generating a signal above LLOQ, calculate the Logit of the signal as

$$\text{Logit}(\text{signal}) = \log\left(\frac{\text{signal} - \min \text{signal}}{\max \text{signal} - \text{signal})}\right)$$

Min and max signals in this formula [13] correspond to the calculated lower and upper asymptotes (top and bottom) of the calibration curve.

3. Calculate the reciprocal relative dilution:

$$\text{relative dilution} = \frac{\text{actual sample dilution}}{\text{maximum dilutions in series}} \times 100$$

$$\text{reciprocal relative dilution} = \frac{1}{\text{relative dilution}}$$

4. Log transform the reciprocal relative dilution (log 10).

5. Plot the Logit of the measured signals against the logs of the corresponding reciprocal relative dilution for each sample and the calibrator.

6. Calculate the slopes for each sample dilution series and the calibrator dilutions by linear regression.

7. Calculate "% in range" as follows:

$$\%\text{in range} = \frac{\text{slope of sample dilution series}}{\text{slope of calibrator dilution series}} \times 10 \ [14]$$

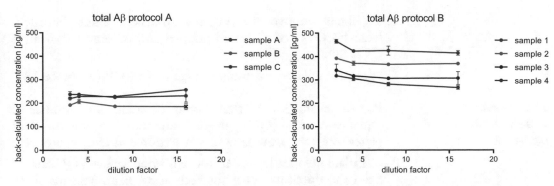

Fig. 1 Impact of sample dilution on back-calculated total Aβ levels. For the assessment of assay protocol A (left-hand side), three different EDTA-plasma samples were analyzed in duplicate reads after 3-, 4-, 8-, and 16-fold dilution. The indicated values represent mean ± SD of two technical replicates for each dilution. The signal obtained with 16-fold diluted sample "B" was below LLOQ (indicated by X). To evaluate the modified protocol B (right-hand side), four different EDTA-plasma samples were measured in duplicates after 2-, 4-, 8-, and 16-fold dilution. All measurements were above LLOQ. Note that different plasma samples were used with protocols A and B

8. Average the "% in range" values of all tested samples and express as mean ± SD.

9. We predefined an acceptance range of ±15% (between 85 and 115% in range) (*see* **Note 12**).

3.5.4 Spike Recoveries (from Experiment 2 "Spike Recoveries")

1. Calculate the "% recovery" for each spike level (low, medium, and high with the following formula, in which c = concentration) [10]:

$$\% \text{ recovery} = \frac{(c \text{ spiked sample} - c \text{ neat sample})}{\text{theoretical } c \text{ spike}} \times 100$$

2. Average the recoveries at the three different spiking levels for each sample to obtain mean "% recovery."

3. Average the mean "% recovery" of all tested samples and present as overall "% recovery ± SD."

4. We predefined an acceptance range of ±15% (between 85 and 115% recovery) (*see* **Note 12**).

3.5.5 Intra-Assay Variance (from Experiment 3 "Intra-Assay Variance")

1. To calculate the intra-assay variance, all samples are measured in multiple technical replicates on the same assay plate.

2. Calculate the mean concentration and standard deviation for each sample.

3. Calculate "% CV" for each sample as follows:

$$\% \text{ CV} = \frac{\text{standard deviation}}{\text{mean}} \times 100$$

4. To obtain the overall intra-assay variance, average the calculated "% CVs" of all tested samples and present as "mean % CV ± SD."

5. We predefined an acceptance range of 15% CV (*see* **Note 12**).

3.5.6 Inter-Assay Variance (from All Experiments)

1. For the evaluation of the inter-assay variance, a number of "quality control (QC) samples" are measured on different plates using the same sample preparation and assay protocol.

2. Calculate the mean total Aβ concentration for each QC sample from the duplicate reads for each assay plate. The mean Aβ concentrations from each assay plate are used to calculate overall mean concentrations, SDs, and % CV for each plasma QC sample under investigation. Finally, the mean inter-assay coefficient of variation is calculated by averaging the % CVs of the QC samples tested.

3. To obtain the mean inter-assay variance, average the calculated % CV of all tested QC samples and present as "mean % CV ± SD."

4. We predefined an acceptance range of 15% CV (*see* **Note 12**).

3.5.7 Impact of Sample Preparation and Assay Variations:

1. If the asvsay validation parameters are not satisfying or do not meet the predefined acceptance range, the pre-analytical sample preparation or the assay protocol can be modified. Note that for all changes, a new assay validation needs to be performed, respectively.

4 Results

4.1 Lower Limits of Detection (LLODs) and Lower Limits of Quantification (LLOQs)

LLODs and LLOQs were calculated for each assay plate with the Discovery Workbench 4.0 Software with the option "use minimum error estimates" activated. In line with the recommendations of the International Union of Pure and Applied Chemistry (IUPAC), LLOD and LLOQ were defined as the lowest concentrations producing a signal 3 and 10 standard deviations, respectively, above the mean zero calibrator (blank) signal [15]. Mean LLODs and LLOQs for the two different assay protocols were obtained by averaging the plate LLODs and LLOQs of the respective experiments. For the assay protocol A, we obtained a mean LLOD of 9.79 pg/mL ± 1.92 (mean ± SD; $n = 7$ plates) and a mean LLOQ of 13.34 pg/mL ± 5.53. With the modified assay protocol (protocol B), the mean LLOD was 9.67 pg/mL ± 0.98 (mean ± SD, $n = 3$ plates) and the mean LLOQ 13.06 pg/mL ± 2.85.

4.2 Impact of Sample Dilution, Parallelism, and Choice of a Suitable Dilution Factor

With protocol A, signals above LLOQ were obtained with three-, four-, and eightfold diluted plasma with all three tested plasma samples. Using assay protocol B, we obtained signals above LLOQ for all tested samples (n = 4) with dilutions up to 16-fold. The impact of sample dilution on the back-calculated total Aβ plasma concentrations is shown in Fig. 1. It appears that with the modified assay procedure (protocol B) the dilution-corrected total Aβ plasma concentrations (back-calculated concentrations) were essentially stable between 8- and 16-fold dilution. Parallelism was assessed with a Logit-log model [13]. The calculated slope of the sample dilution series was 100.0 ± 6.9% in range with the slope of the standard curve with assay protocol A and 107.0 ± 4.3% with assay protocol B. In both cases, the predefined acceptance criterion of 85–115% in range was met.

4.3 Spike Recoveries

Analytical spike recoveries were studied at three different spike levels in four (protocol A) or five plasma samples (protocol B). The final sample dilutions in the assay were 8-fold with assay protocol A and 16-fold with protocol B. In both cases, the chosen dilutions represented the highest dilutions expected to produce signals above LLOQ (*see* above). The mean overall spike recoveries were 51.9% ± 3.8 (mean ± SD) for protocol A and 113.2% ± 5.2 (mean ± SD) for protocol B.

A summary of the results of our partial assay validation with the two different protocols is shown in Table 1.

Table 1
Summary of the assay performance with protocols A and B[a]

	Assay protocol A	Assay protocol B
Sample dilution	8-fold	16-fold
Parallelism (% in range)	100.0 ± 6.9	107 ± 4.3
Mean spike recovery (%)	51.9 ± 3.8[b]	113.2 ± 5.2
LLOD (pg/mL)	9.79 ± 1.92	9.67 ± 0.98
LLOQ (pg/mL)	13.34 ± 5.53	13.06 ± 2.85
Intra-assay variance (% CV)	2.83 ± 0.72	11.63 ± 3.87
Inter-assay variance (% CV)	13.62 ± 0.45	13.9 ± 4.64

[a]Data are presented as mean ± SD if not indicated otherwise
[b]Analytical spike recoveries obtained with assay protocol A did not meet the predefined acceptance range of 85–115%

4.4 Repeatability   Intra-assay variance was assessed by measuring four EDTA-plasma samples after 8-fold dilution in 3 technical replicates (protocol A) or 16-fold dilution (protocol B) in 13 technical replicates on one assay plate for each one of the two assay protocols. In both cases, the predefined acceptance criteria (<15% CV) were met: With protocol A, we observed a mean intra-assay coefficient of variation (% CV) of 2.83 ± 0.72 (mean ± SD, $n = 4$ samples, 3 replicates) and with protocol B 11.63 ± 3.87 (mean ± SD, $n = 4$ samples, 13 replicates). For studying the inter-assay repeatability with protocol A, two different QC plasma samples were measured after eightfold dilution on four different assay plates within 8 weeks. For the assessment of protocol B, two different QC samples were measured after 16-fold dilution on three different assay plates within 7 weeks. Overall mean total Aβ concentrations, standard deviations, and % CVs for each tested sample were calculated from the means of the duplicate reads on each plate. The mean inter-assay coefficient of variation was calculated by averaging the % CVs of all plasma samples that were investigated. The resulting inter-assay % CVs were 13.62 ± 0.45 (mean ± SD) for protocol A and 13.90 ± 4.64 for protocol B.

5 Discussion

Two different assay protocols for measuring total Aβ in human EDTA plasma with a commercial custom chemiluminescence immunoassay were evaluated in partial assay validation campaigns. Protocol A, which was essentially identical to the manufacturer's recommendations, passed predefined acceptance criteria regarding parallelism as well as intra- and inter-assay variance. LLOD and LLOQ were 9.79 pg/mL ± 1.92 (mean ± SD) and 13.34 pg/mL ± 5.53, respectively. Analytical spike recoveries in eightfold diluted EDTA-plasma were poor and out of the predefined acceptance range. As a consequence, we elaborated an optimized assay procedure. The modified assay protocol B, in which we reduced the number of steps and included an additional "Aβ$_{40}$ blocker," allowed for obtaining signals above LLOQ with 16-fold diluted blood plasma. Under these conditions, predefined acceptance criteria regarding parallelism, spike recoveries, and intra- and inter-assay variance were fulfilled. One limitation of this study is that the two different assay protocols were evaluated, not in parallel but consecutively and with a lag of several months in between. For the validation of the original assay protocol A and the optimized protocol B, different plasma samples, different sample numbers, and replicate numbers were used. Thus, direct comparisons of at least some of the assay results are difficult. Additional experiments will be required to define the most appropriate plasma dilution factor for research routine, representing a compromise between assay sensitivity and minimizing interference ("matrix") effects by dilution. Depending on the specific questions to be addressed in future studies, additional performance parameters, e.g., pre-analytical sample handling, sample stability, and between-lot and between-laboratory variance, should be investigated. A comprehensive instruction to full and partial immunoassay validation has been published, recently by Andreasson and colleagues [10].

6 Notes

1. For the analysis of Aβ in blood, we normally use EDTA blood plasma. Avoid hemolysis and make sure that the EDTA is mixed well with the blood sample by gently inverting the monovette eight to ten times immediately.

2. The collection of blood and preparation of plasma or other blood fractions should be performed according to highly standardized protocols to decrease pre-analytic variability [16]. Several different standard operating procedures (SOPs) for that purpose have been published (see, e.g., [17, 18]) which complicates direct comparisons between different studies [16].

3. It is very useful to generate at least five to six aliquots of blood plasma to make sure to have enough material available for repeated measurements. Repeated freezing and thawing should be avoided. Human plasma samples can be stored for several months or years at −80 °C or below.

4. The assay plate can be washed using a plate washer or by hand. In the latter case, dump the liquid with a quick motion into a suitable waste container and immediately tap the plate several times upside down on a stack of blotting paper or paper towels to remove all of the residual liquid.

5. Samples should be pre-diluted or processed in an appropriate way. The determination of an appropriate dilution factor for measuring the specific biological sample under investigation is, among other things, part of the partial assay validation and is discussed later.

6. All samples and standards should be measured in duplicates. Bubble formation can be avoided by reverse pipetting [19].

7. Since bubbles might influence the signal measurement, the reading buffer should always be pipetted by reverse pipetting.

8. For studying the impact of pre-analytical sample dilution using assay protocol A, we tested three different EDTA blood plasma samples after 3-, 4-, 8-, and 16-fold dilution with sample diluent. For assessing the modified assay protocol B, we measured four different plasma samples after 2-, 4-, 8-, and 16-fold dilu-

tion. In general, the dilution factors to be tested should be chosen according to available information regarding expected analyte concentration in the biomaterial under investigation, assay sensitivity, etc. Some EDTA-plasma samples form a smear after dilution with dilution buffer. Therefore we recommend all samples to be initially diluted with the same volume of dilution buffer (1:2 dilution) and centrifuged at $10,000 \times g$ for 10 min at room temperature. Transfer the supernatant carefully into another tube and continue the dilution series with the 1:2 pre-dilution. We recommend performing this pre-dilution step for all experiments.

9. It is well known that blood plasma and other biological fluids may contain components, so-called interference or matrix effects, which can interfere with the immunological detection of Aβ peptides or other analytes [20]. Matrix effects can be detected, for example, by measuring a series of dilutions of the sample and plotting back-calculated concentrations against the dilution factors. Sample dilution is a simple way to minimize matrix effects by reducing the amount of interfering compounds in the measured sample.

10. The spike levels should be adapted to the expected Aβ concentration in the sample under investigation. In the example presented here, the low spike level was chosen close to the expected total Aβ concentration at the tested dilution. The medium spike concentration was twice the lowest spike level. The high spike level was equivalent to $3 \times$ the medium spike level. For the assessment of the analytical spike recoveries with the optimized assay protocol, we measured plasma samples at a final dilution of 1:16 (see also **Note 8**). All samples were prepared in a final volume of 500 μL. A pipetting scheme is shown in Table 2.

11. To assess intra-assay variance of assay protocol A, we measured four different plasma samples after eightfold dilution in three replicates, each. For evaluating protocol B, we measured 13 replicates of four different samples after 16-fold dilution.

Table 2
Pipetting scheme for the assessment of analytical spike recoveries (assay protocol B)

Spike level	μL of 1:2 prediluted plasma	μL of Aβ standard (1940 pg/mL)	μL of sample dilution buffer	Final concentration of spike (pg/mL)
Neat plasma	62.5	–	437.5	0
Low	62.5	2.6	434.9	10.1
Medium	62.5	5.2	432.2	20.2
High	62.5	15.5	422	60.1

12. It appears that there is no general consensus regarding acceptance ranges of specific assay performance parameters (*see*, e.g., [10]). The acceptance ranges that were applied in this study represent the authors' personal views. Other acceptance criteria may be eligible, depending on the assay under investigation and the intended use.

Acknowledgments

This work was supported by the BioPharma-Neuroallianz (grant 16GW0096). Prof. Jens Wiltfang is supported by an Ilídio Pinho professorship and iBiMED (UID/BIM/04501/2013), at the University of Aveiro. We thank Anke Jahn-Brodmann for technical assistance and Ulrike Heinze for the collection and preparation of EDTA-plasma samples.

References

1. Olsson B, Lautner R, Andreasson U, Öhrfelt A, Portelius E, Bjerke M, Hölttä M, Rosén C, Olsson C, Strobel G, Wu E, Dakin K, Petzold M, Blennow K, Zetterberg H (2016) CSF and blood biomarkers for the diagnosis of Alzheimer's disease: a systematic review and meta-analysis. Lancet Neurol 15:673–684. https://doi.org/10.1016/S1474-4422(16)00070-3

2. Wiltfang J, Esselmann H, Bibl M et al (2007) Amyloid beta peptide ratio 42/40 but not A beta 42 correlates with phospho-Tau in patients with low- and high-CSF A beta 40 load. J Neurochem 101(4):1053–1059. https://doi.org/10.1111/j.1471-4159.2006.04404.x

3. Janelidze S, Zetterberg H, Mattsson N et al (2016) CSF Abeta42/Abeta40 and Abeta42/Abeta38 ratios: better diagnostic markers of Alzheimer disease. Ann Clin Transl Neurol 3(3):154–165. https://doi.org/10.1002/acn3.274

4. Klafki HW, Hafermann H, Bauer C et al (2016) Validation of a commercial chemiluminescence immunoassay for the simultaneous measurement of three different amyloid-beta peptides in human cerebrospinal fluid and application to a clinical cohort. J Alzheimers Dis 54(2):691–705. https://doi.org/10.3233/JAD-160398

5. Lewczuk P, Matzen A, Blennow K et al (2017) Cerebrospinal fluid Abeta42/40 corresponds better than Abeta42 to amyloid PET in Alzheimer's disease. J Alzheimers Dis 55(2):813–822. https://doi.org/10.3233/JAD-160722

6. Hansson O, Stomrud E, Vanmechelen E et al (2012) Evaluation of plasma Abeta as predictor of Alzheimer's disease in older individuals without dementia: a population-based study. J Alzheimers Dis 28(1):231–238. https://doi.org/10.3233/JAD-2011-111418

7. Gronewold J, Todica O, Klafki HW et al (2016) Association of plasma beta-amyloid with cognitive performance and decline in chronic kidney disease. Mol Neurobiol. https://doi.org/10.1007/s12035-016-0243-2

8. Zetterberg H, Mattsson N, Blennow K et al (2010) Use of theragnostic markers to select drugs for phase II/III trials for Alzheimer disease. Alzheimers Res Ther 2(6):32. https://doi.org/10.1186/alzrt56

9. Song L, Lachno DR, Hanlon D et al (2016) A digital enzyme-linked immunosorbent assay for ultrasensitive measurement of amyloid-beta 1-42 peptide in human plasma with utility for studies of Alzheimer's disease therapeutics. Alzheimers Res Ther 8(1):58. https://doi.org/10.1186/s13195-016-0225-7

10. Andreasson U, Perret-Liaudet A, van Waalwijk van Doorn LJ et al (2015) A practical guide to immunoassay method validation. Front Neurol 6:179. https://doi.org/10.3389/fneur.2015.00179

11. Long GL, Winefordner JD (1983) Limit of detection. Anal Chem 55(7):A712–A724. https://doi.org/10.1021/Ac00258a001

12. Thomsen V, Schatzlein D, Mercuro D (2003) Limits of detection in spectroscopy. Spectroscopy 18(12):112–114

13. Plikaytis BD, Holder PF, Pais LB et al (1994) Determination of parallelism and nonparallelism in bioassay dilution curves. J Clin Microbiol 32(10):2441–2447

14. van Waalwijk van Doorn LJ, Koel-Simmelink MJ, Haussmann U et al (2016) Validation of soluble APP assays as diagnostic CSF biomarkers for neurodegenerative diseases. J Neurochem 137:112–121. https://doi.org/10.1111/jnc.13527

15. Whitcomb BW, Schisterman EF (2008) Assays with lower detection limits: implications for epidemiological investigations. Paediatr Perinat Epidemiol 22(6):597–602. https://doi.org/10.1111/j.1365-3016.2008.00969.x

16. Watt AD, Perez KA, Rembach AR et al (2012) Variability in blood-based amyloid-beta assays: the need for consensus on preanalytical processing. J Alzheimers Dis 30(2):323–336. https://doi.org/10.3233/JAD-2012-120058

17. Lewczuk P, Kornhuber J, Wiltfang J (2006) The German competence net dementias: standard operating procedures for the neurochemical dementia diagnostics. J Neural Transm 113(8):1075–1080. https://doi.org/10.1007/s00702-006-0511-9

18. Alzheimer's Disease Neuroimaging Initiative 2 (ADNI 2) procedures manual. https://adni.loni.usc.edu/wp-content/uploads/2008/07/adni2-procedures-manual.pdf. Accessed 6 Jan 2017

19. Thermo Fisher Scientific, Good Laboratory Pipetting Guide (2010). https://fscimage.fishersci.com/images/D16542~.pdf. Accessed 6 Jan 2017

20. Wood WG (1991) Matrix effects in immunoassays. Scand J Clin Lab Invest 51:105–112. https://doi.org/10.3109/00365519109104608

Mass Spectrometry-Based Metabolomic Multiplatform for Alzheimer's Disease Research

Raúl González-Domínguez, Álvaro González-Domínguez, Ana Sayago, and Ángeles Fernández-Recamales

Abstract

The integration of complementary analytical platforms has emerged as a suitable strategy to perform a comprehensive metabolomic characterization of complex biological systems. In this work, we describe the most important issues to be considered for the application of a mass spectrometry multiplatform in Alzheimer's disease research, which combines direct analysis with electrospray and atmospheric pressure photoionization sources, as well as orthogonal hyphenated approaches based on reversed-phase ultrahigh-performance liquid chromatography and gas chromatography. These procedures have been optimized for the analysis of multiple biological samples from human patients and transgenic animal models, including blood serum, various brain regions (e.g., hippocampus, cortex, cerebellum, striatum, olfactory bulbs), and other peripheral organs (e.g., liver, kidney, spleen, thymus). It is noteworthy that the metabolomic pipeline here detailed has demonstrated a great potential for the investigation of metabolic perturbations underlying Alzheimer's disease pathogenesis.

Key words Metabolomics, Mass spectrometry, Multiplatform, Alzheimer's disease, Direct MS analysis, Ultrahigh-performance liquid chromatography, Gas chromatography

1 Introduction

1.1 The Utility of Metabolomics in Alzheimer's Disease Research

The elucidation of pathological mechanisms underlying to Alzheimer's disease (AD) is nowadays a very active research field due to the great incidence of this disorder, accounting for up to 70% of dementia cases among the elderly population worldwide [1]. The etiology of this neurodegenerative disease has traditionally been associated with multiple impaired pathways, including abnormal metabolism of the amyloid precursor protein, tau hyperphosphorylation, mitochondrial dysfunction, neuro-inflammatory processes, oxidative stress, altered metal homeostasis, and many others [2–4]. However, the exact causes behind the early onset of AD are still unknown, so that diagnosis can only be performed via exclusion of other pathologies by using a combination of

Robert Perneczky (ed.), *Biomarkers for Alzheimer's Disease Drug Development*, Methods in Molecular Biology, vol. 1750, https://doi.org/10.1007/978-1-4939-7704-8_8, © Springer Science+Business Media, LLC 2018

neuropsychological and laboratory tests [5]. Thus, the discovery of novel AD biomarkers is crucial in order to monitor molecular alterations associated with disease pathogenesis and progression, as well as to develop new diagnostic protocols and drug treatments. In this context, the application of metabolomics has emerged in the last years because of its potential to accomplish a comprehensive characterization of functionally interrelated biochemical changes, as recently reviewed [6]. Metabolomics can be defined as the non-targeted characterization of metabolites present in a biological sample, as well as the identification of metabolic alterations produced in response to external (e.g., drug administration) or internal (e.g., disease development) stimuli. Metabolites are low-molecular-weight compounds (<1500 Da) that directly participate in enzyme-mediated reactions occurring in the organism, so that their homeostasis is tightly regulated by the proper functioning of higher biochemical organization levels as a consequence of the directional flow of genetic information within biological systems, as reflected in the omics cascade represented in Fig. 1. Accordingly, the metabolome is usually considered as the most reliable indicator of the organism's phenotype, reflecting changes downstream of the genomic, transcriptomic, and proteomic levels [7]. However, the great complexity and physicochemical heterogeneity of the human metabolome considerably hinders the simultaneous determination the entire set of these metabolites. Thus, the most common strategy in metabolomic research is the application of analytical multiplatforms based on the combination of complementary profiling techniques with the aim to maximize metabolome coverage.

1.2 Complementary Analytical Platforms to Unravel the Metabolome's Complexity

Global non-targeted metabolomic fingerprinting is only affordable by using powerful analytical tools, with high sensitivity and selectivity, in order to obtain accurate metabolic profiles with the maximum number of detected and subsequently identified metabolites. In this sense, a large number of analytical techniques have traditionally been proposed in metabolomic research, being nuclear magnetic resonance (NMR) and mass spectrometry (MS) the two predominant tools applied in this field. The use of NMR is widely spread in metabolomics because of its high reproducibility, reduced analysis time, and simple annotation of discriminant signals, thus enabling high-throughput analysis of samples in a few minutes [8]. However, this technique also shows very important drawbacks including low spectral resolution, which hinders the identification of individual metabolites in complex samples, and especially low sensitivity, which limits its applicability to the detection of high-abundance metabolites. On the other hand, mass spectrometry is a more sensitive analytical platform that allows the detection of

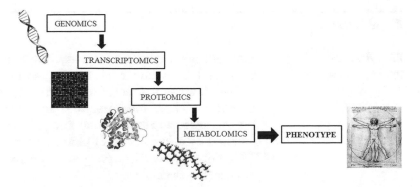

Fig. 1 The omics cascade, which illustrates the directional flow of information within biological systems. Reprinted from González-Domínguez et al. [10] with permission from Future Science

numerous metabolite classes at physiological levels, and their subsequent identification via fragmentation experiments. Furthermore, a wide array of sample introduction systems and ionization sources can be employed, thus significantly expanding the analytical coverage of MS-based approaches [9]. Thereby, MS is nowadays the main workhorse for metabolomic characterization of complex systems. The simplest instrumental configuration is direct mass spectrometry analysis, based on direct introduction of sample extracts into the mass spectrometer without prior chromatographic or electrophoretic separation, which stands out as a suitable platform for fast and comprehensive metabolomic screening [10]. Complementarily, the mass spectrometer can also be hyphenated with a separation technique in order to reduce the complexity of metabolic profiles and thus facilitate the identification of individual metabolites [11]. The interfacing of gas chromatography with mass spectrometry (GC-MS) is a robust tool that provides high sensitivity and good resolution for low-molecular-weight metabolites [12], including organic and amino acids, carbohydrates, amines, fatty acids, and some lipids, among others. Alternatively, liquid chromatography (LC) plays a pivotal role in metabolomics for the simultaneous determination of metabolites with very diverse chemical nature, extending from low-molecular-weight compounds detectable by GC-MS to nonvolatile metabolites, through the use of complementary retention mechanisms (e.g., reversed phase, RP; hydrophilic interaction liquid chromatography, HILIC) and ionization techniques (e.g., electrospray ionization, ESI; atmospheric pressure chemical ionization, APCI; atmospheric pressure photoionization, APPI) [11]. Accordingly, the combination of complementary analytical approaches has become the most suitable strategy to accomplish global metabolomic characterizations.

2   Materials

2.1   Reagents and Standards

High-purity solvents and reagents have to be used for sample treatment and subsequent chromatographic separation, including methanol, ethanol, chloroform, formic acid, ammonium formate, toluene, pyridine, methoxyamine hydrochloride, and *N*-methyl-*N*-trimethylsilyl-trifluoroacetamide (MSTFA). Deionized water is obtained by using a Milli-Q Gradient system (Millipore, Watford, UK). For identification purposes, metabolite standards must be purchased if available.

2.2   Sample Collection

2.2.1   Human Population

Blood samples are obtained from AD patients and healthy controls by venipuncture of the antecubital region. All samples must be collected after 8 h of fasting in the morning (9:00–12:00 a.m.) in order to avoid the influence of postprandial changes and the circadian rhythm. Blood is immediately cooled and protected from light for 30 min to allow clot retraction, and then centrifuge at $1578 \times g$ for 10 min. The resulting serum is divided into aliquots and frozen at −80 °C until analysis (*see* **Note 1**). The study population recruitment is performed following the criteria defined by the National Institute of Neurological and Communicative Disorders and Stroke and the Alzheimer's Disease and Related Disorders Association (NINCDS-ADRDA), as well as in accordance with the principles contained in the Declaration of Helsinki. Alzheimer's disease patients must be newly diagnosed of sporadic AD according to the NINCDS-ADRDA criteria [5], including only subjects that have not received any type of medication. On the other hand, matched healthy controls in sex and age are also enrolled after examination by neurologists to confirm the absence of neurological disorders by means of neuropsychological tests (MMSE, Pfeiffer), who had not more than two reported cases of AD in their families (*see* **Note 2**).

2.2.2   APP × PS1 Transgenic Mice

Transgenic APP × PS1 mice, expressing the Swedish mutation of the amyloid precursor protein (APP) together with deleted presenilin 1 (PS1) in exon 9 [13], as well as age-matched wild-type mice of the same genetic background (C57BL/6) are also employed in order to accomplish a global metabolomic investigation of Alzheimer's disease by analyzing multiple biological samples (*see* **Note 3**), which is inviable in human studies. These animals must be acclimated for 3 days after reception in rooms with a 12-h light/dark cycle at 20–25 °C, with water and food available ad libitum. Then, mice are anesthetized by isoflurane inhalation and blood is extracted by cardiac puncture. Blood samples are immediately cooled and protected from light for 30 min to allow clot retraction, and then centrifuged at $1578 \times g$ for 10 min at 4 °C (*see* **Note 1**). Subsequently, brain and other peripheral organs (liver, kidney, spleen, and thymus) are rapidly removed and rinsed with saline solution (0.9% NaCl, w/v). Furthermore, brains are dissected into hippocampus, cortex, cerebellum, striatum, and olfactory bulbs. Finally, all these samples are snap-frozen in liquid nitrogen and stored at −80 °C until analysis. Handling of animals must be performed according to the directive 2010/63/EU stipulated by the European Community.

3   Methods

3.1 Sample Extraction

3.2.1 Blood Serum Samples

Serum samples are treated following a two-step extraction procedure with the aim to fractionate the serum metabolome in two extracts: (a) a polar extract containing low-molecular-weight metabolites and phospholipids, and (b) a lipophilic extract mainly composed by neutral lipids [14].

1. Mix 100 μL of serum with 400 μL of methanol/ethanol (1:1, v/v).

2. Shake vigorously during 5 min using a vortex mixer in order to precipitate proteins.

3. Centrifuge samples at 2061 × g for 10 min at 4 °C.

4. Transfer the supernatant to a new tube, and keep the precipitate for further treatment.

5. Dry the supernatant under nitrogen stream (*see* **Note 4**), and reconstitute the resulting residue with 100 μL of methanol/ water (80:20, v/v) containing 0.1% formic acid (*polar extract*).

6. Add 400 μL of chloroform/methanol (1:1, v/v) to the protein precipitate.

7. Shake vigorously during 5 min using a vortex mixer.

8. Centrifuge at 12880 × g for 10 min at 4 °C.

9. Dry the supernatant under nitrogen stream (*see* **Note 4**) and reconstitute with 100 μL of dichloromethane/methanol (60:40, v/v) containing 0.1% formic acid and 10 mM ammonium formate (*lipophilic extract*).

3.1.1 Tissue Samples

Tissue samples, including hippocampus, brain cortex, cerebellum, striatum, olfactory bulbs, liver, kidney, spleen, and thymus, are extracted following the methodology previously optimized by González-Domínguez et al. [15–17].

1. Homogenize tissues using a cryogenic homogenizer SPEX SamplePrep (Freezer/Mills 6770) during 30 s at rate of ten strokes per second (*see* **Note 5**).

2. Exactly weight 30 mg of homogenized tissue (or the entire sample for smaller organs) in 1.5 mL Eppendorf tubes.

3. Add 10 μL mg^{-1} of precooled 0.1% formic acid in methanol (−20 °C).

4. Homogenize the mixture during 2 min in an ice bath, using a pellet mixer for cell disruption (VWR International, Lutterworth, Leicestershire, UK).

5. Centrifuge at 12880 × g for 10 min at 4 °C.

6. Transfer the supernatant to a new tube (*polar extract*).

7. Add 10 μL mg^{-1} of precooled chloroform/methanol (2:1, v/v), containing 0.1% formic acid and 10 mM ammonium formate, to the previously obtained pellet (*see* **Note 6**).

8. Repeat **steps 4–6** to obtain the corresponding *lipophilic extracts*.

3.1.2 Quality Control Samples

Prepare quality control (QC) samples by pooling equal volumes of each sample, which allows monitoring the stability and performance of the system along the analysis period [18]. These samples must be analyzed at the start of the run in order to equilibrate the analytical system as well as at intermittent points throughout the sequence to monitor system stability.

3.2 Sample Derivatization

Metabolomic profiling by gas chromatography coupled to mass spectrometry requires the application of a derivatization protocol in order to increase the volatility of metabolites. For this purpose, polar extracts previously obtained from blood and tissue samples must be treated according to the following two-step methodology [19] (*see* **Note 7**).

1. Take 50 μL from the previous polar extracts and dry under nitrogen stream (*see* **Note 4**).

2. Add 50 μL of 20 mg mL^{-1} methoxyamine hydrochloride in pyridine to carry out the protection of carbonyl groups by methoxymation (*see* **Note 8**).

3. After briefly vortexing, incubate the sample at 80 °C for 15 min using a water bath.

4. Add 50 μL of the silylation agent (*N*-methyl-*N*-trimethylsilyl-trifluoroacetamide, MSTFA) (*see* **Note 8**).

5. Incubate at 80 °C for a further 15 min using a water bath.

6. Centrifuge at 2061 × g for 1 min and collect the supernatant for analysis.

3.3 Metabolomic Fingerprinting: Direct MS Analysis

High-resolution mass spectrometry is used to carry out direct MS fingerprinting of polar and lipophilic extracts from serum and tissue samples. Protocols described in this chapter have previously been validated in a quadrupole-time-of-flight (Q-TOF) mass spectrometer, model QSTAR XL Hybrid system (Applied Biosystems,

Foster City, CA, USA). For accurate mass measurement, the TOF analyzer is daily calibrated using renin and taurocholic acid in positive and negative ion modes, respectively.

3.3.1 Direct Infusion Electrospray Mass Spectrometry (DI-ESI-MS)

Sample extracts are directly infused into the mass spectrometer by using a syringe pump operating at 5 μL min⁻¹ flow rate. Mass spectra are obtained by electrospray ionization (ESI) in both positive and negative ionization modes, as previously described [14, 17, 20]. Full-scan spectra are acquired for 0.2 min in the m/z range 50–1100 Da, with 1.005 s scan time. The source temperature is maintained at 60 °C, and high-purity nitrogen is used as curtain and nebulizer gas at flow rates about 1.13 L min⁻¹ and 1.56 L min⁻¹, respectively. The ion spray voltage (IS), declustering potential (DP), and focusing potential are set at 3300/−4000 V, 60/−100 V, and 250/−250 V in positive and negative ion modes, respectively. To acquire MS/MS spectra, nitrogen is used as collision gas.

3.3.2 Flow Injection Atmospheric Pressure Photoionization Mass Spectrometry (FI-APPI-MS)

For FI-APPI analysis, sample extracts are introduced into the mass spectrometer by flow injection using a LC system (injection volume: 10 μL). Furthermore, a syringe pump is also employed to deliver the dopant reagent for photospray ionization. According to the previously validated protocol, methanol is used as flow injection solvent at 50/100 μL min⁻¹ in positive and negative ion modes, respectively [21, 22]. On the other hand, toluene is delivered at 20/40 μL min⁻¹ as photoionization dopant, in both ionization modes. Mass spectra are obtained in positive and negative ion modes, acquiring full-scan spectra in the m/z range of 50–1100 Da, with 1.005 s of scan time. The ion spray voltage (IS) is set at 1500 V and −2300 V in positive and negative modes, while declustering and focusing potentials are set at ±50 V and ±250 V, respectively. The source temperature is maintained at 400 °C, and the gas flows (high-purity nitrogen) are fixed at 1.13 L min⁻¹ for curtain gas, 1.50 L min⁻¹ for nebulizer gas, 3.0 L min⁻¹ for heater gas, and 1 L min⁻¹ for lamp gas. To acquire MS/MS spectra, nitrogen is used as collision gas.

3.4 Metabolomic Profiling: Hyphenated MS-Based Approaches

The combination of liquid and gas chromatography has been established as the most common strategy for comprehensive MS-based metabolomic analysis. Protocols described under this section are based on the use of the following instrumentation, in accordance with previously published papers [15, 23–25] (*see* **Note 9**).

1. Ultra-high-performance liquid chromatograph (Accela LC system, Thermo Fisher Scientific) coupled to a quadrupole-time-of-flight mass spectrometry system equipped with electrospray source (QSTAR XL Hybrid system, Applied Biosystems).

2. Trace GC ULTRA gas chromatograph coupled to an ion trap mass spectrometer detector ITQ 900 (Thermo Fisher Scientific).

3.4.1 Ultrahigh-Performance Liquid Chromatography-Mass Spectrometry (UHPLC-MS)

Chromatographic separations are performed in a reversed-phase column (Hypersil Gold C18, 2.1 × 50 mm, 1.9 μm) thermostated at 50 °C, with an injection volume of 5 μL. Solvents are delivered at 0.5 mL min^{-1} flow rate, using methanol (solvent A) and water (solvent B), both containing 10 mM ammonium formate and 0.1% formic acid. The gradient elution program is 0–1 min, 95% B; 2.5 min, 25% B; 8.5–10 min, 0% B; and 10.1–12 min, 95% B. Full-scan spectra are acquired in positive and negative polarities within the m/z range of 50–1000 Da, with 1.005 s scan time. The ion spray voltage (IS) is set at 5000 V and −2500 V, and high-purity nitrogen is used as curtain, nebulizer, and heater gas at flow rates of about 1.48 L min^{-1}, 1.56 L min^{-1} and 6.25 L min^{-1}, respectively. The source temperature is fixed at 400 °C, with a declustering potential (DP) of 100/−120 V, and a focusing potential (FP) of ±350 V. To acquire MS/MS spectra, nitrogen is used as collision gas.

3.4.2 Gas Chromatography-Mass Spectrometry (GC-MS)

A Factor Four capillary column (VF-5MS 30 m × 0.25 mm ID, 0.25 μm film thickness) is used for GC-based profiling. The column temperature is set at 100 °C for 0.5 min, and programmed to reach 320 °C at a rate of 15 °C per min. Finally, this temperature is maintained for 2.8 min, the total time of analysis being 18 min. The injector temperature is kept at 280 °C, and helium is used as carrier gas at a constant flow rate of 1 mL min^{-1}. For mass spectrometry detection, electron ionization is carried out by using a voltage of 70 eV, and the ion source temperature is set at 200 °C. Data are obtained acquiring full-scan spectra in the m/z range of 35–650 Da. For analysis, 1 μL of sample is injected in splitless mode.

3.5 Data Processing

3.5.1 DI-ESI-MS and FI-APPI-MS Data

Metabolomic data obtained by DI-ESI-MS and FI-APPI-MS analysis are submitted to peak detection by using the Markerview™ software (Applied Biosystems) in order to convert raw files into a two-dimensional data matrix of spectral peaks and their intensities. To this end, all peaks above the noise level (10 counts, determined empirically from experimental spectra) are selected and binned in intervals of 0.1 Da. For FI-MS fingerprints, this processing step is limited to scans within the apex of infusion profiles [21]. Then, preprocessed data are normalized according to the total area sum and exported as a .csv file for further statistical analysis.

3.5.2 UHPLC-MS and GC-MS Data

Raw data obtained by means of hyphenated metabolomic approaches must be processed following the pipeline described by González-Domínguez et al., which proceeds through multiple stages including feature detection, alignment of peaks, and normalization [15, 23–25]. For this purpose, the freely available software XCMS included in the R platform is used (http://www.r-project.org). First, UHPLC-MS files are converted into the mzXML format using the msConvert tool (ProteoWizard), while GC-MS files are converted into netCDF using the Thermo File Converter tool (Thermo Fisher Scientific). Subsequently, data are extracted using the matchedFilter method. This algorithm slices data into extracted ion chromatograms (XIC) on a fixed step size (default 0.1 m/z), and then each slice is filtered with matched filtration using a second-derivative Gaussian as the model peak shape [26]. The XCMS parameters must be optimized according to the characteristics of datasets obtained in order to extract the maximum information as possible. Thereby, the settings applied for UHPLC-MS data are S/N threshold 2 and full width at half-maximum (fwhm) 10, while for GC-MS data the fwhm is set at 3. After peak extraction, grouping and retention time correction of peaks (i.e., alignment) are accomplished in three iterative cycles with descending bandwidth (bw) from 10 to 1 s in UHPLC-MS, and descending bw from 5 to 1 s for GC-MS. Then, imputation of missing values is performed by returning to the raw spectral data and integrating the areas of the missing peaks which are below the applied signal-to-noise ratio threshold, by using the fillPeaks algorithm. For data normalization, the locally weighted scatter plot smoothing (LOESS) normalization method is used, which adjusts the local median of log fold changes of peak intensities between samples in the dataset to be approximately zero across the whole peak intensity range [27]. Finally, pre-processed data are exported as a .csv file for further analysis.

3.6 Statistical Analysis

Processed data are subjected to multivariate statistical analysis by principal component analysis (PCA) and partial least squares discriminant analysis (PLS-DA) in order to compare metabolomic profiles between the study groups (i.e., AD patients vs. healthy controls, APP × PS1 transgenic mice vs. wild-type mice), using the SIMCA-P™ software (version 11.5, UMetrics AB, Umeå, Sweden). Before performing statistical analysis, data are submitted to Pareto scaling for reducing the relative importance of larger values, and logarithmic transformation in order to approximate a normal distribution [28]. Quality of the models is assessed by the R^2 and Q^2 values, supplied by the software, which provide information about the class separation and predictive power of the model, respectively. These parameters are ranged between 0 and 1, and they indicate the variance explained by the model for all the data analyzed (R^2) and this variance in a test set by cross-validation (Q^2). Finally, potential biomarkers are selected according to the variable importance in the projection, or VIP (a weighted sum of squares of the PLS weight, which indicates the importance of the variable in the model), considering only variables with VIP values higher than 1.0, indicative of significant differences among groups. Furthermore, these metabolites can be subsequently validated by t-test with Bonferroni correction for multiple testing (p-values below 0.05), using the STATISTICA 8.0 software (StatSoft, Tulsa, USA).

3.7 Identification of Discriminant Metabolites

The identification of discriminant metabolites detected by GC-MS is made by using the NIST Mass Spectral Library. On the other hand, the identity of potential markers from DI-ESI-MS, FI-APPI-MS, and UHPLC-MS profiles can be elucidated by matching the experimental accurate mass and tandem mass spectra (MS/MS) with those available in metabolomic databases (HMDB, METLIN, and LIPIDMAPS). In the latter case, the knowledge of fragmentation patterns for the most important lipid classes also facilitates this annotation step. Fragmentation of glycerolipids (i.e., mono-, di-, and triglycerides) occurs through the release of fatty acids from the glycerol backbone and subsequent generation of different types of ions (named A, B, C, and D ions), which show characteristic m/z values according to the released fatty acid [29]. Phosphatidylcholines present characteristic fragments in positive ionization mode at m/z 184, 104, and 86, and two typical neutral losses due to the breakage of trimethylamine and phosphocholine head group. Alternatively, product-ion spectra of ethanolamine-, serine-, and glycerol-derived phospholipids are dominated by $[M + H-141]^+$, $[M + H-185]^+$, and $[M + H-172]^+$ ions, arising from the elimination of the phosphoethanolamine, phosphoserine, and phosphoglycerol moiety, respectively. By contrast, these distinctive signals are found in negative-ion mode at m/z 153, 168, 196, 241, 171, and $[M-H-87]^-$, for phosphatidic acids, choline-, ethanolamine-, inositol-, glycerol-, and serine-derived lipids, respectively [30]. Moreover, tandem MS fragmentation of ester linkages enables the identification of individual species of phospholipids by means of the interpretation of ions B, C, and D generated in positive-ion mode, as well as the corresponding carboxylate anions released under ESI(−)-MS ionization [31, 32]. For sphingolipids, typical product ions appear at m/z 264 and 282 due to the fragmentation in the sphingosine moiety, while the cleavage of the phosphocholine head group from sphingomyelins generates characteristic fragments at m/z 184 and 168 in positive- and negative-ion mode, respectively [33]. Cholesterol derivatives are readily annotated thanks to the abundant fragment ion corresponding to the cholesterol moiety (m/z 369) [34], while acylcarnitines can be confirmed based on characteristic fragments at m/z 60 and 85 [35]. Finally, standards must be injected if available to confirm these identifications according to the experimental retention time.

4 Notes

1. Plasma samples can be used instead of serum. For this, blood must be collected in anticoagulant-containing tubes.

2. Patients affected by mild cognitive impairment (MCI), which is normally considered as a preclinical stage of Alzheimer's dis-

ease, can also be enrolled in order to investigate metabolomic changes occurring in the early onset of this neurodegenerative disorder, as previously reported [36, 37].

3. Metabolomic procedures described in this chapter are focused on the investigation of blood and tissue samples, but these methods are also applicable with minor modifications to other biological fluids, such as urine [38].

4. The evaporation of sample extracts can also be carried out by using vacuum concentrators (e.g., SpeedVac), if available.

5. Smaller organs (e.g., hippocampus, striatum, olfactory bulbs) can be directly extracted without prior cryo-homogenization.

6. This second extraction step is of great interest for studying peripheral organs (i.e., liver, kidney, spleen, thymus), due to the high content of neutral lipids in these tissues. However, **steps 7** and **8** can be omitted when brain tissue is analyzed, as previously reported [15, 20].

7. Derivatization must only be accomplished in polar extracts containing low-molecular-weight metabolites. Neutral lipids present in lipophilic extracts present very low volatilities, so they are not readily analyzable by gas chromatography-mass spectrometry.

8. Derivatization reagents here employed (i.e., methoxyamine and MSTFA) are very sensitive to moisture. The methoxyamine solution in pyridine must be daily prepared. With regard to MSTFA, authors recommend the purchase of sealed glass ampoules, which should be used within the day of its opening.

9. Metabolomic methods based on UHPLC-MS and GC-MS described in this chapter are only applicable for polar extracts (*see* Subheading 3.1). As previously stated in **Note 7**, lipophilic extracts are mainly composed by neutral lipids that are not readily analyzable by GC-MS due to their low volatilities. Moreover, the separation of these lipids by reversed-phase liquid chromatography requires the use of very long elution programs. For these reasons, lipophilic extracts are only fingerprinted by direct MS analysis.

References

1. Reitz C, Brayne C, Mayeux R (2011) Epidemiology of Alzheimer disease. Nat Rev Neurol 7:137–152

2. Blennow K, de Leon MJ, Zetterberg H (2006) Alzheimer's disease. Lancet 368:387–403

3. Maccioni RB, Muñoz JP, Barbeito L (2001) The molecular bases of Alzheimer's disease and other neurodegenerative disorders. Arch Med Res 32:367–381

4. González-Domínguez R, García-Barrera T, Gómez-Ariza JL (2014) Characterization of metal profiles in serum during the progression of Alzheimer's disease. Metallomics 9:292–300

5. Dubois B, Feldman HH, Jacova C, Dekosky ST, Barberger-Gateau P, Cummings J, Delacourte A, Galasko D, Gauthier S, Jicha G, Meguro K, O'Brien J, Pasquier F, Robert P, Rossor M, Salloway S, Stern Y, Visser PJ, Scheltens P (2007) Research criteria for the diagnosis of Alzheimer's disease: revising the NINCDS–ADRDA criteria. Lancet Neurol 6:734–746

6. González-Domínguez R, Sayago A, Fernández-Recamales A (2017) Metabolomics in Alzheimer's disease: the need of complementary analytical platforms for the identification of biomarkers to unravel the underlying pathology. J Chromatogr B Analyt Technol Biomed Life Sci 1071:75–92

7. Dunn WB, Broadhurst DI, Atherton HJ, Goodacre R, Griffin JL (2011) Systems level studies of mammalian metabolomes: the roles of mass spectrometry and nuclear magnetic resonance spectroscopy. Chem Soc Rev 40:387–426

8. Emwas AHM, Salek RM, Griffin JL, Merzaban J (2013) NMR-based metabolomics in human disease diagnosis: applications, limitations, and recommendations. Metabolomics 9:1048–1072

9. Theodoridis G, Gika HG, Wilson ID (2011) Mass spectrometry-based holistic analytical approaches for metabolite profiling in systems biology studies. Mass Spectrom Rev 30:884–906

10. González-Domínguez R, Sayago A, Fernández-Recamales A (2017) Direct infusion mass spectrometry for metabolomic phenotyping of diseases. Bioanalysis 9:131–148

11. Kuehnbaum NL, Britz-McKibbin P (2013) New advances in separation science for metabolomics: resolving chemical diversity in a postgenomic era. Chem Rev 113:2437–2468

12. Pasikanti KK, Ho PC, Chan EC (2008) Gas chromatography/mass spectrometry in metabolic profiling of biological fluids. J Chromatogr B Analyt Technol Biomed Life Sci 871:202–211

13. Jankowsky JL, Fadale DJ, Anderson J, GM X, Gonzales V, Jenkins NA, Copeland NG, Lee MK, Younkin LH, Wagner SL, Younkin SG, Borchelt DR (2004) Mutant presenilins specifically elevate the levels of the 42 residue beta-amyloid peptide in vivo: evidence for augmentation of a 42-specific g secretase. Hum Mol Genet 13:159–170

14. González-Domínguez R, García-Barrera T, Gómez-Ariza JL (2014) Using direct infusion mass spectrometry for serum metabolomics in Alzheimer's disease. Anal Bioanal Chem 406:7137–7148

15. González-Domínguez R, García-Barrera T, Vitorica J, Gómez-Ariza JL (2014) Region-specific metabolic alterations in the brain of the APP/PS1 transgenic mice of Alzheimer's disease. Biochim Biophys Acta 1842:2395–2402

16. Gago-Tinoco A, González-Domínguez R, García-Barrera T, Blasco-Moreno J, Bebianno MJ, Gómez-Ariza JL (2014) Metabolic signatures associated with environmental pollution by metals in Doñana National Park using *P. clarkii* as bioindicator. Environ Sci Pollut Res Int 21:13315–13323

17. González-Domínguez R, García-Barrera T, Vitorica J, Gómez-Ariza JL (2015) High throughput multi-organ metabolomics in the APP/PS1 mouse model of Alzheimer's disease. Electrophoresis 36:2237–2249

18. Sangster T, Major H, Plumb R, Wilson AJ, Wilson ID (2006) A pragmatic and readily implemented quality control strategy for HPLC-MS and GC-MS-based metabonomic analysis. Analyst 131:1075–1078

19. González-Domínguez R, García-Barrera T, Gómez-Ariza JL (2015) Metabolite profiling for the identification of altered metabolic pathways in Alzheimer's disease. J Pharm Biomed Anal 107:75–81

20. González-Domínguez R, García-Barrera T, Vitorica J, Gómez-Ariza JL (2015) Metabolomic screening of regional brain alterations in the APP/PS1 transgenic model of Alzheimer's disease by direct infusion mass spectrometry. J Pharm Biomed Anal 102:425–435

21. González-Domínguez R, García-Barrera T, Gómez-Ariza JL (2015) Application of a novel metabolomic approach based on atmospheric pressure photoionization mass spectrometry using flow injection analysis for the study of Alzheimer's disease. Talanta 131:480–489

22. González-Domínguez R, García-Barrera T, Vitorica J, Gómez-Ariza JL (2015) Application of metabolomics based on direct mass spectrometry analysis for the elucidation of altered metabolic pathways in serum from the APP/PS1 transgenic model of Alzheimer's disease. J Pharm Biomed Anal 107:378–385

23. González-Domínguez R, García-Barrera T, Vitorica J, Gómez-Ariza JL (2015) Deciphering metabolic abnormalities associated with Alzheimer's disease in the APP/PS1 mouse model using integrated metabolomic approaches. Biochimie 110:119–128

24. González-Domínguez R, García-Barrera T, Vitorica J, Gómez-Ariza JL (2015) Metabolomic investigation of systemic manifestations associated with Alzheimer's disease

in the APP/PS1 transgenic mouse model. Mol BioSyst 11:2429–2440

25. González-Domínguez R, García-Barrera T, Vitorica J, Gómez-Ariza JL (2015) Metabolomics reveals significant impairments in the immune system of the APP/PS1 transgenic mice of Alzheimer's disease. Electrophoresis 36:577–587

26. Smith CA, Want EJ, O'Maille G, Abagyan R, Siuzdak G (2006) XCMS: processing mass spectrometry data for metabolite profiling using nonlinear peak alignment, matching, and identification. Anal Chem 78:779–787

27. Veselkov KA, Vingara LK, Masson P, Robinette SL, Want E, Li JV, Barton RH, Boursier-Neyret C, Walther B, Ebbels TM, Pelczer I, Holmes E, Lindon JC, Nicholson JK (2011) Optimized preprocessing of ultra-performance liquid chromatography/mass spectrometry urinary metabolic profiles for improved information recovery. Anal Chem 83:5864–5872

28. van den Berg RA, Hoefsloot HCJ, Westerhuis JA, Smilde AK, van der Werf MJ (2006) Centering, scaling, and transformations: improving the biological information content of metabolomics data. BMC Genomics 7:142

29. González-Domínguez R, García-Barrera T, Gómez-Ariza JL (2012) Iberian ham typification by direct infusion electrospray and photospray ionization mass spectrometry fingerprinting. Rapid Commun Mass Spectrom 26:835–844

30. Pulfer M, Murphy RC (2003) Electrospray mass spectrometry of phospholipids. Mass Spectrom Rev 22:332–364

31. Wang C, Xie S, Yang J, Yang Q, Xu G (2004) Structural identification of human blood phospholipids using liquid chromatography/quadrupole-linear ion trap mass spectrometry. Anal Chim Acta 525:1–10

32. González-Domínguez R, García-Barrera T, Gómez-Ariza JL (2014) Combination of metabolomic and phospholipid-profiling approaches for the study of Alzheimer's disease. J Proteome 104:37–47

33. Haynes CA, Allegood JC, Park H, Sullards MC (2009) Sphingolipidomics: methods for the comprehensive analysis of sphingolipids. J Chromatogr B 877:2696–2708

34. Liebisch G, Binder M, Schifferer R, Langmann T, Schulz B, Schmitz G (2006) High throughput quantification of cholesterol and cholesteryl ester by electrospray ionization tandem mass spectrometry (ESI-MS/MS). Biochim Biophys Acta 1761:121–128

35. Vernez L, Hopfgartner G, Wenk M, Krahenbuhl S (2003) Determination of carnitine and acyl-carnitines in urine by high-performance liquid chromatography-electrospray ionization ion trap tandem mass spectrometry. J Chromatogr A 984:203–213

36. González-Domínguez R, García A, García-Barrera T, Barbas C, Gómez-Ariza JL (2014) Metabolomic profiling of serum in the progression of Alzheimer's disease by capillary electrophoresis-mass spectrometry. Electrophoresis 35:3321–3330

37. González-Domínguez R, Rupérez FJ, García-Barrera T, Barbas C, Gómez-Ariza JL (2016) Metabolomic-driven elucidation of pathological mechanisms associated with Alzheimer's disease and mild cognitive impairment. Curr Alzheimer Res 13:641–653

38. González-Domínguez R, Castilla-Quintero R, García-Barrera T, Gómez-Ariza JL (2014) Development of a metabolomic approach based on urine samples and direct infusion mass spectrometry. Anal Biochem 465:20–27

Chapter 9

Blood-Based Biomarker Screening with Agnostic Biological Definitions for an Accurate Diagnosis Within the Dimensional Spectrum of Neurodegenerative Diseases

Filippo Baldacci, Simone Lista, Sid E. O'Bryant, Roberto Ceravolo, Nicola Toschi, Harald Hampel, and for the Alzheimer Precision Medicine Initiative (APMI)

Abstract

The discovery, development, and validation of novel candidate biomarkers in Alzheimer's disease (AD) and other neurodegenerative diseases (NDs) are increasingly gaining *momentum*. As a result, evolving diagnostic research criteria of NDs are beginning to integrate biofluid and neuroimaging indicators of pathophysiological mechanisms. More than 10% of people aged over 65 suffer from NDs. There is an urgent need for a refined two-stage diagnostic model to first initiate an early, sensitive, and noninvasive process in primary care settings. Individuals that meet detection criteria will then be channeled to more specific, costly (positron-emission tomography), and invasive (cerebrospinal fluid) assessment methods for confirmatory biological characterization and diagnosis.

A reliable and sensitive blood test for AD and other NDs is not yet established; however, it would provide the golden screening gate for an efficient primary care management. A limitation to the development of a large-scale blood-screening biomarker-based test is the traditional application of clinically descriptive criteria for the categorization of single late-stage ND constructs. These are genetically and biologically heterogeneous, reflected in multiple pathophysiological mechanisms and subsequent pathologies throughout a dimensional *continuum*. Evidence suggests that a shared, "open-source" integrated multilevel categorization of NDs that clusters individuals based on descriptive clinical phenotypes and pathophysiological biomarker signatures will provide the next incremental step toward an improved diagnostic process of NDs. This intermediate objective toward unbiased biomarker-guided early detection of individuals at risk for NDs is currently carried out by the international pilot Alzheimer Precision Medicine Initiative Cohort Program (APMI-CP).

Key words Neurodegenerative diseases, Alzheimer's disease, Biomarkers, Pathophysiology, Alzheimer precision medicine initiative, Systems biology, Systems neurophysiology, Precision medicine, Blood, Screening

Robert Perneczky (ed.), *Biomarkers for Alzheimer's Disease Drug Development*, Methods in Molecular Biology, vol. 1750, https://doi.org/10.1007/978-1-4939-7704-8_9, © Springer Science+Business Media, LLC 2018

1 Toward Biomarker-Based Diagnostic Criteria in Neurodegenerative Diseases

The pathology term of neurodegeneration refers to a multifaceted family of nervous system diseases developing a plethora of late-stage behavioral, cognitive, motor, and sensory symptoms and syndromes on the pathological background of progressive neuronal cell loss [1, 2]. The lack of qualified biomarkers which can track pathophysiological mechanisms and support both early diagnosis and reliable prognosis has significantly hampered and delayed the successful development of therapeutic strategies for treating neurodegenerative diseases (NDs). While the management of NDs was largely confined within traditional boundaries purely based on clinical criteria [2, 3], during the last two decades, criteria employed in ND research have begun to integrate emerging core feasible candidate biomarkers as relevant diagnostic features to be employed in conjunction with an increasingly detailed and standardized description of the clinical phenotypes.

The Biomarkers Definitions Working Group (BDWG) of the National Institutes of Health (NIH) proposed a standardized definition of a biomarker as "a characteristic that is objectively measured and evaluated as an indicator of normal biological processes, pathogenic processes or pharmacological responses to a therapeutic intervention" [4]. Biomarkers are employed—both in clinical praxis and in clinical trials—for detection, diagnosis, prediction, staging, enrichment, stratification, or outcome assessment. Thus, they have gained a key role in drug development throughout all therapeutic areas [5, 6]. Given the substantial progresses in elucidating the pathophysiological mechanisms of various diseases both from molecular and from a cellular point of view, biomarkers serve as powerful tools to inform and advance all phases of the drug discovery and development process, i.e., by allowing the assessment of successful target engagement or the validation of putative mechanisms of actions (MoA) [7]. The use of biomarkers needs to be integrated into clinical trials in order to increase the diagnostic accuracy as well as to facilitate the enrichment of patient cohorts [6, 8, 9]. Biomarkers are also needed for the stratification of participants to improve clinical response, enhance the processes of monitoring disease progression and response to therapy, identify prognostic signatures, and develop diagnostic assays [6, 8, 9]. As a result, they are increasingly employed in research and development (R&D) strategies which aim to identify novel prospective candidate drugs, from the discovery and validation to the regulatory authorization steps [10, 11]. Biomarkers are categorized into several groups: (1) MoA biomarkers, evaluating downstream biochemical effects; (2) target engagement biomarkers, aiming to test assumptions about the interaction of candidate drugs with their molecular targets; (3) outcome biomarkers, appraising both efficacy and safety of drugs; (4) safety biomarkers, assessing and predicting both tolerability and adverse side effects; and (5) theragnostic biomarkers, supporting the selection of the therapy by predicting both the most appropriate treatment (or response to treatment) and the most suitable dose for the subject [6, 7, 12]. Differently from clinical markers, biomarkers of disease encompass (1) measurements based on biological samples (e.g., namely cerebrospinal fluid (CSF) and blood (plasma/serum))—or (2) neuroimaging methods (including magnetic resonance imaging (MRI), positron-emission tomography (PET), single-photon emission computed tomography (SPECT)). The latter are used to detect in vivo brain alterations associated with neurodegeneration and cognitive decline in human subjects.

2   Integration of Biomarkers in the Diagnostic/Research Criteria of Neurodegenerative Diseases: A Recent History

It seems clear that we are facing a progressive integration phase of biomarkers within the *corpus* of the evolving internationally recognized and applied research diagnostic criteria for the most common NDs. In 1994, the electrophysiological evidence of upper and lower motor neuron disease in the bulbar and spinal regions was recognized as a diagnostic feature of amyotrophic lateral sclerosis (ALS) [13]; however, despite intense research efforts, no additional biomarkers have yet been developed [14, 15]. More recently, in 2007, the measurement of the CSF concentrations of the 42-amino acid-long amyloid beta (Aβ) peptide (Aβ$_{1-42}$), hyperphosphorylated tau (p-tau), and total tau (t-tau) proteins as well as of the cerebral amyloid-PET uptake was proposed [16] and then successfully adopted, later progressed into clinical practice, as prodromal proxies of underlying Alzheimer's disease (AD) pathophysiology [17–21]. In addition, both decrease of the hippocampal volumes—as detected by MRI—and hypometabolism in the parietotemporal and posterior cuneus areas—as measured by 2-deoxy-2-[fluorine-18]fluoro-D-glucose ([^{18}F]-FDG)-PET—are considered core feasible biomarkers of progression in AD. Structural imaging indicators, as compared to CSF markers, are probably less specific and sensitive in later preclinical to prodromal disease stages [22]. Very recently, the presence of cardiac sympathetic denervation on iodine-123-meta-iodobenzylguanidine ([^{123}I]-MIBG) scintigraphy became a supportive diagnostic tool within the updated version of the criteria for the diagnosis of Parkinson's disease (PD). In addition, the normal and active functioning of the presynaptic dopaminergic system, as detected by PET or SPECT approaches, allowed the exclusion of PD diagnosis [23]. Notably, a clear subthreshold tracer uptake of the presynaptic dopaminergic system, as measured by SPECT or PET, and the existence of an enlarged echogenic size ("hyperechogenicity") of the *substantia nigra* on transcranial sonography achieved the *status* of predictive biomarkers of PD (or dementia with Lewy bodies, DLB) diagnosis in subjects with mild symptoms of parkinsonism which do not allow a definitive clinical diagnosis. Therefore, along with the previous statements about the concepts of prodromal AD or mild cognitive impairment (MCI) due to AD [19, 24], the Movement Disorder Society (MDS) group developed research diagnostic criteria to properly identify the novel clinical category of prodromal PD [25]. In this regard, it should be emphasized that, since 2005, the subthreshold tracer uptake of the presynaptic dopaminergic system as well as the cardiac sympathetic denervation on [^{123}I]-MIBG scintigraphy are, respectively, suggestive and supportive diagnostic tools for DLB, and are largely employed for the differential diagnosis between DLB and AD [26]. Similarly to AD, [^{18}F]-FDG-PET hypometabolism and/or MRI atrophy have also been integrated as biomarkers to support the diagnosis of frontotemporal lobar degeneration (FTLD). This was possible once their relevance had been demonstrated in definite brain areas depending on the specific type of FTLD variants [27, 28]. Finally, MRI atrophy detected at the level of putamen, middle cerebellar peduncle, pons, or cerebellum as well as [^{18}F]-FDG-PET hypometabolism measured in putamen, brainstem, or cerebellum have been considered potential additional indicators of multiple system atrophy (MSA) [29], although they normally appear only in advanced disease stages. In contrast, the diagnosis of progressive supranuclear palsy (PSP) [30] and corticobasal degeneration (CBD) [31] is still almost entirely reliant on clinical diagnostic criteria. In summary, while still in the early stages, the discovery and validation process of novel candidate biomarkers as putative surrogate end points of innovative potential therapies for treating NDs are increasingly gaining *momentum*. Unfortunately, although the search for objective and precise surrogates of molecular pathophysiological pathways charting the *spectrum* of NDs is rapidly growing, only few biomarkers of neurodegeneration have been validated and translated into the clinical practice [32]. In addition, in spite of the evidence of the continuous failures of disease-modifying treatments in ND clinical trials, a reductionist and outdated vision of NDs as homogenous clinicopathological entities still exists in biomedical research as well as drug discovery and development programs.

3   Toward the Development of a Novel Working Language for the Definition of the *Spectrum* of Neurodegenerative Diseases

The term NDs indicates a heterogeneous "constellation" of central nervous system (CNS) diseases characterized by abnormal deposits of misfolded proteins. Hence, NDs are designated as CNS proteinopathies [33] and, more precisely, they should be considered as part of a dimensional disease *spectrum* and not as distinct and separate categories [34]. Actually, one proteinopathy may reveal multiple phenotypes and one single phenotype may refer to the combination of abnormal deposits of several misfolded proteins [1, 35]. Additionally, comorbidity of these different pathologies is more the rule rather than the exception and, therefore, a focus on any single pathology rarely provides the complete pathological picture. In addition, the pathophysiological processes driving cerebrovascular diseases may overlap with neurodegeneration mechanisms, thus creating a *continuum* of complex/mixed patterns of converging pathophysiological pathways that are often clinically indiscernible [2, 17, 36, 37]. Interestingly, even the "gold standard" *postmortem* examination utilized for ND diagnosis is not conceptually adequate and satisfactory since it coincides with the final stage of several pathophysiological pathways, which probably begin and progress through multiple and dissimilar longitudinal trajectories but possibly converge to comparable pathophysiological end points [1, 38]. Within this scenario of multilevel and multiscale dynamic complexities, a systems theory-based approach represents the best strategy to explicate the source and timing of the multiple structural/functional perturbations characterizing all neurodegenerative processes at all systems levels, as assessed by the systems biology and systems neurophysiology paradigms [39]. This would allow the development of theoretical and experimental models that need to spatially integrate different scales of magnitude—from micro- to macro-dimensions, e.g., genetic/epigenetic, biochemical, cellular, brain anatomical and functional networks, and environmental—across time [40, 41]. As theoretical consequence, there is no single clinical, imaging, or biological marker able to fully depict the *spectrum* of pathophysiological mechanisms of a given polygenic ND and, therefore, multiple markers should be simultaneously considered to fully elucidate the pathophysiological processes affecting any individual patient. The biomarkers currently employed in AD clinical research criteria—and more recently in other NDs—have been discovered via a hypothesis-driven approach. This is essentially centered on the use of prospective candidate biomarkers resulting from existing knowledge about the pathophysiological mechanisms of NDs. Notably, this approach allowed recognizing the role of CSF the $A\beta_{1-42}$ peptide as well as t-tau and p-tau proteins as core diagnostic indicators of AD. Conversely, in last years, the "omic" tools emerged as alternative a posteriori approaches, i.e., not based on any preexisting assumption. Such a data-driven discovery strategy applies to the high-throughput screening of human biofluids—e.g., CSF, blood (plasma/serum), urine, and saliva—and tissues—e.g., brain, peripheral nerves, and colon mucosa—on large-scale clinical/ research datasets in order to simultaneously identify several potential biomarkers for NDs [3, 32]. These unbiased screening analyses supporting the discovery of potentially novel biomarkers, or biomarker algorithms, and clarifying ND-related pathophysiological mechanisms, mandatorily need substantial interdisciplinary integration, including advanced knowledge in bioinformatics and statistics to manage and decipher huge amounts of data [32]. Indeed, the ultimate goal is the harmonization and integration of large-scale clinical/research information, including "omic" data, with the aim of "turning big data into smart data" [42, 43]. In this regard, the Worldwide Alzheimer's Disease Neuroimaging Initiative (WW-ADNI) [44] and, more recently, the Parkinson's Progression Marker Initiative (PPMI) [45] have been established with the aim of connecting worldwide research by collecting, validating, and sharing multidimensional biomarker data (genetic/epigenetic, biochemical, imaging, and psychometric) as diagnostic surrogates and longitudinal predictors of disease progression and treatment responsiveness. However, since the crucial need to combine interdisciplinary work with constant advancement in bioinformatics still remains, traditional diagnostic boundaries commonly employed for a first collection, classification, and organization of clinical/research datasets are obsolete and, therefore, represent a substantial limitation for precisely and efficiently exploiting big data. In this context, the examination of any particular ND will need a precise multi-modular description in terms of clinical, brain network, and molecular markers. This should also lead to the reconsideration of the best strategies for collecting and categorizing information [2]. From a pragmatic viewpoint, one of the most relevant challenges derived from managing different sources of big data is how to strategically plan their initial collection in order to obtain reliable information. This will be particularly useful to stratify NDs, from the highest to the lowest degrees of complexity, by detecting (1) clinical indicators defining phenotypes—e.g., psychometric evaluations and specific scales describing motor symptoms—(2) surrogates of network disruption tracking structural/functional brain changes—e.g., cortical thickness, diffusion-weighted imaging (DWI), task-free MRI, and [^{18}F]-FDG-PET—(3) theory-driven and unbiased "omic"-based biomarkers tracking pathophysiological mechanisms, and (4) genetic markers (Fig. 1). In addition, given that NDs have intrinsically dynamic nonlinear disease processes, the accurate temporal description of disease evolution, providing detailed anamnestic (or retrospective) and prospective longitudinal information, should be supported by clinical and biological markers. Hence, personal history of exposition to environmental risk factors, such as traumatic brain injury, should be systematically investigated and collected to enrich dataset information. In this direction, details on both onset and duration of the disease should be provided since they are essential to correctly interpret the commonly observed different rate of clinical progression of NDs (Fig. 1). Finally, we believe that one of the key objectives of

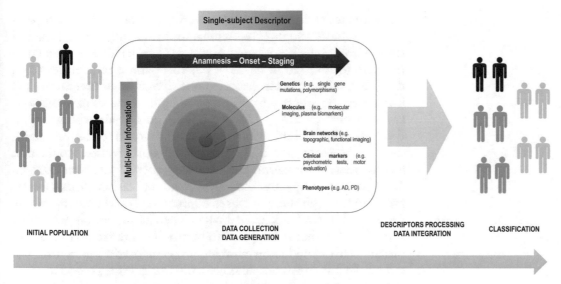

Fig. 1 From data collection to population stratification. Data related to NDs are collected and organized in single-subject descriptors providing multiscale homogenous information on clinical phenotypes and pathophysiological mechanisms. This approach is useful in order to attain the stratification of NDs, from the highest to the lowest degree of complexity, and to combine data according to their similarities or divergences. The final objective is the harmonization and integration of multidimensional information through combined analysis, possibly leading to a redefinition of clinical phenotypes and novel therapeutic strategies of NDs. *Abbreviations*: NDs, neurodegenerative diseases

the recently established international pilot Alzheimer Precision Medicine Initiative (APMI) [39] is the creation of a shared, "opensource" integrated multilevel categorization of NDs able to cluster individuals based on clinical phenotypes, genetic profile, and biomarker signatures. The immediate practical advantage of such an approach will be the combination of data according to their pathophysiological network disruption and phenotypic similarities or divergences, independently of the initial clinical diagnosis. Finally, heterogeneous data from a certain population should be systematically collected and consequently funneled in synthetic, individually based descriptors containing multiscale homogenous information that could be efficiently analyzed to provide a novel data-driven agnostic classification of NDs (Fig. 1).

The idea of identifying novel and more precise disease categories, positioned along a multidimensional *continuum* spanned by a subspace of all available multimodal patient data, falls within the realm of pattern recognition and machine learning. Specifically, once the data are available and have been harmonized, unsupervised pattern recognition methods can be employed detecting higher order, nonlinear associations within the multidimensional data point represented by each patient in the highly heterogeneous space constituted by genetic, imaging, and biohumoral data.

This equates to identifying the effective degrees of freedom present in a subject's augmented biomarker panel and, hence, isolating the variables which are most useful for any particular prediction problem formulated in terms of possible patient trajectories (e.g., drug response, disease progression). Possible strategies would include employing raw patient data as input for a set of evolutionary machine-discovery and model-building algorithms that, through joint optimization approaches, would build predictive models. Notably, this multidimensional optimization could also include meta-information like treatment cost or caregiver burden. As a further step, the knowledge about disease mechanisms acquired through these unbiased approaches could be semantically formalized into a "molecular-imaging-behavioral ontology" which should be specifically designed to be readily understandable by clinicians. This would allow seamless implementation in clinical use cases as well as constant refinement and integration as soon as additional knowledge accrues.

4   The Precision Medicine Paradigm Is Needed for the Treatment of Neurodegenerative Diseases

One of the final objectives is expected to be the amalgamation of individuals displaying very clinical different phenotypes but share comparable pathophysiological mechanisms. In this regard, it is well known that several patients clinically labeled as DLB or frontotemporal dementia (FTD) can exhibit elevated cerebral amyloid-PET uptake [17, 36, 46] and, as a result, they may benefit from clinical trials using anti-Aβ drugs. Furthermore, patients with suspected neurodegenerative mechanisms and brain microglia activation, as detected by PET imaging, might be treated with anti-neuroinflammatory drugs independently of the clinical diagnosis. Given that ND phenotypes can considerably differ and commonly used criteria are frequently inconsistent in terms of diagnostic and categorization accuracy, a clinically based selection of patients for clinical trials is questionable [2]. Interestingly, the increasing identification of concomitant and overlapping pathophysiological mechanisms underlying NDs is far from the "one-size-fits-all" approach employed in drug discovery ("one-drug-fits-all"). Indeed, this strategy showed a very low success rate in the development of therapeutic agents [3, 47]. In opposition to the classical "one-drug-fits-all" system, the exploratory, integrative, and interdisciplinary paradigm of precision medicine aims to substantially enhance the effectiveness of disease therapies as well as prevention. This can be achieved by considering an individual's specific "biological makeup"—such as genetic/epigenetic, biochemical, phenotypic, lifestyle, and psychosocial features—that covers the heterogeneity of all NDs for targeted interventions [3].

It should be stressed that precision medicine is a form of biomarker-guided medicine. Actually, in accordance with the definition of the Food and Drug Administration (FDA) and the NIH Biomarkers, Endpoints, and other Tools (BEST) Resource, biomarkers can be classified into distinct categories, as follows: (1) susceptibility/risk biomarkers, (2) diagnostic biomarkers, (3) monitoring biomarkers, (4) prognostic biomarkers, (5) predictive biomarkers, (6) pharmacodynamic/response biomarkers, and (7) safety biomarkers [48]. Unfortunately, such clear-cut distinctions across the biomarker *spectrum* are difficult to implement in the field of AD. In this regard, amyloid positivity might be regarded—depending on each specific patient—as a diagnostic or predictive biomarker (or both). Nonetheless, the distinction between different biomarker types is paramount for disease treatment and prevention targeted to the individual characteristics [48]. Importantly, high-throughput profiling technologies will allow the identification and differentiation of highly specific biomarkers that can increase our understanding of the heterogeneity of AD and other NDs in terms of disease development and prognosis under comprehensive holistic systems-level approaches, namely the systems biology and systems neurophysiology paradigms [3]. The successful implementation of precision medicine will require the development of optimized infrastructures and technologies to assay biomarkers on the one hand and collaboration between all stakeholders involved in ND care on the other hand.

5 A Blood-Based Model for Patient Screening and Precision Medicine Therapeutics

The discovery and advancement biomarkers of NDs (outlined above) have focused nearly exclusively on CSF and imaging modalities. These markers have been highly effective as confirmatory diagnostics. As highlighted above, there is oftentimes pathological overlap in individual patients suffering from NDs and, therefore, it is likely that a multitiered, multi-marker model will be utilized. The multi-model approach has been outlined and, in this section, we provide a multitiered model that integrates this multi-marker model.

In NDs, there is a tremendous need for a model able to initiate the diagnostic process within primary care clinics and successively refer those who need it most to more costly (PET) and invasive (CSF) biomarker assessment for confirmatory diagnostics. As is the case with other diseases, imaging and CSF modalities are never the first step in the diagnostic process in primary care settings. Given that there are over 40 million people aged 65 and above in the USA alone (and these numbers are growing rapidly), there is an urgent need for a multilevel neurodiagnostic process [49]. A blood test, as the initial step, can be easily integrated into primary settings globally and can be scalable to meet the patient throughput needs. Additionally, as is the case with all primary care screening tools, the primary goal is to rule out those who should not undergo second-level assessment. This is due to the base rates of disease positive. Specifically, it is estimated that approximately 12% of those aged 65 years and over suffer from AD (*see* https://www.alz.org/documents_custom/2016-facts-and-figures.pdf). If approximately 20% suffer from any ND, 80% are disease negative. Therefore, the first step in the multitiered approach is to remove as many of these patients from the neurodiagnostic process as possible in a cost-effective manner. Achieving a 90% negative predictive value would accomplish this goal irrespective of the positive predictive value, which is 20% or less in primary care tools [9]. Such a model will be immediately required once disease-modifying therapies are available (1) because of the global surge that would be seen in primary care of patients seeking medications to treat or prevent disease and (2) because access to medications will require biomarker confirmation of pathology presence for drug prescription. A multitiered approach beginning with a blood test can serve this need with all receiving a positive result being referred for CSF and/or PET scan biomarker assessment for confirmatory diagnostics. As an example of the financial implications, if a blood test costs $100 per test, this would cost $2,000,000,000 if only 20 million people were screened. If the test yielded a sensitivity of 0.80 and specificity of 0.75, the positive predictive and negative predictive values would be 0.48 and 0.93, respectively, with a 20% base rate. This would result in 14,900,000 (only 500,000 false negatives) of the patients immediately being screening out and not referred to confirmatory diagnostics and 5,100,000 being sent for CSF and/or PET examinations. If PET scan costs $5000 per scan the resulting cost would be $25 billion globally. The cost savings by using the blood test as the first step to screen out nearly 15 million patients would be $73 billion annually as compared to using only PET scans to identify those patients who obtain access to disease-modifying therapies for treatment or prevention. It is noteworthy that there were over 600 million people aged 65 and over globally in 2016, so this financial model underestimates the need and cost savings. The availability of a blood-based method for screening patients into a novel precision medicine paradigm for treatments and prevention will drastically open access to disease-modifying therapies, but also provide scientists with a means of identifying patients from community-based settings for enrollment into novel studies and trials.

Notably, in addition to being utilized for screening into regulatory approved therapeutic and novel clinical trials, blood-based biomarkers may also aid in the development of a precision medicine approach to treating and preventing NDs [39]. Blood-based biomarkers may be utilized for the identification of subgroups of patients that exhibit dysfunction of key biological systems. In fact, it has been proposed that the proteomic biomarker profiling approach is a promising method for discovering biomarkers for NDs [50, 51] because a battery of markers covering a range of biological processes may be required to address the needs of such complex disorders [52]. Using a specific example, inflammation has been shown to be altered across a range of NDs, including AD, and it has been proposed that profiling inflammation may provide novel therapeutic interventions for neurodegeneration [53, 54]. Therefore, there may be a subset of patients suffering from NDs where inflammation is the primary pathophysiological process that should be targeted, in addition to Aβ peptides, tau protein, α-synuclein, or other CSF-identified pathologies. In such a scenario, a blood-based tool can be used to screen into CSF and/or PET modalities and, then, further profiling can be employed to refine the underlying pathophysiology of the specific patients for multimodal interventions, as outlined in Fig. 2. The combination of multitier and multimodal biomarker assessment can lead to a cost-effective means for patient identification as well as a refined precision medicine-based model for novel interventions. In such a scenario, clinical phenotypes do not drive therapeutic directions, but rather patients suffering from NDs are provided targeted interventions based on multimodal biomarker profiling. For instance, a patient with both Aβ and α-synuclein pathology would be funneled into multimodal therapy for both, in addition to an anti-inflammatory agent if that pathway was also dysfunctional. The clinical definition of AD versus PD would be irrelevant from a therapeutic standpoint. This is akin to saying that "cancer" is irrelevant to therapeutics as "tissue of origin" is becoming irrelevant, but rather cancer therapeutics are driven by the biology of the presenting patient. As in the case of cancer, moving to this model is predicted to result in drastically improved patient outcomes.

6 Conclusions

Owing to its complex, multifactorial pathogenesis, a deeper knowledge of AD requires the integration of data from different but parallel sources (systems or networks). To achieve this goal, both clinical and basic research is required. The former approach includes (1) high-throughput molecular profiling of AD patients—e.g., genomics/epigenomics, transcriptomics/miRNAomics, proteomics/peptidomics, metabolomics/lipidomics, and interactomics; (2) the use of different structural and functional brain imaging techniques, as well as connectomics—which examines the organization and functioning of the brain across the connectome, namely all the anatomical and functional connections of the brain; (3) detailed neurophysiological assessments; and (4) extensive

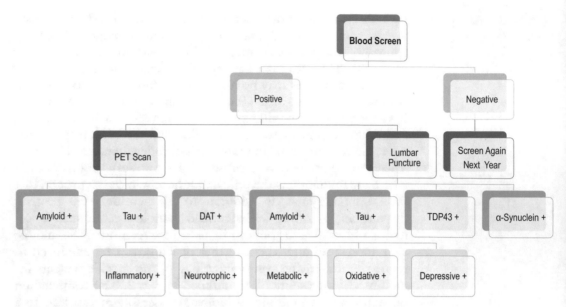

Fig. 2 Schematic depiction of multilevel biomarker-driven diagnostic and therapeutic model. First, a blood screen aids in determining which patients undergo PET or CSF confirmatory diagnostic procedures. If positive, refer, and if negative, evaluate again in the future as needed. Second level is at the CSF and PET confirmatory diagnostics for specific pathophysiological markers (not disease presence, but pathology presence). The third level adds blood-based biomarker profiles of specific biological systems known to be altered in NDs that may be present in addition to the pathophysiological markers identified by PET and/or CSF. The second and third levels guide specific multimodal interventions. As an example, a patient could be positive on blood screen and then undergo both CSF evaluation for amyloid, tau, and α-synuclein. The patient, then, also undergoes blood-biomarker profiling for inflammatory, neurotrophic, metabolic, and oxidative dysfunction. A positive finding for amyloid only would move the patient to amyloid only therapy. A positive finding for amyloid, α-synuclein, and inflammation would move the patient to multimodal therapy targeting amyloid, α-synuclein, and inflammation. *Abbreviations*: CSF, cerebrospinal fluid; NDs, neurodegenerative diseases; PET, positron-emission tomography

psychometric evaluations. With regard to basic science, the availability of high-throughput "-omic" technologies has recently allowed the unbiased identification of new promising biomarkers from different biological sources (e.g., CSF, plasma/serum, tissues, and cells).

Importantly, the eagerly awaited implementation of systems biology and systems neurophysiology strategies aimed at gaining deeper and novel insights into AD pathophysiology will require the combined assessment of big and deep heterogeneous data. The integrated analysis of big data will be necessarily dependent on the availability of adequate tools not only for data storage and management, but also for their modeling according to disease pathophysiology. Highly accurate, sophisticated methods will thus be required to systematically screen for biomarkers related to AD and other NDs, as well as to gain insights into their spatiotemporal interactions.

Because the results obtained with different experimental approaches may provide complementary information on the pathophysiological underpinnings of the disease, their integration is expected to provide deeper insights into our clinical interpretation of its pathophysiology. For this reason, the Big Data Research and Development Initiative (available at https://obamawhitehouse.archives.gov/blog/2012/03/29/big-data-big-deal) announced by the previous Obama Administration should be seen as an important catalyst for the implementation of precision medicine through the integration of big biomedical data. Actually, such an initiative is expected to take the ability to extract knowledge and insights from ample and complex collections of digital data to the next level. Hopefully, this program will promote significant progresses in the field of science and engineering, with major implications both for strengthening the national security and for transforming the current teaching/learning practices. The ability to deal with "big data science," accompanied by the adoption of an integrative disease modeling, is an essential aspect of the recently established international APMI, strictly linked to the US "All of Us Research Program"—formerly known as and evolved from the US PMI Cohort Program (available at https://www.nih.gov/research-training/allofus-research-program)—and other related global initiatives.

Undoubtedly, the last decade has witnessed major advances in the field of blood-based biomarkers of AD and other NDs. Compared with CSF markers, blood-based biomarkers are more cost efficient and easy to measure; in addition, venipuncture is a routine, safe procedure that does not pose any harm to the patient. As such—and differently from CSF sampling—the assessment of blood biomarkers is more easily accepted in the clinical realm [9]. In line with the successful implementation of the precision medicine paradigm in the area of oncology, it is paramount to identify the biomarker signatures of AD before the disease course has reached a point at which a decompensation and potentially irreversible pathological damage have occurred. The hope for the future is that blood-based biomarkers could be helpful to develop a multistep diagnostic approach, according to which only patients who test positive on initial blood tests will be referred to more advanced (and costly) diagnostic modalities, including CSF sampling and PET imaging. Remarkably, such a possibility would also be invaluable for enriching patient recruitment in AD clinical trials. In this scenario, another crucial advancement will be represented by the possibility to identify patients who are most likely to benefit from targeted preventive or therapeutic strategies. Finally, the application of systems biology to blood-based biomarker data obtained through the application of the "omic" techniques will allow to identify specific patient subsets, or "endophenotypes," that share a common pathophysiology (which in turn might potentially be targeted by agents informed by such fine gained knowledge).

The successful introduction of the systems biology and systems neurophysiology paradigms to AD research and development is thus expected to facilitate the use of precision medicine for AD patients toward clinical reality [9].

Acknowledgments

S.E.O. is supported by the National Institute on Aging of the National Institutes of Health under Award Numbers R01AG051848 and R56AG054073. The content is solely the responsibility of the authors and does not necessarily represent the official views of the National Institutes of Health.

H.H. is supported by the AXA Research Fund, the "Fondation Université Pierre et Marie Curie" and the "Fondation pour la Recherche sur Alzheimer," Paris, France. Ce travail a bénéficié d'une aide de l'Etat "Investissements d'avenir" ANR-10-IAIHU-06. The research leading to these results has received funding from the program "Investissements d'avenir" ANR-10-IAIHU-06 (Agence Nationale de la Recherche-10-IA Agence Institut Hospitalo-Universitaire-6).

Disclosure Statement

S.L. received lecture honoraria from Roche. H.H. reports no conflict of interest with the content of the present manuscript. He serves as Senior Associate Editor for the Journal *Alzheimer's & Dementia*; he has been a scientific consultant and/or speaker and/or attended scientific advisory boards of Axovant, Anavex, Eli Lilly and company, GE Healthcare, Cytox Ltd., Jung Diagnostics GmbH, Roche, Biogen Idec, Takeda-Zinfandel, Oryzon Genomics, and Qynapse; and he receives research support from the Association for Alzheimer Research (Paris), Pierre and Marie Curie University (Paris), and Pfizer & Avid (paid to institution); and he has patents, but receives no royalties. F.B., S.E.O., R.C., and N.T. declare no conflicts of interest.

References

1. Kovacs GG (2016) Molecular pathological classification of neurodegenerative diseases: turning towards precision medicine. Int J Mol Sci 17:pii: E189. https://doi.org/10.3390/ijms17020189

2. Baldacci F, Lista S, Garaci F et al (2016) Biomarker-guided classification scheme of neurodegenerative diseases. J Sport Health Sci 5:383–387. https://doi.org/10.1016/j.jshs.2016.08.007

3. Hampel H, O'Bryant SE, Castrillo JI et al (2016) Precision medicine—the golden gate for detection, treatment and prevention of Alzheimer's disease. J Prev Alz Dis 3:243–259. https://doi.org/10.14283/jpad.2016.112

4. Biomarkers Definitions Working Group (2001) Biomarkers and surrogate endpoints: preferred definitions and conceptual framework. Clin Pharmacol Ther 69:89–95. https://doi.org/10.1067/mcp.2001.113989

5. Hampel H, Lista S, Khachaturian ZS (2012) Development of biomarkers to chart all Alzheimer's disease stages: the royal road to cutting the therapeutic Gordian Knot. Alzheimers Dement J Alzheimers Assoc 8:312–336. https://doi.org/10.1016/j.jalz.2012.05.2116

6. Blennow K, Hampel H, Weiner M, Zetterberg H (2010) Cerebrospinal fluid and plasma biomarkers in Alzheimer disease. Nat Rev Neurol 6:131–144. https://doi.org/10.1038/nrneurol.2010.4

7. Hampel H, Lista S (2013) Use of biomarkers and imaging to assess pathophysiology, mechanisms of action and target engagement. J Nutr Health Aging 17:54–63. https://doi.org/10.1007/s12603-013-0003-1

8. Blennow K, Hampel H, Zetterberg H (2014) Biomarkers in amyloid-β immunotherapy trials in Alzheimer's disease. Neuropsychopharmacol Off Publ Am Coll Neuropsychopharmacol 39:189–201. https://doi.org/10.1038/npp.2013.154

9. O'Bryant SE, Mielke MM, Rissman RA et al (2017) Blood-based biomarkers in Alzheimer disease: current state of the science and a novel collaborative paradigm for advancing from discovery to clinic. Alzheimers Dement J Alzheimers Assoc 13:45–58. https://doi.org/10.1016/j.jalz.2016.09.014

10. Hampel H, Frank R, Broich K et al (2010) Biomarkers for Alzheimer's disease: academic, industry and regulatory perspectives. Nat Rev Drug Discov 9:560–574. https://doi.org/10.1038/nrd3115

11. Vellas B, Carrillo MC, Sampaio C et al (2013) Designing drug trials for Alzheimer's disease: what we have learned from the release of the phase III antibody trials: a report from the EU/US/CTAD Task Force. Alzheimers Dement J Alzheimers Assoc 9:438–444. https://doi.org/10.1016/j.jalz.2013.03.007

12. Lista S, Dubois B, Hampel H (2015) Paths to Alzheimer's disease prevention: from modifiable risk factors to biomarker enrichment strategies. J Nutr Health Aging 19:154–163. https://doi.org/10.1007/s12603-014-0515-3

13. Brooks BR (1994) El Escorial World Federation of Neurology criteria for the diagnosis of amyotrophic lateral sclerosis. Subcommittee on Motor Neuron Diseases/Amyotrophic Lateral Sclerosis of the World Federation of Neurology Research Group on Neuromuscular Diseases and the El Escorial "Clinical limits of amyotrophic lateral sclerosis" workshop contributors. J Neurol Sci 124(Suppl):96–107

14. Al-Chalabi A, Hardiman O, Kiernan MC et al (2016) Amyotrophic lateral sclerosis: moving towards a new classification system. Lancet Neurol 15:1182–1194. https://doi.org/10.1016/S1474-4422(16)30199-5

15. Vu LT, Bowser R (2016) Fluid-based biomarkers for amyotrophic lateral sclerosis. Neurother J Am Soc Exp Neurother 14:119–134. https://doi.org/10.1007/s13311-016-0503-x

16. Dubois B, Feldman HH, Jacova C et al (2007) Research criteria for the diagnosis of Alzheimer's disease: revising the NINCDS-ADRDA criteria. Lancet Neurol 6:734–746. https://doi.org/10.1016/S1474-4422(07)70178-3

17. Dubois B, Feldman HH, Jacova C et al (2014) Advancing research diagnostic criteria for Alzheimer's disease: the IWG-2 criteria. Lancet Neurol 13:614–629. https://doi.org/10.1016/S1474-4422(14)70090-0

18. McKhann GM, Knopman DS, Chertkow H et al (2011) The diagnosis of dementia due to Alzheimer's disease: recommendations from the National Institute on Aging-Alzheimer's Association workgroups on diagnostic guidelines for Alzheimer's disease. Alzheimers Dement J Alzheimers Assoc 7:263–269. https://doi.org/10.1016/j.jalz.2011.03.005

19. Albert MS, DeKosky ST, Dickson D et al (2011) The diagnosis of mild cognitive impairment due to Alzheimer's disease: recommendations from the National Institute on Aging-Alzheimer's Association workgroups on diagnostic guidelines for Alzheimer's disease. Alzheimers Dement J Alzheimers Assoc 7:270–279. https://doi.org/10.1016/j.jalz.2011.03.008

20. Jack CR, Bennett DA, Blennow K et al (2016) A/T/N: an unbiased descriptive classification scheme for Alzheimer disease biomarkers. Neurology 87:539–547. https://doi.org/10.1212/WNL.0000000000002923

21. Sperling RA, Aisen PS, Beckett LA et al (2011) Toward defining the preclinical stages of Alzheimer's disease: recommendations from the National Institute on Aging-Alzheimer's Association workgroups on diagnostic guidelines for Alzheimer's disease. Alzheimers Dement J Alzheimers Assoc 7:280–292. https://doi.org/10.1016/j.jalz.2011.03.003

22. Jack CR, Knopman DS, Jagust WJ et al (2013) Tracking pathophysiological processes in Alzheimer's disease: an updated hypothetical model of dynamic biomarkers. Lancet Neurol 12:207–216. https://doi.org/10.1016/S1474-4422(12)70291-0

23. Postuma RB, Berg D, Stern M et al (2015) MDS clinical diagnostic criteria for Parkinson's disease. Mov Disord Off J Mov Disord Soc 30:1591–1601. https://doi.org/10.1002/mds.26424

24. Dubois B, Feldman HH, Jacova C et al (2010) Revising the definition of Alzheimer's disease: a new lexicon. Lancet Neurol 9:1118–1127. https://doi.org/10.1016/S1474-4422(10)70223-4

25. Berg D, Postuma RB, Adler CH et al (2015) MDS research criteria for prodromal Parkinson's disease. Mov Disord Off J Mov Disord Soc 30:1600–1611. https://doi.org/10.1002/mds.26431

26. McKeith IG, Dickson DW, Lowe J et al (2005) Diagnosis and management of dementia with Lewy bodies: third report of the DLB Consortium. Neurology 65:1863–1872. https://doi.org/10.1212/01.wnl.0000187889.17253.b1

27. Gorno-Tempini ML, Hillis AE, Weintraub S et al (2011) Classification of primary progressive aphasia and its variants. Neurology 76:1006–1014. https://doi.org/10.1212/WNL.0b013e31821103e6

28. Piguet O, Hornberger M, Mioshi E, Hodges JR (2011) Behavioural-variant frontotemporal dementia: diagnosis, clinical staging, and management. Lancet Neurol 10:162–172. https://doi.org/10.1016/S1474-4422(10)70299-4

29. Gilman S, Wenning GK, Low PA et al (2008) Second consensus statement on the diagnosis of multiple system atrophy. Neurology 71:670–676. https://doi.org/10.1212/01.wnl.0000324625.00404.15

30. Litvan I, Agid Y, Calne D et al (1996) Clinical research criteria for the diagnosis of progressive supranuclear palsy (Steele-Richardson-Olszewski syndrome): report of the NINDS-SPSP international workshop. Neurology 47:1–9

31. Armstrong MJ, Litvan I, Lang AE et al (2013) Criteria for the diagnosis of corticobasal degeneration. Neurology 80:496–503. https://doi.org/10.1212/WNL.0b013e31827f0fd1

32. Chen-Plotkin AS (2014) Unbiased approaches to biomarker discovery in neurodegenerative diseases. Neuron 84:594–607. https://doi.org/10.1016/j.neuron.2014.10.031

33. Ahmed RM, Devenney EM, Irish M et al (2016) Neuronal network disintegration: common pathways linking neurodegenerative diseases. J Neurol Neurosurg Psychiatry 87:1234–1241. https://doi.org/10.1136/jnnp-2014-308350

34. Pievani M, Filippini N, van den Heuvel MP et al (2014) Brain connectivity in neurodegenerative diseases—from phenotype to proteinopathy. Nat Rev Neurol 10:620–633. https://doi.org/10.1038/nrneurol.2014.178

35. Warren JD, Rohrer JD, Schott JM et al (2013) Molecular nexopathies: a new paradigm of neurodegenerative disease. Trends Neurosci 36:561–569. https://doi.org/10.1016/j.tins.2013.06.007

36. Hyman BT, Phelps CH, Beach TG et al (2012) National Institute on Aging-Alzheimer's Association guidelines for the neuropathologic assessment of Alzheimer's disease. Alzheimers Dement J Alzheimers Assoc 8:1–13. https://doi.org/10.1016/j.jalz.2011.10.007

37. Skrobot OA, Attems J, Esiri M et al (2016) Vascular cognitive impairment neuropathology guidelines (VCING): the contribution of cerebrovascular pathology to cognitive impairment. Brain 139:2957–2969. https://doi.org/10.1093/brain/aww214

38. Kovacs GG, Milenkovic I, Wöhrer A et al (2013) Non-Alzheimer neurodegenerative pathologies and their combinations are more frequent than commonly believed in the elderly brain: a community-based autopsy series. Acta Neuropathol (Berl) 126:365–384. https://doi.org/10.1007/s00401-013-1157-y

39. Hampel H, O'Bryant SE, Durrleman S et al (2017) A precision medicine initiative for Alzheimer's disease: the road ahead to biomarker-guided integrative disease modeling. Climacteric 20:107–118. https://doi.org/10.1080/13697137.2017.1287866

40. Lista S, Khachaturian ZS, Rujescu D et al (2016) Application of systems theory in longitudinal studies on the origin and progression of Alzheimer's disease. Methods Mol Biol Clifton NJ 1303:49–67. https://doi.org/10.1007/978-1-4939-2627-5_2

41. Vidal M (2009) A unifying view of 21st century systems biology. FEBS Lett 583:3891–3894. https://doi.org/10.1016/j.febslet.2009.11.024

42. Geerts H, Dacks PA, Devanarayan V et al (2016) Big data to smart data in Alzheimer's disease: the brain health modeling initiative to foster actionable knowledge. Alzheimers Dement J Alzheimers Assoc 12:1014–1021. https://doi.org/10.1016/j.jalz.2016.04.008

43. Haas M, Stephenson D, Romero K et al (2016) Big data to smart data in Alzheimer's disease: real-world examples of advanced modeling and simulation. Alzheimers Dement

J Alzheimers Assoc 12:1022–1030. https://doi.org/10.1016/j.jalz.2016.05.005

44. Carrillo MC, Bain LJ, Frisoni GB, Weiner MW (2012) Worldwide Alzheimer's disease neuroimaging initiative. Alzheimers Dement J Alzheimers Assoc 8:337–342. https://doi.org/10.1016/j.jalz.2012.04.007

45. Parkinson Progression Marker Initiative (2011) The Parkinson Progression Marker Initiative (PPMI). Prog Neurobiol 95:629–635. https://doi.org/10.1016/j.pneurobio.2011.09.005

46. McCann H, Stevens CH, Cartwright H, Halliday GM (2014) α-Synucleinopathy phenotypes. Parkinsonism Relat Disord 20(Suppl 1):S62–S67. https://doi.org/10.1016/S1353-8020(13)70017-8

47. Reitz C (2016) Toward precision medicine in Alzheimer's disease. Ann Transl Med 4:107. https://doi.org/10.21037/atm.2016.03.05

48. Group F-NBW (2016) FDA-NIH Biomarker Working Group. Food and Drug Administration (US)

49. O'Bryant SE, Edwards M, Johnson L et al (2016) A blood screening test for Alzheimer's disease. Alzheimers Dement (Amst) 3:83–90. https://doi.org/10.1016/j.dadm.2016.06.004

50. Henchcliffe C, Dodel R, Beal MF (2011) Biomarkers of Parkinson's disease and dementia with Lewy bodies. Prog Neurobiol 95:601–613. https://doi.org/10.1016/j.pneurobio.2011.09.002

51. Ho GJ, Liang W, Waragai M et al (2011) Bridging molecular genetics and biomarkers in Lewy body and related disorders. Int J Alzheimers Dis 2011:e842475. https://doi.org/10.4061/2011/842475

52. Shtilbans A, Henchcliffe C (2012) Biomarkers in Parkinson's disease: an update. Curr Opin Neurol 25:460–465. https://doi.org/10.1097/WCO.0b013e3283550c0d

53. Durrenberger PF, Fernando FS, Kashefi SN et al (2015) Common mechanisms in neurodegeneration and neuroinflammation: a BrainNet Europe gene expression microarray study. J Neural Transm (Vienna) 122:1055–1068. https://doi.org/10.1007/s00702-014-1293-0

54. Heneka MT, Kummer MP, Latz E (2014) Innate immune activation in neurodegenerative disease. Nat Rev Immunol 14:463–477. https://doi.org/10.1038/nri3705

Part IV

Magnetic Resonance Imaging Methods

Chapter 10

Functional Magnetic Resonance Imaging in Alzheimer' Disease Drug Development

Stefan Holiga, Ahmed Abdulkadir, Stefan Klöppel, and Juergen Dukart

Abstract

While now commonly applied for studying human brain function the value of functional magnetic resonance imaging in drug development has only recently been recognized. Here we describe the different functional magnetic resonance imaging techniques applied in Alzheimer's disease drug development with their applications, implementation guidelines, and potential pitfalls.

Key words fMRI, Alzheimer's disease, Treatment, Prevention, Biomarker, Dementia

1 Introduction

An important limitation of CNS drug development is the inaccessibility of human brain tissue for evaluation of target engagement and treatment effects. While some techniques like positron-emission tomography can be used to demonstrate such effects their usability is often limited by the unavailability of appropriate tracers and the high cost and time demands associated with such studies [1, 2]. In contrast, functional magnetic resonance imaging (MRI) of metabolic activity provides an easy implementable framework for evaluation of pharmacodynamic (PD) effects [3]. Two major types of such metabolic costs that can be now routinely measured through different functional MRI sequences are blood oxygen level dependence (BOLD) and cerebral blood flow (CBF). While the first reflects relative increases in oxygen consumption following regional neural activity during specific tasks or rest the latter provides quantitative information on regional blood flow associated with the neural activity. For BOLD, a further distinction is made between task-based (fMRI) and task-free magnetic resonance imaging (rsfMRI) measures. In contrast, CBF is typically measured in a task-free setting. The temporal resolution of both types of measures is limited by the slowness of the hemodynamic response, i.e., the peak of oxygen level follows neural activation by 4–8 s [4]. Further limitations of functional MRI measures that are important to consider in particular

Robert Perneczky (ed.), *Biomarkers for Alzheimer's Disease Drug Development*, Methods in Molecular Biology, vol. 1750, https://doi.org/10.1007/978-1-4939-7704-8_10, © Springer Science+Business Media, LLC 2018

in the context of drug development result from their indirect measure of neural activity. As these measures represent a metabolic sum function associated with respective neural activity they do not dissociate between direct and indirect or specific and nonspecific drug effects on the underlying neural activity across different neurotransmitter systems. They can also be confounded by peripheral physiological contributions—such as fluctuations in vascular blood flow—or acquisition-related noise—such as artifacts due to head motion [5–7]. Despite those limitations, metabolic MRI measures have a high potential for improving central nervous system (CNS) drug development. Major applications of metabolic MRI in drug development are the demonstration of PD effects and as potential efficacy or stratification biomarkers.

Different software and analyses packages have been implemented in the past decades for processing and analyses of metabolic MRI data. While some routines may differ between those packages some consensus emerged about the general framework for handling of such imaging data. This framework is outlined below rsfMRI and relevant differences in the analysis of the metabolic markers (BOLD and CBF) as well as in the analysis of the task-based versus task-free MRI are highlighted.

2   Choice of Study Designs

Depending on the expected mechanism of action of respective compounds the choice of an appropriate study design is essential to allow subsequent estimation of drug-induced effects onto respective metabolic MRI biomarkers. More specifically, a key question to be answered prior to the choice of a study design is if the effect of pharmacological treatment on the brain is expected to last after its termination and appropriate washout time. Such effects are in particular expected for treatments with an expected disease-modifying mechanism of action. However, they may occur upon chronic exposure to symptomatic treatment as long-term exposure to such treatments for example with antipsychotics has been shown to have long-lasting effects on brain structure and function [8]. If such effects are expected or cannot be excluded the choice of a parallel arm study design is preferable with a baseline acquisition being recommended to reduce the contribution of between-subject variability. In contrast, if such effects are not expected, i.e., when evaluating the effects of an acute or a short-term administration of a symptomatic treatment, crossover designs are preferable as they allow for a better control of between-session effects.

2.1   Considerations for the Choice of Functional Imaging Modalities

The decision on which metabolic MRI modalities and which primary end points to include can be based on knowledge of disease-specific imaging phenotypes to be modified by the treatment and based on their sensitivity to potential treatment effects. However, most important consideration for the choice of functional MRI modalities to be included into a clinical trial is the goal that is supposed to be achieved by the respective biomarker. More specifically, the goals can be subdivided into the following categories with specific examples:

1. Improving diagnosis: Reduced CBF in specific regions has been shown to be a sensitive diagnostic biomarker for Alzheimer's disease. Inclusion of patients meeting a specific cutoff on this measure may therefore be applied to enrich the clinical trial by reducing the proportion of misdiagnosed patients.

2. Demonstrating pharmacodynamic effects: Drug A has been shown to modify rsfMRI functional connectivity of a network N. Another drug in development with similar mechanism of action could be evaluated if it induces a similar brain response on the respective measurement.

3. Stratification of treatment response: An exploratory analysis of a previous trial revealed that only patients showing a treatment-related pharmacodynamic effect on CBF above a specific threshold also show improvement in clinical symptoms. A new trial is designed with the respective treatment in the same patient population. The identified relationship could be used to define a sensitivity analysis focusing only on patients meeting the respective cutoff.

4. Surrogate efficacy readout: Schizophrenia patients with negative symptoms show a reduced ventral striatal activation in a reward-expectation fMRI task. A drug targeting the respective circuitry could be tested if it normalizes the respective deficit in this patient cohort.

2.2 Preprocessing of Functional MRI Data

While different software packages comprise some differences with respect to specific pre-processing steps or its order, some consensus of major pre-processing steps exists and is outlined below (Fig. 1):

1. Optional step for fMRI and rsfMRI only: An optional slice timing correction for BOLD fMRI data to correct for temporal differences in slice acquisition.

2. Motion correction to reduce the impact of motion on the underlying signal.

3. Optional step for fMRI and rsfMRI only: distortion correction.

4. For CBF only: computation of quantitative CBF maps from pairs of labeled and control images scaled by M0 map.

5. Spatial normalization to a standard space (i.e. Montreal Neurological Institute space) either directly or if no stronger spatial distortions through parameters derived from a co-registered structural scan of the same subject.

6. Smoothing with a Gaussian kernel with a full width at half maximum (FWHM) of about two to three times the voxel size.

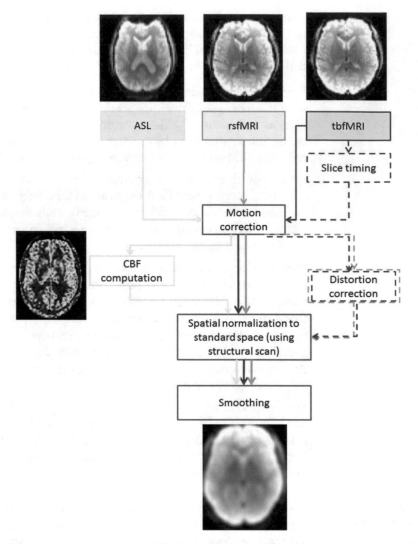

Fig. 1 Schematic overview of functional MRI data processing. ASL—arterial spin labeling, CBF—cerebral blood flow, rsfMRI—resting-state functional magnetic resonance imaging, tbFMRI—task-based functional magnetic resonance imaging

2.3 Statistical Analyses of Metabolic MRI Data

1. For fMRI only: first-level voxel-wise analyses per subject and session contrasting conditions of interest of the respective fMRI task and controlling for six motion regressors.

2. For rsfMRI only: computation of functional or effective connectivity or activity metrics per subject and session controlling for motion, mean global signal, white matter, and cerebrospinal fluid contribution.

3. Group-level statistical hypothesis testing for differences between drug and placebo conditions modeled as within-subject effects for crossover designs and as condition by time interactions for parallel arm designs.

4. Evaluation of dose-response relationships by testing for significant linear or nonlinear associations between imaging changes and dose or exposure measures.

2.4 Further Considerations

1. For validation trials of previous findings or trials focusing on modification of a disease-associated imaging phenotype, the mean of a prespecified region of interest can be used based on respective previous knowledge to restrict the outcome to a single test. Alternatively, a small volume correction within the respective region can be used but is less preferable in case of a specific regional hypothesis unless the region is very large and/or substantial heterogeneity is expected within the region.

2. Cluster extent thresholds corrected for multiple comparisons (defined for example using permutation-based algorithms) combined with less conservative voxel-wise thresholds are more sensitive to pick up drug effects in case of exploratory analyses in particular for CBF and rsfMRI data.

3. For fMRI, paradigms selected based on a phenotype/deficit in activation in a specific patient population restriction of analyses to regions that are known to be activated by the task may be meaningful to reduce the number of multiple comparisons and to facilitate interpretation of potential findings.

References

1. Kapur S, Zipursky RB, Remington G et al (1998) 5-HT2 and D2 receptor occupancy of olanzapine in schizophrenia: a PET investigation. Am J Psychiatry 155(7):921–928. https://doi.org/10.1176/ajp.155.7.921

2. Nordstrom AL, Farde L, Wiesel FA et al (1993) Central D2-dopamine receptor occupancy in relation to antipsychotic drug effects: a double-blind PET study of schizophrenic patients. Biol Psychiatry 33(4):227–235

3. Borsook D, Becerra L, Hargreaves R (2006) A role for fMRI in optimizing CNS drug development. Nat Rev Drug Discov 5(5):411–424. https://doi.org/10.1038/nrd2027

4. Logothetis NK (2008) What we can do and what we cannot do with fMRI. Nature 453(7197):869–878. https://doi.org/10.1038/nature06976

5. Okon-Singer H, Mehnert J, Hoyer J et al (2014) Neural control of vascular reactions: impact of emotion and attention. J Neurosci 34(12):4251–4259. https://doi.org/10.1523/JNEUROSCI.0747-13.2014

6. Van Dijk KR, Sabuncu MR, Buckner RL (2012) The influence of head motion on intrinsic functional connectivity MRI. NeuroImage 59(1):431–438. https://doi.org/10.1016/j.neuroimage.2011.07.044

7. Volkow ND, Wang GJ, Fowler JS et al (2003) Cardiovascular effects of methylphenidate in humans are associated with increases of dopamine in brain and of epinephrine in plasma. Psychopharmacology (Berl) 166(3):264–270. https://doi.org/10.1007/s00213-002-1340-7

8. Fusar-Poli P, Smieskova R, Kempton MJ et al (2013) Progressive brain changes in schizophrenia related to antipsychotic treatment? A meta-analysis of longitudinal MRI studies. Neurosci Biobehav Rev 37(8):1680–1691. https://doi.org/10.1016/j.neubiorev.2013.06.001

Chapter 11

Neuroimaging Methods for MRI Analysis in CSF Biomarkers Studies

Carles Falcon, Grégory Operto, José Luis Molinuevo, and Juan Domingo Gispert

Abstract

Among others, the existence of pathophysiological biomarkers such as cerebrospinal fluid (CSF) Aβ-42, t-tau, and p-tau preceding the onset of Alzheimer's disease (AD) symptomatology have shifted the conceptualization of AD as a *continuum*. In addition, magnetic resonance imaging (MRI) enables the study of structural and functional cross-sectional correlates and longitudinal changes in vivo and, therefore, the combination of CSF data and imaging analyses emerges as a synergistic approach to understand the structural correlates related with specific AD-related biomarkers. In this chapter, we describe the methods used in neuroimaging that will allow researchers to combine data on CSF metabolites with imaging analyses.

Key words Magnetic resonance imaging, ROI-based analysis, Voxel-based morphology, Diffusion Tensor Imaging, Structural and functional connectivity, Functional MRI, Imaging biomarkers, Alzheimer's disease

1 Introduction

A promising approach to increase the accuracy in the diagnosis of Alzheimer's disease (AD) and improve the prognosis of persons with cognitive decline or impairment is the use of AD cerebrospinal fluid (CSF) biomarkers [1]. Furthermore, as the well-established AD CSF biomarkers (Aβ-42, t-tau, and p-tau) represent proxies of pathology, they may be incorporated in research studies to know the underlying biology of a given cohort. An interest approach is combining several of them as a normalized index enabling researchers to study the AD *continuum* even in cross-sectional samples [2, 3]. On the other hand, analysis and interpretation of neuroimaging data are often carried out to investigate on intra-individual longitudinal changes and/or intersubject/group differences, in particular in the context of AD. Magnetic resonance imaging (MRI) allows the study of structural and functional cross-sectional correlates and longitudinal changes in vivo and, therefore, the

Robert Perneczky (ed.), *Biomarkers for Alzheimer's Disease Drug Development*, Methods in Molecular Biology, vol. 1750, https://doi.org/10.1007/978-1-4939-7704-8_11, © Springer Science+Business Media, LLC 2018

combination of CSF data and imaging analyses in AD research stands as a synergistic approach to understand the structural correlates related with specific disease-related biomarkers.

During the last decade, we have followed this approach for studying cerebral correlates of AD biomarkers along the disease *continuum*. In order to do it, the first step was to develop a normalized biomarker index, the AD CSF index, which allowed us to estimate the degree of pathology. This endorsed us to conclude that changes in different brain areas follow a nonlinear pattern along the AD *continuum* also occurring with different degrees of pathological load [4]. This approach also allowed us to study the impact of inflammation, through the study of astroglial and microglial markers, on the structure of the brain along the *continuum* [5, 6]. Furthermore, the use of different MRI sequences enables us not only to define macroscopic structural changes, but also to delve into the cerebral microstructure through Diffusion Tensor Imaging (DTI), which allows us to hypothesize on their physiopathology.

In this chapter, we describe the methods used in neuroimaging in order to combine data on CSF metabolites with imaging analyses. Specifically, we discuss different MRI analysis modalities which are as follows: (1) volumetric region of interest (ROI)-based analysis: As hypotheses are frequently stated in terms of brain structures or ROIs, ROI-based analysis allows to focus data analysis over a number of parcels with homogeneous characteristics; (2) voxel-based morphology (VBM): The aim of VBM is to assess for inter-group morphological differences using a voxel-by-voxel statistical analysis; (3) parametric maps from Diffusion Tensor Imaging (DTI): DTI has gained interest in AD for its ability to characterize white matter integrity; (4) structural and functional connectivity: Parametric maps give quantitative measures about white matter integrity but hides anatomical and topological information. With respect to this, recent tractography techniques are now able to extract models of the fiber tracts connecting nuclei of the central nervous system, giving detailed descriptions of the structural connectome and opening the way to their analysis at the group level; and (5) functional MRI (fMRI): The goal of fMRI is to detect the voxels in the brain related to the task the subject performs during the scanning time [7–9].

2 Materials

This section is organized as follows: First, a brief introduction on the different MRI modalities is presented. Then, the fundamental image processing tools are described. Finally, pipelines for typical neuroimaging analyses are presented.

2.1 Magnetic Resonance Imaging Modalities

MRI combines radiofrequency (RF) pulses and magnetic gradients to explore magnetic properties of tissues, such as the longitudinal (T1) and transversal (T2) magnetic relaxation times [10]. Each particular combination of RF pulses and gradients is referred to as MRI sequence, and provides different information about the morphology, physiology, and functionality of tissues [11]. The main sequences used in neuroimaging are three-dimensional T1-weighted structural images (3dT1w), BOLD-contrast images (fMRI), and Diffusion Tensor Imaging (DTI).

2.1.1 Three-Dimensional T1-Weighted (3dT1w) Images

A 3dT1w sequence provides detailed information about the morphology of the brain, offering a good contrast between gray and white matter. It accounts for differences in longitudinal relaxation parameter T1 across the brain (Fig. 1a). Analyses benefit from the voxel (contraction of "*volume*" and "*elements*") to be isotropic (i.e., with the same size in all three spatial directions). Voxel size depends on the scanner capability and the time to spend on the acquisition. Standard value ranges from 0.5 to 1.2 mm, and values tend to get lower as scanner technology improves. Other important parameters to be fixed are repetition time (TR), echo time (TE), inversion time (TI), and flip-angle. Their optimal values depend on the scanner and image resolution. The acquisition time extends from 3 to 9 min.

2.1.2 Blood Oxygen Level Dependent (BOLD) Contrast Imaging

The echo planar imaging (EPI) sequence is an ultrafast sequence that can be sensitive to the oxyhemoglobin–deoxyhemoglobin ratio in blood, the so-called blood-level oxygenation dependent (BOLD) signal, which is related to the brain function. Images are acquired while the subject is performing a cognitive-sensitive task (fMRI, functional MRI) or during a rest period (rs-fMRI, resting-

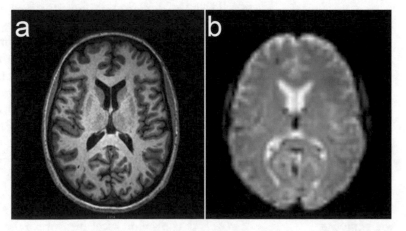

Fig. 1 Example of 3dT1w (**a**) and fMRI (**b**) images from the same subject

state functional MRI). Neural activation cannot be detected itself but its physiological effects: a local increase of perfusion, which does not entail an increase in oxygen consumption that produces a rise of the oxyhemoglobin–deoxyhemoglobin ratio, the so-called hemodynamic response function (HRF). The whole brain is scanned in 1–4 s (TR) (Fig. 1b). As the change in contrast due to brain activation is very low (below 3%), images are noisy and the intensity of each voxel also depends on other uncontrolled variables, several images have to be acquired (from 60 to few hundreds) during a scan period that ranges from 3 up to 30 min and posterior statistical analyses should be done to determine the voxels related to the brain function in study. Relevant acquisition parameters, apart from TR, are TE, flip-angle, voxel size, and slice thickness and inter-slice gap. To correct for geometrical distortion of EPI due to Eddy currents and field inhomogeneity related to different magnetic susceptibility of tissues, it is necessary to acquire a B0-map or few images with reverse phase encoding direction [12].

2.1.3 Diffusion Tensor Imaging (DTI)

DTI is a processed image derived from a T2-weighted image, referred to as b0 (Fig. 2a), and a set of diffusion-weighted images with the same geometrical prescription. Diffusion-weighted images are obtained by adding two opposite gradients between the magnetic excitation and the signal readout to the b0 image. The double gradient produces a drop of signal, with respect to b0 image, proportional to the amount of water diffusion in its direction (Fig. 2b). From DTI data can be derived various diffusivity parametric maps, e.g., mean diffusivity (MD) (Fig. 2c), radial diffusivity (RD), fractional anisotropy (FA) (Fig. 2d), and axial diffusivity (AD). These parameters measure specific microstructural alterations that are related to relevant biological factors such as cytotoxic edema (cell swelling) that is associated to restricted water diffusivity or demyelination (axonal loss) that reduces FA. On top of this, it must be noted that the direction of higher diffusion follows the main direction of the axons since myelin bands restrict diffusion across them. This property enables the tracking of white matter fibers in the so-called "fiber-tracking" (Fig. 2e) (see Note 1). The main acquisition parameters for DTI are TR, TE, flip-angle, voxel size (must be cubic with inter-slice gap zero to perform tractography), and the intensity of the diffusion weighting monitored by the parameter b. Like BOLD-contrast images, DTI is an EPI sequence. Therefore, B0-map or a b0 image with reverse phase encoding directions can be useful to correct for image distortion that highly improves the quality of the derived images.

2.2 Fundamental Neuroimaging Processing Tools

The raw signal in images is presented as a three-dimensional grid of voxels that provide local measures related to structure or function. Signal variations can be analyzed either at the region level or at the *voxel* level.

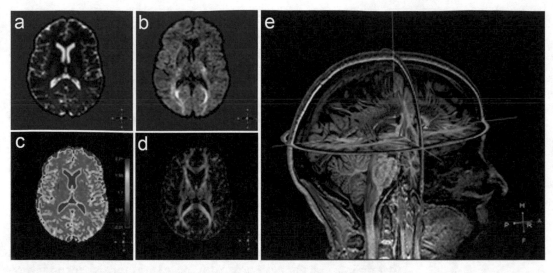

Fig. 2 b0 image (**a**), diffusion-weighted image (**b**), mean diffusivity map (**c**), fractional anisotropy map (**d**) from the same subject. Partial tractography of white matter bundles through corpus callosum and cortico-spinal path overlaid on a 3dT1w image (**e**)

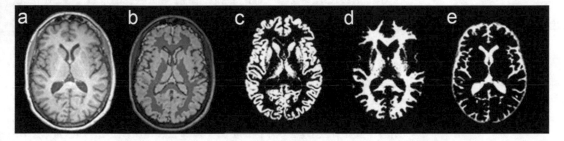

Fig. 3 Segmentation of a 3dT1w images (**a**): labeling voxels according their gray level and position in the brain (**b**), and creating a 0–1 tissue probabilistic map of GM (**c**), WM (**d**), and CSF (**e**)

2.2.1 Segmentation

Segmentation techniques are used to identify voxels that belong to the same tissue (typically, gray matter, white matter, and cerebrospinal fluid) or brain structure. By doing so, volume and other morphometric features of these tissues or structures can be obtained and analyzed. The partitioning of the voxels can be "hard" (i.e., each voxel is assigned a single label) or "probabilistic" (i.e., each voxel is assigned a probability of belonging to one label). Tissue probability maps are extracted from structural images by means of tissue segmentation algorithms. This step converts 3dT1w images, which have arbitrary units and scaling factor, to 0 to 1 maps (Fig. 3). Voxel values can be interpreted as the probability of the voxel belonging to the mapped tissue and account for its gray level, location, and partial volume effects (edge voxels containing more than one tissue). Sometimes, the outcome of the segmentation is the boundary separating the different tissues or brain regions. Segmentation algorithms may be specialized and focus on a specific structure or may cover a full range of regions (e.g., FSL, FreeSurfer, SPM, volBrain) and the nature of their results can vary from voxel-based clusters for volumetric structures to cortical surface 3d meshes or patches, fiber bundles, and cortical folds models, among many others. Resulting objects are likely to be closer to the individual anatomical truth, and by focusing on the signal of interest tend to improve sensitivity [13]. Depending on the accuracy of the method, this opens the way to shape analysis techniques or object-based morphometry as opposed to standard voxel-based methods. As a logical consequence, using individually segmented structures rather than warping data onto a reference atlas is advocated for the study of intersubject variability.

2.2.2 Coregistration and Spatial Normalization

Coregistration is the process of geometrically aligning two images: one is defined as the "target" or "reference" image (i.e., the one that defines the target geometrical space) and the other the "moving" image (i.e., the one that is going to be spatially transformed to be aligned with the target image). Depending on whether the two images belong to the same modality and/or subject different algorithms apply. The easiest situation is intersubject registration of images of the same modality. For instance, in fMRI acquisitions, slight head movements can be corrected using these techniques by aligning all the images in the series to the first or to the mean image. In these cases, the algorithm first estimates the "rigid" spatial transformation (three rotations and three displacements along the x, y, z directions) so that the matching of the two images is optimal. Then, two options are normally available: the moving image can be resampled to the voxel size and dimensions of the target image or the transformation can be stored in the header of the moving image for displaying purposes, but without altering the actual data in the images. Images of different modalities can also be aligned using multimodal registration techniques. A typical example would be to coregister a 3dT1w image with a PET image of the same individual. The first image conveys detailed structural information on the brain anatomy and the PET image provides the functional information.

Coregistration can also be performed between images of different individuals. Generally, this step is referred to as spatial normalization or warping, since the moving image needs to be distorted to match the target image. In spatial normalization, the target image is usually a "template," that is, a representative image, which can be provided by the normalization method or computed from the sample under study. On a first instance, spatial normalization enables the voxel-wise analysis of the images. Since individual morphological features are removed, the same anatomical locations fall into the same voxels and group comparisons or correlation analyses can be implemented without having to define regions of interest a priori. But spatial normalization techniques also enable morphometric studies by analyzing the different deformation fields that characterize the individual anatomy. Deformation fields establish a mapping between each voxel of the moving image to their corresponding location in the reference space. Therefore, they can be analyzed as three-dimensional mappings (i.e., tensor- or deformation-based morphometry) or a spatially varying scalar property of the deformation can be computed to drive the morphometric analysis. This is the case in voxel-based morphometry, where the relative changes in volume are computed by calculating the Jacobian determinants or the divergence of the individual deformation maps. Many normalization methods exist and differ in nature and degree of the applied spatial transformation. Many reference templates are also available; the mostly used is MNI stereotactic frame. Selecting the right one amounts to finding the most representative of the population under study, e.g., in the context of the aging brain [14]. Diffeomorphic transformations have been shown to provide the best performance among non-affine transformations [15].

The warping of images of different modalities across different individuals is not straightforward at all and does not constitute a typical requirement of brain image processing pipelines. Thus, it exceeds the scope of this chapter.

2.2.3 Smoothing and Denoising

Smoothing solves three problems. First, it reduces noise and increases the correlation across neighboring voxels. From the physiological point of view, it makes no sense one voxel showing a significant difference and not the surrounding ones. There is an implicit prior that involved brain areas should have a minimum extension. Secondly, it makes the information on the voxels being slightly expanded to ensure certain degree of interaction of misaligned voxels due to subtle normalization inaccuracies. Third, the main one, it ensures parametric statistics can be applied in the voxel-based statistical analysis. Under certain assumptions, not always verified, a smoothed map behaves as a Gaussian Field, and, then, Random Field Theory can be used to determine statistical thresholds of significance.

MR images come with signal properties/quality that depend on the type and parameters of the acquisition sequence. Some algorithms are efficient at improving the signal-to-noise ratio of the images, and as such form part of the analysis pipeline as standard preprocessing steps. Such techniques generally rely on a distribution model of the noise (e.g., Rician) and apply corrections based on the information found either locally around every voxel [16] or on similar patches elsewhere in the image [17].

3 Methods

3.1 Region of Interest (ROI)-Based Volumetric Analysis

ROI-based analysis allows focusing the analysis over a number of parcels with homogeneous characteristics. ROIs are thus often defined over anatomical data and then used to filter the signal from other modalities.

Two approaches are generally available, as two opposite ways of addressing the core obstacle represented by anatomical variability. The first one consists in warping all the subjects to a common reference space and using ROIs defined from a brain atlas (*see* **Note 2**). The other one consists in delineating ROIs individually in every subject, e.g., using segmentation algorithms. Countless methods are able to perform automatic or semiautomatic segmentation of an exhaustive variety of brain structures, which may then be used as ROIs on any individual data. The following section gives a template of a standard ROI-based analysis workflow.

3.1.1 ROI-Based Analysis Using an Atlas

- Coregister the image of interest (image modality, parametric map) with a structural image (3dT1w) for every subject.

- Perform spatial normalization on every subject's 3dT1w, save the registration parameters, and calculate the inverse transformation. Select a brain atlas of ROIs in standard space matching the interest of the study and apply the *inverse* transformation to the brain atlas in order to warp the atlas to the subject's native space.

- Alternatively to **step 2**, select a segmentation method of a specific or a variety of structure(s) and run it on every subject's anatomy to obtain subject-matched ROIs.

- Alternatively to **steps 2** and **3**, perform the spatial normalization and apply the parameters to the image of interest to match it to the atlas in the standard space.

- Extract numerical features from every ROI over every image of interest in the subject's native space.

- Perform statistical analyses on these features.

3.1.2 Alternatives

It is possible also to perform shape and other geometrical property analyses of regions themselves, not on their content [18].

3.2 Voxel-Based Morphology (VBM)

Prior to statistical analysis, images should be processed to normalize their intensity (tissue segmentation), and morphometry (spatial normalization) and to ensure parametric statistics could be applied (smoothing). Preprocessing steps are slightly different for cross-sectional and longitudinal studies.

3.2.1 Cross-sectional VBM Processing Pipeline

1. Segmentation of 3dT1w image in tissues: Gray matter (GM), white mater (WM), and cerebrospinal fluid (CSF) maps and, optionally, others.

2. Spatial normalization of tissue maps.

3. Normalized maps are multiplied by the Jacobian determinant of the spatial normalization (modulation), which encodes the differences of volume on the original images as differences on intensity on normalized images.

4. Smoothing images by convolution with a Gaussian kernel. The standard range of size of the kernel is 6–12 mm FWHM (Full Width at Half Maximum).

3.2.2 Longitudinal Studies Processing Pipeline

- Linear and nonlinear registration of pre and post images. Linear registration helps nonlinear registration to converge. Nonlinear registration results in the pre-post average, Jacobian determinant (JD) (or alternatively divergence of deformations) images.

- Pre-post average images are segmented.

- From GM, WM, and CSF maps the subject's GM/WM mask (depending on the tissue in study) is obtained by selecting those voxels whose probability of belonging to GM/WM is bigger to the probability of being part of any other tissue.

- GM/WM mask are applied to JD map.

- Spatial normalization of average images is performed. The modulation of spatial normalization to template is not applied to avoid mixing cross and longitudinal effects.

- Smoothing of normalized JD images with a 6–12 mm FWHM Gaussian Kernel.

3.2.3 Getting Statistical Mappings

Once preprocessed, the proper statistical test to accept or reject the hypothesis in study is performed voxel by voxel (Fig. 4a) resulting in a statistical parametric map (T or F value for all the voxels on analysis). After choosing a statistical criterion to determine what difference is considered as significant (Fig. 4b), surviving voxels can be overlaid to an anatomical template or an anatomically labeled atlas to report the affected regions (Fig. 4c). It is important to note the high risk of false positives, due to massive number of analyses, and the way to deal with it.

3.2.4 Alternatives

There are several other alternative analyses of 3dT1w images, for instance, cortical thickness analysis [19], shape analysis of substructures [18, 20], analysis of sulci [21] or machine learning and other multivariate methods [22, 23].

3.3 Parametric Diffusion Tensor Imaging (DTI) Analysis

The typical workflow includes the processing in parallel of DTI data and 3dT1w images. 3dT1w images provide structural anatomical resolution at a higher resolution than DTI and therefore are used both for intersubject normalization and by some methods to guide the processing of DTI data. Yet some integrated software

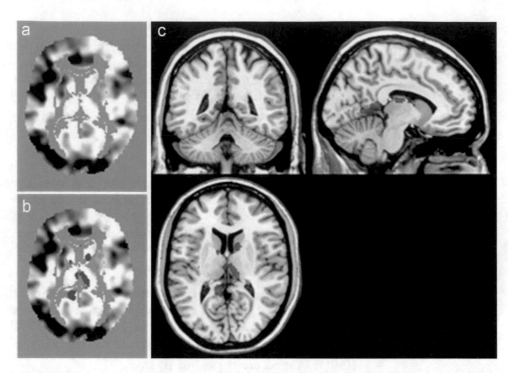

Fig. 4 Statistical parametric map of a voxel-wise T-test (T-value of the T-test performed voxel by voxel) (**a**), significant voxels in red (T-value over the statistical threshold of significance) (**b**), and overlaid of significant areas over a 3dT1w image as reference (**c**)

solutions, e.g., TBSS (Tract-Based Spatial Statistics) from FSL toolbox drive the intersubject spatial matching based on pure DTI data and rely on no other modality. In particular, this approach applies nonlinear registration across subjects on diffusion data and then perform a group-level analysis along skeletons modeling the main fiber tracts [24].

3.3.1 Preprocessing and Generation of Parametric Maps from DTI Data

1. Apply denoising algorithm on both the 3dT1w and the DTI data, e.g., a nonlocal means (NL-means) Rician denoising method on all DTI and 3dT1w to increase image quality.

2. Apply bias correction on 3dT1w.

3. Apply eddy current correction to adjust the DTI data for distortion and motion using affine registration to the non-weighted diffusion volume (B0 map).

4. Run model estimation on corrected DTI data. This will generate red-green-blue (RGB) color-coded maps showing diffusion local directions as well as maps of the first eigenvalues of every local model.

5. Generate parametric maps MD, FA, RD, and AD obtained from the local combination of the various eigenvalues.

3.3.2 Spatial Normalization Through Anatomical Images and Statistical Analyses

The following part of the workflow warps every subject into a normalized space to then allow an exploratory whole-brain voxel-level group analysis. Anatomical normalization is applied to all subjects' anatomical data (e.g., 3dT1w). This solves the core problem of localization [25] and spatial correspondence between subjects at the cost of geometric distortion. A number of reference templates or atlases are available. Selecting the right one amounts to finding the most representative of the population under study, e.g., in the context of the aging brain [14]. As a result of this step combined by the previous one, DTI data undergo a two-step transformation, first from native DTI space to the subject's 3dT1w space, then from the subject's 3dT1w space to reference space (*see* Subheading 3.2 for this last step).

1. Perform a segmentation task to extract the brain mask out from the b0 image.

2. Perform a segmentation task to extract a mask of the white matter from the b0 image.

3. Repeat these two operations on the 3dT1w to get a brain mask and a white matter mask map from 3dT1w.

4. Apply coregistration from the b0-image white matter mask to the 3dT1w white matter mask and save registration parameters.

5. Apply transformation to every parametric map using these same registration parameters in order to warp it to the 3dT1w space.

6. Normalize 3dT1w as described in Subheading 3.2 and apply the transformation to DTI maps.

7. Standard ROI-based analyses are applicable from this step on. It is also possible to run a voxel-based statistical analysis on every set of smoothed normalized parametric maps (FA, MD, RD, AD), e.g., based on General Linear Models using the standard Statistical Parametric Mapping software for neuroimaging.

3.4 Structural Connectivity

Structural connectivity between cortical areas and subcortical structures can be represented as a non-oriented graph made of nodes (i.e., the whole set of areas and structures) and edges (i.e., connections, or the absence thereof, between two areas/structures) with a weight measuring the strength of connection (i.e., in numbers of fibers) between any two nodes. Such a graph has an equivalent matrix representation, called adjacency matrix in graph theory, and connectivity matrix in the neuroimaging context (Fig. 5). The first step consists in generating parametric maps, which was described in Subheading 3.3. In this context actually, parametric maps are essentially used for quality assurance purposes after the preprocessing steps. The following pipeline describes how to achieve a structural connectivity analysis using tractography and automatic segmentation of anatomical structures:

1. Generate parametric maps (FA maps in particular) for every subject in their native DTI space, following Subheading 3.3.

2. Visually inspect FA and RGB maps for quality control. This step is crucial to ensure the right orientations of the fibers and possibly spot errors in the gradients used for the modeling. It is especially recommended to check for any possible axis swap from one subject to another.

3. Run anatomical segmentation pipeline on every subject's anatomy. Maps of the interface between gray and white matter (GM maps) and/or CSF are generally helpful to create constraints and boundaries for the tractography. A large variety of algorithmic tools provide such representations as segmentation maps or triangulated meshes. Besides, any other segmented structure may be used as a *seed* by the tractography step. Such seeds correspond to ROIs from/to which the streamlines will start/end, be either cortical or subcortical structures. The resulting information about structural connectivity hence depends on the definition of such cortical or subcortical ROIs to be taken as nodes of the connectome.

4. Check the quality of the resulting segmentation maps by overlaying these over the subject's anatomy.

5. Warp the segmentation maps (GM, CSF, and *seeds*) to the subject's DTI space using the same 3dT1w-to-b0 image coregistration parameters estimated during the prior generation of parametric maps (Fig. 5a).

6. Run the tractography step taking the segmentation map as *seed map* to generate both the streamline tracks and the connectivity matrix. Provide GM and CSF masks as constraints to guide the process (fibers do not cross the ventricles or sulci) (Fig. 5b).

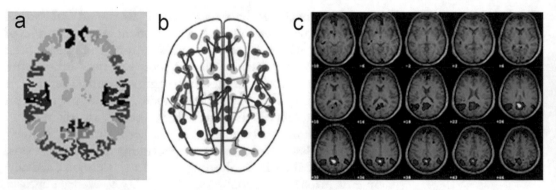

Fig. 5 Atlas adapted to the subject's anatomy (**a**), structural connectivity graph (**b**), and map of regions correlated with precuneus in a resting-state functional connectivity study (**c**)

7. Estimate a connectivity matrix with respect to the ROIs used as *seeds*, measuring the number of existing connecting fibers for each pair. According to the study and the corresponding ROIs, the matrix hence describes cortico-cortical and/or cortico-subcortical connections. It may be symmetrical, of size the number of seed regions: in this case each row/column would give the estimated numbers of connections from every seed to any other.

8. Perform statistical analysis on the connectivity matrices. Statistical analysis can be performed at the group level over the entire set of matrices once estimated for every subject. It is important to check for normality in order to properly apply parametric or nonparametric statistical tests.

3.5 Functional Connectivity (fMRI)

fMRI preprocessing pipeline is different in fMRI and rs-fMRI studies. fMRI requires a model of the expected activation pattern (task/stimulus onset and duration convolved with the HRF) and to check, voxel by voxel, if temporal variations of intensity are independent (random/physiological) or related to the task. rs-fMRI looks for inter-region correlations of the spurious activity of the brain when no specific task is performed.

3.5.1 Processing fMRI

1. If available, BOLD images are corrected for EPI distortions.

2. The set of fMRI-volumes are aligned to correct for involuntary small movements during the acquisition. The mean image of the fMRI series is created.

3. Mean fMRI image is registered to structural anatomical image 3dT1w and the transformation is applied to the rest of volumes.

4. 3dT1w images are spatially normalized to a standard template (mainly in MNI stereotactic space) using affine and non-affine transformations. fMRI are spatially normalized by applying the transformation calculated during the 3dT1w spatial normalization.

5. fMRI are smoothed with a Gaussian filter (6–12 mm FWHM kernel).

6. GLM statistical analyses are performed to check voxel by voxel if its temporal evolution is related to the model. GLM results in a statistical parametric mapping (T-value voxel by voxel) that provides activated areas once a proper statistical threshold is applied.

3.5.2 Processing of rs-fMRI

It is not as fixed as in fMRI. Depending on the images characteristics and the posterior statistical analyses to be performed, it could be convenient to add, suppress, or change the order of the steps to get more reliable results. Next, a standard pipeline is shown

- Slice-timing correction (*see* **Note 3**).

- Correction for EPI distortions, realign of time series, register to 3dT1w and spatially normalization, as done in fMRI.

- Detection of outliers, bad volumes or dark slices, due to sudden movements of the subject during the exploration (due to cough, for instance).

- Detrending the time series (up to third-order polynomials) to flattener the base line and to make next step more efficient.

- Regress out the mean WM and CSF signal, the values obtained in the realign procedure (three rotations and three translations for each volume to correct for involuntary head movements during the scanning time), the mean value of the image (optional), and the nulling regressors to avoid the effect of the outliers [26].

- Smoothing of images with a Gaussian Kernel of 8–12 mm (FWHM).

- Band-pass filtering images to remove non-relevant intensity variations. The frequencies of interest, from the physiological point of view, are in the range of 0.1–0.01 Hz. Each study can use customized cutoff frequencies to select the appropriate information to answer specific questions.

- Voxel-based analysis of functional connectivity, i.e., determination of functional networks of areas of the brain working conjointly, requires the selection of the area (ROI) whose functional connectivity is investigated, to take the mean value of the image and evaluate the correlation, voxel by voxel, the correlation of its time series with the ROI time series (first-order analysis, seed-based connectivity) (Fig. 5c).

3.5.3 Second-Order Statistics, Group Comparison

Both fMRI and seed-based functional connectivity studies allow a second-order analysis to determine differences of statistical maps between groups. The main second-order analysis is the random effects analysis (RFX) (*see* **Note 4**).

3.5.4 Functional Connectivity

Alternatively, GM can be parceled as described previously. Then, the correlation of the temporal series of each ROI with the rest of ROI's time series will result in a functional connectivity matrix for each subject [27]. Fisher transformation is used to convert correlation coefficients to z-scores to make possible the parametric statistical analysis of functional connectivity matrices between groups (*see* **Note 5**).

3.5.5 Alternatives

There are alternatives to fMRI analyses, mainly the free-model multivariate analyses such as principal component analysis (PCA) and independent component analysis (ICA). Functional connectivity can be also assessed by alternative analyses such as matching learning or neural networks methods [28].

4 Notes

1. Tractography techniques produce streamlines paths that model anatomical tracts found in the white matter. The validation of these (millions of) streamlines is a tough problem due to factors such as the difficult access to ground truth or some complex patterns, e.g., fanning and crossing fibers. White matter tractography is generally done either with a method known as "deterministic" tractography or with a "probabilistic" method. Advantages of the probabilistic method include the ability to explicitly represent uncertainty in the data and a higher reliable reconstruction of crossing fibers at higher computational costs [29]. In both approaches, prior knowledge of the anatomy of fiber tracts is important for distinguishing between fiber tracts of interest and streamline tracks that follow improbable routes or suggest nonexistent connections between brain areas.

2. In this context, *brain atlases* come into play to provide a set of ROIs that cover the brain volume. However, an atlas provides regions that generally account for a certain state of the current knowledge while the targeted effect of the study might not fit the grain of the atlas ROIs. Moreover, an atlas is constructed and used to represent a certain population, therefore possibly failing at capturing individual anatomical traits. The most widely used atlas is AAL [30].

3. Statistical analyses require each volume to be scanned at once, in the same time point. However, slices are acquired sequentially and in an interleaved way. Slices-timing correction uses temporal interpolation to guess the slice intensity as it was acquired at the same time of a reference slice. It is necessary to know the order of slice acquisition beforehand.

4. RFX performs voxel-by-voxel analyses on contrast images (difference of intensity among rest and activation in fMRI and degree of correlation in rs-fMRI) with the hypothesis that, if the difference in a voxel is random (false positive) it would not appear in the other subjects and the mean value among subjects should tend to zero. If the mean value of the contrast in one voxel is significantly different from zero, it can be concluded that there is an effect of interest. The surrounding hypothesis is that all subjects use the same network (strategy) to perform the cognitive task. It is fundamentally a good experiment design to ensure that it happens.

5. It is important to note that both signal and noise can be correlated. Image artifacts can derive in great correlations values that don't reveal real functional connectivity. A good quality assurance of rs-fMRI images is mandatory to get reliable functional matrices [31, 32].

5   Conclusions

Neuroimaging techniques are increasingly being used in scientific areas (epidemiology, population genetics, etc.) other than the traditional research fields where they used to play a central role (neurology, psychiatry, neuroscience, etc.). Noteworthy, these research fields are characterized by conducting research in much larger sample sizes. This interest has fostered the use of neuroimaging-derived outcome variables, neuroimaging modalities, and analytical methods. It has also spurred the development of technological solutions for acquiring, storing, transferring, analyzing, and sharing large neuroimaging datasets. Neuroimaging analysis is a highly "technified" field with analytical tools and software suites that have been developed and used for decades, which have created their own scientific environments and user communities. It falls beyond the scope of this text to recommend any of the publicly available tools for a particular application or to perform a detailed analysis of their characteristics. On the other hand, we intended to present and describe the most common image processing tools and pipelines for investigators from outside the neuroimaging field to better understand the way images are processed and analyzed and common pitfalls and limitations in neuroimaging analyses.

In this regard, we would like to put the emphasis on three aspects: (1) knowing what the "hidden" algorithms do is critical to correctly interpret has the results, (2) quality control of the images is mandatory, and (3) pitfalls and limitations in the statistical analysis of neuroimages.

It is necessary to have an intimate understanding the image processing tools in order to correctly interpret the results of a neuroimaging analysis. Even though the neuroimaging software tools are progressively easier to use, the implications of the technical underpinnings of the underlying algorithms are critical to understand the scope and limitations of the results. For this reason, we intentionally avoided to take one particular neuroimaging analysis suite and provide step-by-step instructions to make typical analyses. Novel users may find several of these "recipes" online. On the other hand, we intended to present the rationale under some standard pipelines for novel users to better understand neuroimaging results on their labs and/or on the literature. For instance in VBM analyses, knowing whether images have been modulated to code for changes in volume, whether the modulation takes into account global brain volume or it has to be regressed out in the design matrix or the way variance is partitioned in a design matrix where columns are orthogonalized to the previous ones are common examples that have triggered endless discussions, even among experts. All the major neuroimaging platforms have supporting forums that gather users and developers. In case of doubt, it is strongly recommended to resort to these forums. Even in the event of not having any concerns on a particular study, regular consultation of these forums may help identifying pitfalls in our own analyses.

State-of-the-art automatic imaging processing tools are highly robust and refined. However, users have to be aware that there is no guarantee that the result of the processing will be of sufficient quality for the ensuing analysis. Therefore, quality control of the raw and intermediate images is mandatory. Unfortunately, the development of quality control tools has not received the same amount of attention as that of novel analytical or processing tools. Development of aids to streamline the quality control of the images and the adoption of common quality control standards are impending needs to improve the reproducibility of neuroimaging results. Examples in the good direction are quantitative quality control tools and metrics developed for monitoring raw images on the XNAT platform (http://cbs.fas.harvard.edu/science/core-facilities/neuroimaging/information-investigators/qc) or, for processed images, the Quality Assessment (QA) tool in the Computational Anatomy Toolbox for SPM (http://www.neuro.uni-jena.de/cat/index.html#QA).

Of course, a preliminary consideration is the detection of any incidental findings that may constitute exclusion criteria for the study or compromise the correct processing or analysis of the image. Depending on the age, the acquired image modalities, and other clinical characteristics of the study participants, a significant percentage of incidental findings have been reported in the literature even when scanning asymptomatic individuals and up to 15% of them may actually require referral for clinical follow-up [33]. In this regard, neuroradiological review of all the images should be mandatory but, unfortunately, it is not as commonly performed for research studies as it probably should.

Finally, voxel-wise statistical analysis of neuroimages present with some limitations that are important to bear in mind for interpreting our own results or those in the literature. The most notorious pitfall is the multiple comparisons problem. Typically, an unbiased, whole-brain voxel-wise analysis simultaneously tests hundreds of thousands of voxels. In this scenario, the probability of detecting some false positives is almost certain. However, some features in the images alleviate this situation. First, neighboring voxels present with very similar information that originally stem from the inherent limitation of the spatial extent of the homologies that can be established between the brain anatomies of different individuals. Based on this assumption, spatial normalization algorithms implement regularization terms that penalize gross fine-detail deformations, and smoothing algorithms are applied to remove high spatial frequency noise while not affecting the signal to the same extent. The correlation observed among neighboring voxels make the Bonferroni correction far too conservative for neuroimaging analyses and several methods have been developed to estimate the actual number of independent observations in the images, taking into account the cumulative effect of all preprocessing steps. Please note that the degree of smoothing in the preprocessing step will have a critical impact on this estimation and, hence, on the corrected p-value of the analysis. Larger smoothing kernels result in more significant corrected p-values at the cost of decreased sensitivity to detect small-localized effects. Therefore, a tradeoff between statistical power and the spatial resolution of the analysis is inherently being performed. However, even though the impact on the expected number of false positives under the null hypothesis is estimated by the multiple comparison correction, the loss of sensitivity to detect regionally small effects is only controlled indirectly through the size of the smoothing kernel as no Type-II error (false negative) estimation is typically performed. In addition, it is common to establish a minimum cluster size in order for a positive result to be considered as significant. Several of these strategies have been put into question recently [34], but it must be noted that the major neuroimaging analysis suites have improved their methods accordingly. Some of them implement Monte-Carlo permutation strategies that minimize the assumptions in the correction for multiple comparisons.

Other general statistical considerations are also prominent sources of worry in the analyses of neuroimages: dealing with outliers, overfitting, highly correlated predictor variables, the impact of the order of their inclusion and the way that different software packages deal with this situation, etc. In this regard, it must be noted that neuroimaging analysis packages are generally not equipped with diagnostic tools to neither check the validity of the statistical assumptions nor implement nonparametric alternatives in the event that these are not met in certain cases. They do not include either tools to estimate the attained statistical power of the analysis.

In conclusion, neuroimaging analysis suites provide with an armory of state-of-the-art tools to render high-quality and reliable data and analyses. Their continuous development and testing by thousands of researches over the last decades result in extremely robust open-source algorithms and highly specialized user communities that welcome and are eager to help novel users. In addition, the standardization of the major processing steps, analytical criteria, and even algorithmic implementations has a positive impact on the comparability of different studies. Since the analysis can be scripted, source data and analytical methods can be stored for future reference or shared with the community for additional analyses and meta-analyses. Together with publicly available datasets, enabling the access of proprietary data together with the scripts used for attaining published results greatly contribute to enhance the reproducibility of neuroimaging research. No particular analytical platform or algorithm can be regarded as superior to the rest in general terms, and comparison studies are required to rationally selecting one implementation for a particular application. Overall, users should be aware of the implications and limitations of the different processing and analysis options for a correct interpretation of their own results and that of the existing literature.

References

1. Balasa M, Sánchez-Valle R, Antonell A et al (2014) Usefulness of biomarkers in the diagnosis and prognosis of early-onset cognitive impairment. J Alzheimers Dis 40:919–927. https://doi.org/10.3233/JAD-132195

2. Molinuevo JL, Gispert JD, Dubois B et al (2013) The AD-CSF-index discriminates Alzheimer's disease patients from healthy controls: a validation study. J Alzheimers Dis 36:67–77. https://doi.org/10.3233/JAD-130203

3. Struyfs H, Molinuevo JL, Martin J-J et al (2014) Validation of the AD-CSF-index in autopsy-confirmed Alzheimer's disease patients and healthy controls. J Alzheimers Dis 41:903–909. https://doi.org/10.3233/JAD-131085

4. Gispert JD, Rami L, Sánchez-Benavides G et al (2015) Nonlinear cerebral atrophy patterns across the Alzheimer's disease continuum: impact of APOE4 genotype. Neurobiol Aging 36:2687–2701. https://doi.org/10.1016/j.neurobiolaging.2015.06.027

5. Gispert JD, Monté GC, Suárez-Calvet M et al (2017) The APOE ε4 genotype modulates CSF YKL-40 levels and their structural brain correlates in the continuum of Alzheimer's disease but not those of sTREM2. Alzheimers Dement 6:50–59. https://doi.org/10.1016/j.dadm.2016.12.002

6. Gispert JD, Suárez-Calvet M, Monté GC et al (2016) Cerebrospinal fluid sTREM2 levels are associated with gray matter volume increases and reduced diffusivity in early Alzheimer's disease. Alzheimers Dement 12:1259–1272. https://doi.org/10.1016/j.jalz.2016.06.005

7. Friston KJ et al (2007) Statistical parametric mapping : the analysis of funtional brain images. Elsevier/Academic Press, Cambridge. Print. ISBN: 9780123725608

8. Mazziotta JC, Toga AW (2002) Brain mapping: the methods. Academic, New York

9. Toga AW, Mazziotta JC (2000) Brain mapping: the systems, vol 2. Academic, New York

10. Stark DD, Bradley WG (1999) Magnetic resonance imaging. Mosby, Maryland Heights

11. Bernstein MA, King KE, Zhou XJ, Fong W (2005) Handbook of MRI pulse sequences. Med Phys 32. https://doi.org/10.1118/1.1904597

12. Hutton C, Bork A, Josephs O et al (2002) Image distortion correction in fMRI: a quantitative evaluation. NeuroImage 16:217–240. https://doi.org/10.1006/nimg.2001.1054

13. Mangin JF, Rivière D, Cachia A et al (2004) Object-based morphometry of the cerebral cortex. IEEE Trans Med Imaging 23:968–982

14. Samanez-Larkin GR, D'Esposito M (2008) Group comparisons: imaging the aging brain. Soc Cogn Affect Neurosci 3:290–297. https://doi.org/10.1093/scan/nsn029

15. Klein A, Andersson J, Ardekani BA et al (2009) Evaluation of 14 nonlinear deformation algorithms applied to human brain MRI registration. NeuroImage 46:786–802. https://doi.org/10.1016/j.neuroimage.2008.12.037

16. Manjón JV, Coupé P, Concha L et al (2013) Diffusion weighted image denoising using overcomplete local PCA. PLoS One 8:e73021. https://doi.org/10.1371/journal.pone.0073021

17. Coupe P, Yger P, Prima S et al (2008) An optimized blockwise nonlocal means denoising filter for 3-D magnetic resonance images. IEEE Trans Med Imaging 27:425–441. https://doi.org/10.1109/TMI.2007.906087

18. Scher AI, Xu Y, Korf ESC et al (2007) Hippocampal shape analysis in Alzheimer's disease: a population-based study. NeuroImage 36:8–18. https://doi.org/10.1016/j.neuroimage.2006.12.036

19. Fischl B (2012) FreeSurfer. NeuroImage 62:774–781. https://doi.org/10.1016/j.neuroimage.2012.01.021

20. Tondelli M, Wilcock GK, Nichelli P et al (2012) Structural MRI changes detectable up

to ten years before clinical Alzheimer's disease. Neurobiol Aging 33:825.e25–825.e36. https://doi.org/10.1016/j.neurobiolaging.2011.05.018

21. Rametti G, Junqué C, Bartrés-Faz D et al (2010) Anterior cingulate and paracingulate sulci morphology in patients with schizophrenia. Schizophr Res 121:66–74. https://doi.org/10.1016/j.schres.2010.05.016

22. Habeck CG (2010) Basics of multivariate analysis in neuroimaging data. J Vis Exp:1–6. https://doi.org/10.3791/1988

23. Ziegler G, Dahnke R, Gaser C (2012) Models of the aging brain structure and individual decline. Front Neuroinform 6:3. https://doi.org/10.3389/fninf.2012.00003

24. Smith SM, Jenkinson M, Johansen-Berg H et al (2006) Tract-based spatial statistics: voxelwise analysis of multi-subject diffusion data. NeuroImage 31:1487–1505. https://doi.org/10.1016/j.neuroimage.2006.02.024

25. Devlin JT, Poldrack RA (2007) In praise of tedious anatomy. NeuroImage 37:1033–1041. https://doi.org/10.1016/j.neuroimage.2006.09.055

26. Lemieux L, Salek-Haddadi A, Lund TE et al (2007) Modelling large motion events in fMRI studies of patients with epilepsy. Magn Reson Imaging 25:894–901. https://doi.org/10.1016/j.mri.2007.03.009

27. KR a VD, Hedden T, Venkataraman A et al (2010) Intrinsic functional connectivity as a tool for human connectomics: theory, properties, and optimization. J Neurophysiol 103:297–321. https://doi.org/10.1152/jn.00783.2009

28. Mourão-Miranda J, Bokde ALW, Born C et al (2005) Classifying brain states and determining the discriminating activation patterns: Support Vector Machine on functional MRI data. NeuroImage 28:980–995. https://doi.org/10.1016/j.neuroimage.2005.06.070

29. Hagler DJ, Ahmadi ME, Kuperman J et al (2009) Automated white-matter tractography using a probabilistic diffusion tensor atlas: application to temporal lobe epilepsy. Hum Brain Mapp 30:1535–1547. https://doi.org/10.1002/hbm.20619

30. Tzourio-Mazoyer N, Landeau B, Papathanassiou D et al (2002) Automated anatomical labeling of activations in SPM using a macroscopic anatomical parcellation of the MNI MRI single-subject brain. NeuroImage 15:273–289. https://doi.org/10.1006/nimg.2001.0978

31. KR a v D, Sabuncu MR, Buckner RL (2012) The influence of head motion on intrinsic functional connectivity MRI. NeuroImage 59:431–438. https://doi.org/10.1016/j.neuroimage.2011.07.044

32. Cole (2010) Advances and pitfalls in the analysis and interpretation of resting-state FMRI data. Front Syst Neurosci. https://doi.org/10.3389/fnsys.2010.00008

33. Brugulat-Serrat A, Rojas S, Bargalló N et al (2017) Incidental findings on brain MRI of cognitively normal first-degree descendants of patients with Alzheimer's disease: a cross-sectional analysis from the ALFA (Alzheimer and Families) project. BMJ Open 7:e013215. https://doi.org/10.1136/bmjopen-2016-013215

34. Eklund A, Nichols TE, Knutsson H (2016) Cluster failure: why fMRI inferences for spatial extent have inflated false-positive rates. Proc Natl Acad Sci U S A 113:7900–7905. https://doi.org/10.1073/pnas.1602413113

Chapter 12

Hybrid PET-MRI in Alzheimer's Disease Research

Ismini C. Mainta, Maria I. Vargas, Sara Trombella, Giovanni B. Frisoni, Paul G. Unschuld, and Valentina Garibotto

Abstract

Multiple factors, namely amyloid, tau, inflammation, metabolic, and perfusion changes, contribute to the cascade of neurodegeneration and functional decline occurring in Alzheimer's disease (AD). These molecular and cellular processes and related functional and morphological changes can be visualized in vivo by two imaging modalities, namely positron emission tomography (PET) and magnetic resonance imaging (MRI). These imaging biomarkers are now part of the diagnostic algorithm and of particular interest for patient stratification and targeted drug development.

In this field the availability of hybrid PET/MR systems not only offers a comprehensive evaluation in a single imaging session, but also opens new possibilities for the integration of the two imaging information. Here, we cover the clinical protocols and practical details of FDG, amyloid, and tau PET/MR imaging as applied in our institutions.

Key words PET-MRI, Hybrid imaging, Amyloid, FDG, Tau, fMRI

---

1 Introduction

In the current view, the etiology of Alzheimer's disease (AD) is the result of multiple molecular and cellular factors contributing to a cascade of phenomena leading to neurodegeneration, dysfunction, and finally cell death, exceeding compensatory mechanisms and finally reaching the clinical expression of dementia. These multiple processes, namely the molecular hallmarks of AD, amyloid and tau deposition, are the target of experimental drugs tested in number of clinical trials under way.

This field has been significantly impacted by the availability of biomarkers able to measure directly or indirectly these molecular processes in vivo. Indeed, in the first amyloid-targeting trials, the inclusion criteria based solely on a clinical diagnosis of probable AD had insufficient specificity, with over 20% of the subjects treated lacking amyloid pathology. Currently, all trials targeting the synthesis, accumulation or removal of amyloid, use a biomarker of

Robert Perneczky (ed.), *Biomarkers for Alzheimer's Disease Drug Development*, Methods in Molecular Biology, vol. 1750,
https://doi.org/10.1007/978-1-4939-7704-8_12, © Springer Science+Business Media, LLC 2018

amyloidosis as inclusion criteria. Clinical trials are also increasingly introducing biomarkers as secondary outcome, as a measure of target engagement and possibly of biological efficacy. This second use requires specific quantitative approaches, guaranteeing that the biomarker accuracy is not biased by the treatment itself.

Among AD biomarkers, imaging, namely magnetic resonance imaging (MRI) and positron emission tomography (PET), play a pivotal role. MRI is characterized by high soft tissue contrast, which in addition to a qualitative analysis, also allows good distinction between the different cerebral structures and therefore quantification of the cerebral cortex thickness as well as the volume of most cerebral structures. This is an interesting feature in this type of diseases because localized atrophy can be detected in earlier stages and compared with functional information from PET. Furthermore, longitudinal studies of each patient's cerebral volume are made possible.

Currently, sequences such as MP2RAGE can provide a morphometric analysis of the brain in the form of an automatic morphometric report with the volume of all cerebral structures [1, 2]. Other sequences such as 3DT1 also allow a quantitative analysis but they are not automatic and require post-processing.

As for molecular PET imaging, various tracers have been and are still being developed, approaching in vivo from every angle, the issue of neurodegeneration. The most common radiopharmaceutical used in daily practice is 18-Fluoro-2-deoxy-glucose (FDG), an analogue of glucose, the main energy substrate of the brain. Brain glucose metabolism is tightly connected to synaptic activity and integrity [3]. Furthermore, it has been shown that amyloid-β, a hallmark of AD, is a competitive inhibitor of insulin binding and action [4], which may place the reduced metabolism in an even earlier step of the degeneration cascade.

Extracellular neuritic amyloid plaques and intraneuronal hyperphosphorylated tau neurofibrillary tangles are the basis of the two main causative hypotheses, and both can nowadays be imaged in vivo.

Three tracers are currently FDA- and EMA-approved for the assessment of the density and distribution of amyloid plaques, with sensitivities and specificities above 90%, validated against postmortem pathology: 18F-florbetapir (18F-AV-45), 18F-flutemetamol, and 18F-florbetaben (18F-AV-1).

Although a negative scan has high diagnostic value, reducing the likelihood of having AD as the underlying pathology, a positive scan does not establish the diagnosis of AD, as amyloid neuritic plaques are present in normal older people and in other neurologic conditions as well.

Tau PET imaging is still in a phase of development, with a few tracers currently evaluated in clinical cohorts. Their sensitivity, specificity, and affinity profile for the different tau isoforms, as well as the affinity for β-amyloid, α-synuclein [5], and other off-target binding, such as MAO inhibitors [6], are still to be validated. 18-F-FDDNP lacks of selectivity, showing Aβ and α-synuclein binding as well. 11-C-PPB3 apart from a light-sensitive labeling with the short-lived 11C (half-life 20 min), which limits its widespread use, it has been shown to convert in vivo into a blood–brain crossing radiometabolite. 18-F-THK523, 18-F-THK5105, and 18-F-THK5117 demonstrated in vitro high affinity and specificity for tau binding in AD patients, but high white matter retention and variable tau binding in non-AD pathologies. A more recent derivative, 18-F-THK5351, exhibits promising kinetics with lower white matter retention. 18-F-T808, besides its good in vitro and in vivo properties, with tracer's uptake pattern consistent with Braak stages, it presents, because of defluorination, high bone uptake in the skull. 18-F-T807 (AV-1451) has relatively slower kinetics, but it shows no defluorination and the pattern of tracer's uptake is consistent with Braak stages, as well, making it the most widely used tracer so far [7–11].

Measures of tracer distribution derived from amyloid and tau tracer early imaging have also been tested as an indirect measure of perfusion, another relevant biomarker in AD, and represent a promising additional information [12].

Hybrid PET/MRI offers the unique opportunity to combine MRI and PET information in a single imaging session. This technology is available in clinical practice since less than a decade: its feasibility in patients investigated for AD has been consistently shown, with the different types of PET/MR tomographs currently in use [13].

A prerequisite for valid quantification of PET data is attenuation correction. This process is less straightforward in hybrid PET/MR systems, lacking a direct measure of tissue attenuation. However, while some of the current vendor-implemented MR-based attenuation correction (MR-AC) techniques for the brain are not accounting for bone attenuation, introducing quantification errors, various prototype methods recently tested provided results within acceptable quantitative limits (±5% of CT-corrected data) [14, 15].

The added value of hybrid PET/MRI against the standard of PET and MR images acquired separately is currently under investigation. The availability of an accurate measure of atrophy systematically available and acquired at the same time point could facilitate a larger use of partial volume corrected PET measures.

In addition, the use of MR-derived input function could further improve PET quantification [16, 17].

2 Materials

2.1 Hybrid PET/MR Tomographs

There are three different designs of hybrid PET/MR systems currently available: one with sequential acquisition of PET and MR data and two with simultaneous acquisition. The technical characteristics of each tomograph are summarized in Table 1 [18–23].

2.2 Tracer for Glucose Metabolism Assessment

1. Radioisotope: Fluorine 18.
2. Radiopharmaceutical: 18-Fluoro-2-deoxy-glucose.
3. Activity: 200 MBq.
4. Mode of administration: intravenous injection.
5. Mechanism of uptake: facilitated transport and metabolic trapping.
6. Interpretation: visual analysis and quantification (*see* **Note 2**(g) and (h)).

2.3 Tracer for Amyloid Imaging

1. Radioisotope: Fluorine 18.
2. Radiopharmaceutical: 18-F-florbetapir (18-F-AV-45).
3. Activity: 370 MBq.
4. Mode of administration: intravenous injection.
5. Mechanism of uptake: selective binding.
6. Interpretation: visual analysis and quantification (*see* **Note 3**(d), (e) and (f)).

2.4 Tracer for Tau Imaging

1. Radioisotope: Fluorine 18.
2. Radiopharmaceutical: 18-F-AV1451.
3. Activity: 185 MBq.
4. Mode of administration: intravenous injection.
5. Mechanism of uptake: selective binding.
6. Interpretation: visual analysis and quantification (*see* **Note 4**(a) and (b)).

3 Methods

3.1 MRI Protocol (See Note 1)

The standard protocol includes morphological sequences such as T2 FSE, T1, FLAIR, and T2 GRE and advanced sequences such as diffusion tensor imaging (DTI), while additional sequences, such as ASL and resting state functional MRI, are used for research purposes (*see* **Note 1**). The protocols described below have been designed for the Philips Ingenuity:

Table 1
Main technical characteristics of the three hybrid PET/MR systems that have been commercialized

	Philips ingenuity TF PET/MR	Siemens biograph mMR	GE SIGNA PET/MR
PET			
Scintillator	LYSO	LSO	LBS
Photodetector	PMT	APD	SiPM
Scintillator size (mm³)	4 × 4 × 22	4 × 4 × 20	4 × 5.3 × 25
Total detector elements	28.336	28.672	20.160
Energy resolution (%)	11.6	14.5	11
Lower energy threshold (keV)	440	430	425
Scatter fraction (%)	26	37.9	43.6 at peak NECR
Sensitivity (cps/kBq)	7.0	13.2	21
Coincidence window (ns)	6	5.86	4.57
Peak NEC (kcps at kBq/mL)	88.5 at 13.7	175 at 21.8	210 at 17.5
Time of flight	Yes	No	Yes
TOF resolution (ps)	525	–	400
Axial FOV (mm)	180	258	250
MR			
Filed strength (T)	3	3	3
Bore size (cm)	60	60	60
Max FOV (cm³)	50 × 50 × 45	50 × 50 × 45	50 × 50 × 50
Field homogeneity (40 cm³)	0.5 ppm	0.25 ppm	NA
PET/MR			
Acquisition	Sequential (same room)	Simultaneous	Simultaneous
PET attenuation correction for brain	MR-based (3D T1-weighted spoiled gradient echo)	MR-based (Dixon, Dixon-VIBE)	Atlas-based (co-registration of 2 point Dixon)

1. 3D Flair: sagittal orientation, in-plane resolution 1 × 1 mm, slice thickness 1.12 mm reconstructed every 0.56 mm, TE/TR 281/4800 ms, TI 1650 ms, parallel imaging acceleration factor 2(AP) × 2(RL), FOV 250 × 250 mm, 340 slices, two averages, acquisition time 7 min 36 s.

2. T2 TSE: transverse orientation, in-plane resolution 0.45 × 0.53 mm (reconstruction 0.4 × 0.4 mm), slice thickness 4 mm, TE/TR 100/4025 ms, parallel imaging acceleration factor 1.5, FOV 220 × 177 mm, 35 slices, two averages, acquisition time 3 min 53 s.

3. T2* GRE: transverse orientation, in-plane resolution 0.75 × 0.83 mm (reconstruction 0.4 × 0.4 mm), slice thickness 4 mm, TE/TR 16/1077 ms, flip angle 18°, parallel imaging acceleration factor 1.5, FOV 230 × 191 mm, 35 slices, acquisition time 2 min 50 s.

4. 3D T1 TFE: sagittal orientation, inversion pre-pulse, in-plane resolution 0.9 × 0.9 mm (reconstruction 0.45 × 0.45 mm), slice thickness 0.90 mm reconstructed every 0.45 mm, TE/TR 3.1/6.4 ms, flip angle 8°, FOV 240 × 240 mm, 390 slices, acquisition time 6 min 50 s.

5. Diffusion tensor imaging (DTI): transverse orientation, in-plane resolution 1.97 × 2 mm (reconstruction 1.7 × 1.7 mm), slice thickness 2 mm, b0 and b1000 with 30 diffusion directions, TE/TR 69/8315 ms, parallel imaging acceleration factor 2.3, FOV 244 × 244 mm, 75 slices, two averages, acquisition time 8 min 44 s.

3.2 PET Protocols

Basic elements of patient management and tracer administration are recapitulated in Subheading 3.1 and apply also for the following protocols. The details provided here, namely for activity to administer, uptake phase duration, and acquisition duration, reflect the practice established in our institutions.

3.2.1 Glucose Metabolism (See Note 2)

1. Patient's preparation is mandatory, 6 h (minimum 4 h) of fasting (nothing per os except for water) (*see* **Note 2**(a) and (c)).

2. Serum glucose level is checked, if glucose is higher than 160 mg/dL, consider rescheduling the exam under more proper conditions (*see* **Note 2**(b)).

3. An intravenous catheter is placed (*see* **Note** 2(d)).

4. The patient is instructed to rest in a comfortable position for 30 min (20 min minimum) before the programmed FDG administration. He/she is instructed to keep the eyes open but not to talk, read, listen to music, etc. The room should be warm, silent, and dimly lit. The patient should be under continuous supervision but with minimal interaction in order to avoid any functional activation [3].

5. Intravenous administration of 200 MBq of 18-Fluoro-2-deoxyglucose followed by flushing of the line with 10 mL of normal saline 0.9%, with minimal interaction with the patient.

6. After the injection, the patient is left to rest for 20 more minutes during the FDG brain uptake, following the same instructions as mentioned in **step 5**. If the patient is uncooperative, sedation may be applied (*see* **Note 2**(e)).

7. Just before the scan, the patient should be encouraged to void the bladder, in order to minimize discomfort during the acquisition.

8. 25 min post injection the patient is positioned on the camera, as comfortably as possible, with head restrains to minimize motion artifacts.

9. The acquisition starts with the MR localizer and MR sequence for the attenuation correction.

10. 30 min post injection the PET data are acquired for 15 min in 3-D mode (*see* **Note 2**(f)) (Fig. 1).

11. Specific MRI sequences, as detailed above, are acquired simultaneously or subsequently.

3.2.2 Amyloid Imaging
(See **Note 3**)

1. No special preparation of the patient (neither fasting nor drug interruption) is required.

2. Bolus IV administration of 18-F-florbetapir on the camera bed, followed by a flush of 0.9% sterile sodium chloride (*see* **Note 3**(a)).

3. Early 5 min acquisition of PET data, 1–6 min pi (*see* **Note 3**(b)).

4. MRI sequences, as detailed above.

5. 50 min post injection delayed 15 min brain PET acquisition in 3-D list mode (50–65 min) (*see* **Note 3**(c)) (Fig. 2).

3.2.3 Tau Imaging
(See **Note 4**)

1. No special preparation of the patient (neither fasting nor drug interruption) is required.

2. IV administration of 185 MBq of 18-F-AV1451.

3. 75 min post injection starts the acquisition of PET data for 30 min in 3-D list mode (75–105 min) (*see* **Note 4**) (Fig. 3).

4. MR sequences, as detailed above.

4 Notes

1. Additional research MRI sequences: Currently, there are several ongoing studies using imaging protocols that include arterial spin labeling (ASL) [24]. This allows cerebral blood flow to be measured as an attempt to detect early changes in cerebral perfusion and compare the information obtained with morphologic MR sequences and PET alone. The advantages of

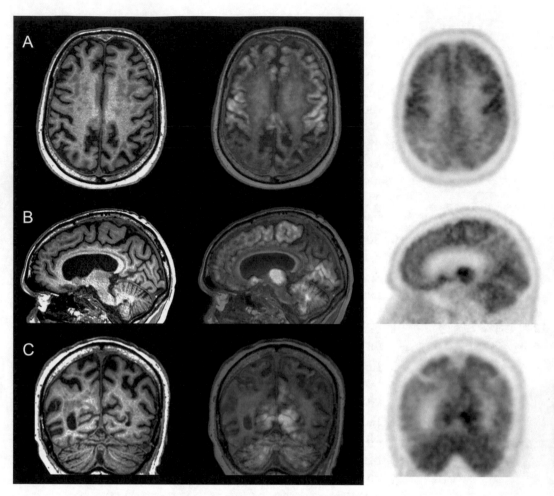

Fig. 1 T1 MP-RAGE, PET/MRI fusion, and PET-FDG, in axial (**a**), coronal (**b**), and sagittal plane (**c**) of an AD patient, showing decreased bilateral parietal and posterior temporal metabolism, as well as hypometabolism of the posterior cingulate and the precuneus; with sparing of sensorimotor and occipital cortices

this technique are that no intravenous contrast is needed, studies can be repeated, and longitudinal follow-up is possible. The main disadvantage is that even at the high field strengths (3 T) the resolution is lower. Resting state functional MRI (or task-free functional MRI), a technique that measures low-frequency fluctuations of BOLD signal, allows the assessment of changes of functional connectivity within the default mode network (DMN) related to AD throughout the course of the disease, with an initial, probably compensatory, increase of the posterior DMN (posterior cingulum and precuneus) in amnestic MCI patients, followed by a decrease of connectivity in posterior regions and increase in the frontal regions in AD patients, progressing eventually to a global decrease of connectivity of the DMN. Rs-fMRI appears to be a promising biomarker for AD on a group level, but the experience on a single-subject

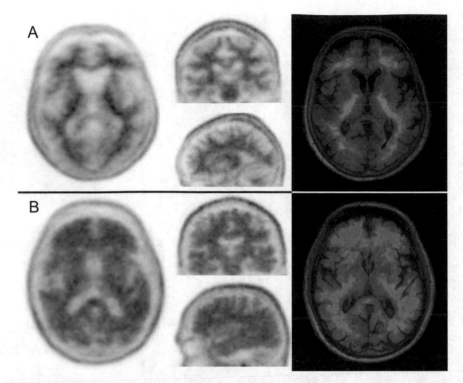

Fig. 2 PET-18F-AV45 in axial, coronal, and sagittal view and PET/MRI fusion of a negative case (**a**) without gray matter uptake (SUVR of 0.66) and a positive case (**b**) with uptake in gray matter equal to the adjacent white matter in frontal, temporal, and parietal cortices (SUVR of 1.52)

level is limited. Preprocessing methods need to be standardized, analysis methods may further be improved to increase sensitivity, and functional databases should be established, before validation for clinical use [25, 26]. Lately, an animal study has illustrated the advantages of utilizing combined systems such as PET/MR. The paper explains a new method that uses the segmentation of cervical arteries obtained with 3DTOF-MR. This is used as an anatomical mask to clearly depict the supra-aortic vessels in the cervical region and perform a true spatial alignment for correction of partial volume effects (PVE) and point spread. This method allows an entirely automatic calculation to obtain the image-derived input function (IDIF) in one single session using PET/MR [16].

2. Glucose Metabolism:

  (a) *Patient's preparation.* Meticulous preparation is mandatory for glucose metabolism studies. Fasting for 6 h (minimum 4 h) is instructed, including intravenous dextrose and parenteral nutrition. Good hydration with water is encouraged. Stimulating beverages, such as coffee, tea, etc., should be avoided. Medication may be continued

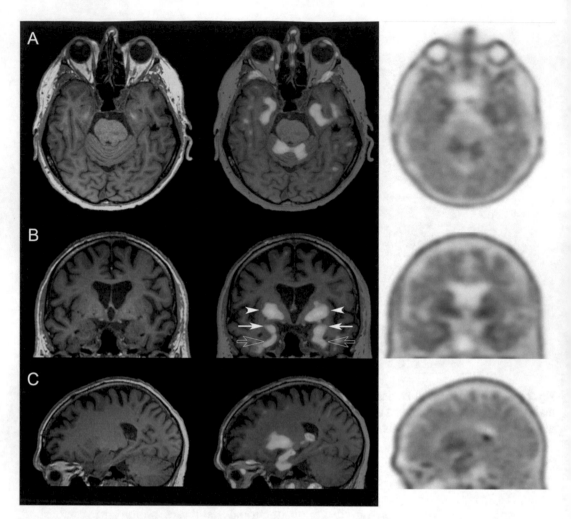

Fig. 3 T1 MP-RAGE PET/MRI fusion and PET 18-F-AV 1451 in axial (**a**), sagittal, (**b**) and coronal display (**c**), showing increased uptake of the hippocampus and the transentorhinal regions (blank arrows) (Braak stage II). Beware of off-target binding of the tracer in the choroid plexus of the ventricles (arrows) and the striatum (arrow heads)

normally (except for insulin and psychotropic drugs, as mentioned below) and is to be taken only with water [27, 3, 28].

(b) *Serum glucose.* Concerning FDG, both hyperglycemia and hyperinsulinemia are equally disturbing. With hyperglycemia, there is increased competition for GLUT and hexokinase, while hyperinsulinemia decreases FDG bioavailability, because of increased muscle uptake. Fast serum glucose correction, with IV insulin administration, is not recommended. There is a lag phase between the correction of intracellular glucose levels and plasma glucose. If fast correction protocol is applied, check insulin's leaflet to ensure that it can be used for IV administration. FDG administration should be delayed for at least 1-h post IV insulin, preferably 90 min [3]. In type II diabetes controlled with per os treatment, medication is continued normally. In insulin-dependent type I and type II diabetes, the management depends on the type of insulin used. Patients on regular insulin are instructed to take insulin with their breakfast and are scheduled for the late morning/early afternoon slots, while patients on evening long-acting insulin should be scheduled early in the morning, after an overnight fast. For patients with uncontrolled hyperglycemia, consult the endocrinology department for treatment arrangement [28].

(c) *Psychotropic drugs.* Psychotropic drugs alter brain metabolism. Discontinuation of drugs on the day of the scan is recommended, but if this is not possible, it should be noted on the report [3]. Benzodiazepines induce significant global cortical metabolic decrease, mostly on the occipital cortex and the cerebellum. Neuroleptics have been associated with increased striatal and thalamic activity and decreased activity of the frontal cortex and the anterior cingulate cortex [29].

(d) *IV catheter.* It is recommended to position the IV catheter as early as possible, at least 10 min before FDG administration, in order to minimize stimuli [3].

(e) *Sedation.* In uncooperative patients, conscious sedation may be applied with short-acting benzodiazepines (midazolam) administered at least 20 min after the FDG administration (preferably a few minutes before data acquisition), with appropriate monitoring and emergency chariot directly available [3].

(f) *3-D mode of PET acquisition.* 3-D mode is preferred over 2-D, in order to decrease scan's duration and consequently patient's discomfort and the probability of motion artifacts. When PET data are acquired in 3-D mode, appropriate scatter correction has to be applied [3].

(g) *Image interpretation.* The typical FDG distribution in Alzheimer's disease is decreased metabolic activity in the precuneus and posterior cingulum and bilateral parieto-temporal cortex, with sparing of the sensorimotor and visual cortex. The hypometabolism can be asymmetric, especially in early stages.

(h) *Quantification.* Several software are available for automated or semiautomated voxel-wise statistical analysis compared to a normal database providing objective measures and a threshold for abnormality. In case of a ready-to-use database of normal subjects, obtain information about the machines used and the reconstruction to use; otherwise, if an in-house normal database is used, use a standard protocol.

3. Amyloid imaging:

   (a) *Injection.* As instructed by the manufacturer, in order to minimize potential adherence of the drug to the catheter, use a short intravenous catheter (approximately 1.5 in. or less). Administrate as a single intravenous bolus and then flush the line with 10 mL of 0.9% sterile sodium chloride.

   (b) *Early PET acquisition.* An early 5 min acquisition of PET data, from the first to the sixth minute post injection, is potentially useful providing an FDG-like image [30].

   (c) *Delayed PET acquisition.* The delayed 15 min PET acquisition can start from 30 to 50 min post injection. The average SUVR increases rapidly from 0 to 30 min post injection, with gradual increase of the gap between the healthy controls and the AD patients. Thereafter, only minimal changes are noticed, reaching a plateau at 40–50 min p.i. [31].

   (d) *Image interpretation.* For the visual assessment the black and white scale is recommended by the manufacturer, with the maximum intensity of the scale set to the maximum intensity of the whole brain. The brain is analyzed on the axial plane, with periodic reference to the coronal and sagittal plane for verification. Image interpretation is binary, either negative or positive comparing the radioactivity of gray matter with the adjacent white matter. A positive result corresponds to moderate or frequent presence of amyloid plaques according to the CERAD score. The criteria for a positive Amyvid scan are:

   • Two or more areas, larger than one cortical gyrus, with reduced or absent contrast between gray and white matter.

   • One or more areas of intense gray matter uptake, more than the adjacent white matter.

   (e) Although the principle of image interpretation remains the same for the other PET amyloid tracers, each manufacturer recommends its own color scale and criteria for the visual analysis [7].

   (f) *Quantification.* As an adjunct to the visual analysis, a simple semiquantitative approach has been proposed in the literature. Using a dedicated software with predefined ROIs (precuneus, anterior and posterior cingulate, and frontal median, temporal, parietal, and occipital cortex), we calculate the global SUVR, which is defined as the mean uptake of the tracer within these regions normalized to the uptake of the whole cerebellum. With a cutoff value of 1.122, global SUVR shows 92.3% sensitivity and 90.5% specificity (AUC 0.894) [32]. This protocol instructed by the manufacturer is intended for diagnostic purposes, but it seems insufficient for longitudinal studies especially in case of disease-modifying drugs, as recently shown. For this purpose, subtle differences cannot be assessed visually and SUVR being sensitive to perfusion changes, which are more prominent in AD patients, does not permit accurate quantification for the follow-up, constituting dynamic imaging and kinetic analysis essential, with the distribution volume ratio (DVR) being more reliable compared to SUVR [33]. Another recent study found that for longitudinal purposes, it was more optimal to calculate the SUVR using partial volume correction and a composite reference region containing voxels in the white matter and the whole cerebellum [34].

4. Tau imaging:

   (a) *Image interpretation.* Increased cortical uptake is noticed in AD patients, as well as in MCI stage, in a pattern consistent with the Braak stages, starting from increased uptake in the transentorhinal regions for the earliest stages (Braak stages I/II) and involving increasingly the lateral temporal and occipital cortices in advanced stages (Braak stages IV–VI) [35]. Increased off-target uptake has been demonstrated in the striatum (putamen) and the choroid plexus in AD, MCI patients, and older healthy controls [7, 36], as well as in blood vessels, iron-associated regions, leptomeningeal melanin, and the pituitary [37].

   (b) *Quantification.* In a recent kinetic modeling study, it was shown that a late acquisition as the one described here is a reasonable alternative to 0–100 min dynamic imaging [36, 11].

Acknowledgment

This work was supported by the Swiss National Science Foundation under grant SNF 320030_169876.

References

1. Fujimoto K, Polimeni JR, van der Kouwe AJ, Reuter M, Kober T, Benner T, Fischl B, Wald LL (2014) Quantitative comparison of cortical surface reconstructions from MP2RAGE and multi-echo MPRAGE data at 3 and 7T. NeuroImage 90:60–73. https://doi.org/10.1016/j.neuroimage.2013.12.012

2. Marques JP, Kober T, Krueger G, van der Zwaag W, Van de Moortele PF, Gruetter R (2010) MP2RAGE, a self bias-field corrected sequence for improved segmentation and T1-mapping at high field. NeuroImage 49(2):1271–1281. https://doi.org/10.1016/j.neuroimage.2009.10.002

3. Varrone A, Asenbaum S, Vander Borght T, Booij J, Nobili F, Nagren K, Darcourt J, Kapucu OL, Tatsch K, Bartenstein P, Van Laere K (2009) EANM procedure guidelines for PET brain imaging using [18F]FDG, version 2. Eur J Nucl Med Mol Imaging 36(12):2103–2110. https://doi.org/10.1007/s00259-009-1264-0

4. Xie L, Helmerhorst E, Taddei K, Plewright B, Van Bronswijk W, Martins R (2002) Alzheimer's beta-amyloid peptides compete for insulin binding to the insulin receptor. J Neurosci 22(10):RC221. 20026383 [pii]

5. Kantarci K, Lowe VJ, Boeve BF, Senjem ML, Tosakulwong N, Lesnick TG, Spychalla AJ, Gunter JL, Fields JA, Graff-Radford J, Ferman TJ, Jones DT, Murray ME, Knopman DS, Jack CR Jr, Petersen RC (2016) AV-1451 tau and beta-amyloid positron emission tomography imaging in dementia with Lewy bodies. Ann Neurol 81:58. https://doi.org/10.1002/ana.24825

6. Hostetler ED, Walji AM, Zeng Z, Miller P, Bennacef I, Salinas C, Connolly B, Gantert L, Haley H, Holahan M, Purcell M, Riffel K, Lohith TG, Coleman P, Soriano A, Ogawa A, Xu S, Zhang X, Joshi E, Della Rocca J, Hesk D, Schenk DJ, Evelhoch JL (2016) Preclinical characterization of 18F-MK-6240, a promising PET tracer for in vivo quantification of human neurofibrillary tangles. J Nucl Med 57(10):1599–1606. https://doi.org/10.2967/jnumed.115.171678

7. Aleksandar Jovalekic NK, Mueller A, Stephens AW (2016) New protein deposition tracers in the pipeline. EJNMMI Radiopharm Chem 1(11). https://doi.org/10.1186/s41181-016-0015-3

8. Harada R, Okamura N, Furumoto S, Tago T, Yanai K, Arai H, Kudo Y (2016) Characteristics of tau and its ligands in PET imaging. Biomol Ther 6(1):7. https://doi.org/10.3390/biom6010007. biom6010007 [pii]

9. Shah M, Seibyl J, Cartier A, Bhatt R, Catafau AM (2014) Molecular imaging insights into neurodegeneration: focus on alpha-synuclein radiotracers. J Nucl Med 55(9):1397–1400. https://doi.org/10.2967/jnumed.113.136515

10. Villemagne VL, Okamura N (2014) In vivo tau imaging: obstacles and progress. Alzheimers Dement 10(3 Suppl):S254–S264. https://doi.org/10.1016/j.jalz.2014.04.013

11. Wooten D, Guehl NJ, Verwer EE, Shoup TM, Yokell DL, Zubcevik N, Vasdev N, Zafonte RD, Johnson KA, El Fakhri G, Normandin MD (2016) Pharmacokinetic evaluation of the tau PET radiotracer [18F]T807 ([18F]AV-1451) in human subjects. J Nucl Med, vol 58, p 484. https://doi.org/10.2967/jnumed.115.170910

12. Rodriguez-Vieitez E, Leuzy A, Chiotis K, Saint-Aubert L, Wall A, Nordberg A (2017) Comparability of [18F]THK5317 and [11C]PIB blood flow proxy images with [18F]FDG positron emission tomography in Alzheimer's disease. J Cereb Blood Flow Metab 37(2):740–749. https://doi.org/10.1177/0271678X16645593

13. Mainta IC, Perani D, Delattre BM, Assal F, Haller S, Vargas MI, Zekry DS, Frisoni GB, Zaidi H, Ratib O, Garibotto V (2017) FDG PET/MR imaging in major neurocognitive disorders. Curr Alzheimer Res 14(2):186–197. CAR-EPUB-76693 [pii]

14. Ladefoged CN, Law I, Anazodo U, St Lawrence K, Izquierdo-Garcia D, Catana C, Burgos N, Cardoso MJ, Ourselin S, Hutton B, Merida I, Costes N, Hammers A, Benoit D, Holm S, Juttukonda M, An H, Cabello J, Lukas M, Nekolla S, Ziegler S, Fenchel M, Jakoby B, Casey ME, Benzinger T, Hojgaard L, Hansen AE, Andersen FL (2016) A multi-centre evaluation of eleven clinically feasible brain PET/MRI attenuation correction techniques using a large cohort of patients. NeuroImage 147:346–359. https://doi.org/10.1016/j.neuroimage.2016.12.010

15. Werner P, Rullmann M, Bresch A, Tiepolt S, Jochimsen T, Lobsien D, Schroeter ML, Sabri O, Barthel H (2016) Impact of attenuation correction on clinical [(18)F]FDG brain PET in combined PET/MRI. EJNMMI Res 6(1):47. https://doi.org/10.1186/s13550-016-0200-0

16. Jochimsen TH, Zeisig V, Schulz J, Werner P, Patt M, Patt J, Dreyer AY, Boltze J, Barthel H, Sabri O, Sattler B (2016) Fully automated calculation of image-derived input function in simul-

taneous PET/MRI in a sheep model. EJNMMI Phys3(1):2.https://doi.org/10.1186/s40658-016-0139-2

17. Loeb R, Navab N, Ziegler SI (2015) Direct parametric reconstruction using anatomical regularization for simultaneous PET/MRI data. IEEE Trans Med Imaging 34(11):2233–2247. https://doi.org/10.1109/TMI.2015.2427777

18. Delso G, Furst S, Jakoby B, Ladebeck R, Ganter C, Nekolla SG, Schwaiger M, Ziegler SI (2011) Performance measurements of the Siemens mMR integrated whole-body PET/MR scanner. J Nucl Med 52(12):1914–1922. https://doi.org/10.2967/jnumed.111.092726

19. Grant AM, Deller TW, Khalighi MM, Maramraju SH, Delso G, Levin CS (2016) NEMA NU 2-2012 performance studies for the SiPM-based ToF-PET component of the GE SIGNA PET/MR system. Med Phys 43(5):2334. https://doi.org/10.1118/1.4945416

20. Juttukonda MR, Mersereau BG, Chen Y, Su Y, Rubin BG, Benzinger TL, Lalush DS, An H (2015) MR-based attenuation correction for PET/MRI neurological studies with continuous-valued attenuation coefficients for bone through a conversion from R2* to CT-Hounsfield units. NeuroImage 112:160–168. https://doi.org/10.1016/j.neuroimage.2015.03.009

21. Khalil MM (ed) (2017) Basic science of PET imaging. Springer, Cham

22. Vandenberghe S, Mikhaylova E, D'Hoe E, Mollet P, Karp JS (2016) Recent developments in time-of-flight PET. EJNMMI Phys 3(1):3. https://doi.org/10.1186/s40658-016-0138-3

23. Zaidi II, Ojha N, Morich M, Griesmer J, Hu Z, Maniawski P, Ratib O, Izquierdo-Garcia D, Fayad ZA, Shao L (2011) Design and performance evaluation of a whole-body ingenuity TF PET-MRI system. Phys Med Biol 56(10):3091–3106. https://doi.org/10.1088/0031-9155/56/10/013

24. Drzezga A, Barthel H, Minoshima S, Sabri O (2014) Potential clinical applications of PET/MR imaging in neurodegenerative diseases. J Nucl Med 55(Suppl 2):47S–55S. https://doi.org/10.2967/jnumed.113.129254

25. Damoiseaux JS (2012) Resting-state fMRI as a biomarker for Alzheimer's disease? Alzheimers Res Ther 4(2):8. https://doi.org/10.1186/alzrt106

26. Vemuri P, Jones DT, Jack CR Jr (2012) Resting state functional MRI in Alzheimer's disease. Alzheimers Res Ther 4(1):2. https://doi.org/10.1186/alzrt100

27. Alan D, Waxman MKH, Lewis DH, Herscovitch P, Minoshima S, Ichise M, Drzezga AE,Devous MD, Mountz JM (2009) Society of Nuclear Medicine Procedure Guideline for FDG PET Brain Imaging Version 1.0, approved February 8, 2009

28. Surasi DS, Bhambhvani P, Baldwin JA, Almodovar SE, O'Malley JP (2014) (1)(8)F-FDG PET and PET/CT patient preparation: a review of the literature. J Nucl Med Technol 42(1):5–13. https://doi.org/10.2967/jnmt.113.132621

29. Berti V, Mosconi L, Pupi A (2014) Brain: normal variations and benign findings in fluorodeoxyglucose-PET/computed tomography imaging. PET Clin 9(2):129–140. https://doi.org/10.1016/j.cpet.2013.10.006

30. Hsiao IT, Huang CC, Hsieh CJ, Hsu WC, Wey SP, Yen TC, Kung MP, Lin KJ (2012) Correlation of early-phase 18F-florbetapir (AV-45/Amyvid) PET images to FDG images: preliminary studies. Eur J Nucl Med Mol Imaging 39(4):613–620. https://doi.org/10.1007/s00259-011-2051-2

31. Wong DF, Rosenberg PB, Zhou Y, Kumar A, Raymont V, Ravert HT, Dannals RF, Nandi A, Brasic JR, Ye W, Hilton J, Lyketsos C, Kung HF, Joshi AD, Skovronsky DM, Pontecorvo MJ (2010) In vivo imaging of amyloid deposition in Alzheimer disease using the radioligand 18F-AV-45 (florbetapir [corrected] F 18). J Nucl Med 51(6):913–920. https://doi.org/10.2967/jnumed.109.069088

32. Camus V, Payoux P, Barre L, Desgranges B, Voisin T, Tauber C, La Joie R, Tafani M, Hommet C, Chetelat G, Mondon K, de La Sayette V, Cottier JP, Beaufils E, Ribeiro MJ, Gissot V, Vierron E, Vercouillie J, Vellas B, Eustache F, Guilloteau D (2012) Using PET with 18F-AV-45 (florbetapir) to quantify brain amyloid load in a clinical environment. Eur J Nucl Med Mol Imaging 39(4):621–631. https://doi.org/10.1007/s00259-011-2021-8

33. van Berckel BN, Ossenkoppele R, Tolboom N, Yaqub M, Foster-Dingley JC, Windhorst AD, Scheltens P, Lammertsma AA, Boellaard R (2013) Longitudinal amyloid imaging using 11C-PiB: methodologic considerations. J Nucl Med 54(9):1570–1576. https://doi.org/10.2967/jnumed.112.113654

34. Schwarz CG, Senjem ML, Gunter JL, Tosakulwong N, Weigand SD, Kemp BJ, Spychalla AJ, Vemuri P, Petersen RC, Lowe VJ, Jack CR Jr (2017) Optimizing PiB-PET SUVR

change-over-time measurement by a large-scale analysis of longitudinal reliability, plausibility, separability, and correlation with MMSE. Neuroimage 144(Pt A):113–127. https://doi.org/10.1016/j.neuroimage. 2016.08.056

35. Schwarz AJ, Yu P, Miller BB, Shcherbinin S, Dickson J, Navitsky M, Joshi AD, Devous MD Sr, Mintun MS (2016) Regional profiles of the candidate tau PET ligand 18F-AV-1451 recapitulate key features of Braak histopathological stages. Brain 139(Pt 5):1539–1550. https://doi.org/10.1093/brain/aww023

36. Shcherbinin S, Schwarz AJ, Joshi A, Navitsky M, Flitter M, Shankle WR, Devous MD Sr, Mintun MA (2016) Kinetics of the tau PET tracer 18F-AV-1451 (T807) in subjects with normal cognitive function, mild cognitive impairment, and Alzheimer disease. J Nucl Med 57(10):1535–1542. https://doi.org/10.2967/jnumed.115.170027

37. Lowe VJ, Curran G, Fang P, Liesinger AM, Josephs KA, Parisi JE, Kantarci K, Boeve BF, Pandey MK, Bruinsma T, Knopman DS, Jones DT, Petrucelli L, Cook CN, Graff-Radford NR, Dickson DW, Petersen RC, Jack CR Jr, Murray ME (2016) An autoradiographic evaluation of AV-1451 Tau PET in dementia. Acta Neuropathol Commun 4(1):58. https://doi.org/10.1186/s40478-016-0315-6

Part V

Molecular Imaging Approaches

Chapter 13

Amyloid PET Imaging: Standardization and Integration with Other Alzheimer's Disease Biomarkers

Silvia Morbelli and Matteo Bauckneht

Abstract

Amyloid plaques are a neuropathologic hallmark of Alzheimer's disease (AD), which can be imaged through positron emission tomography (PET) technology using radiopharmaceuticals that selectively bind to the fibrillar aggregates of amyloid-β plaques (Amy-PET). Several radiotracers for amyloid PET have been investigated, including ^{11}C-Pittsburgh compound B and the ^{18}F-labeled compounds such as ^{18}F-florbetaben, ^{18}F-florbetapir, and ^{18}F-flutemetamol. Besides the injected radiotracer, images can be interpreted by means of visual/qualitative, semiquantitative, and quantitative criteria. Here we summarize the main differences between the available radiotracers for Amy-PET, the proposed interpretation criteria, and analytical methods.

Key words Amyloid PET, Biomarkers, Alzheimer's disease, Brain

1 Introduction

Over the past two decades, one of the major breakthroughs for the approach to Alzheimer's disease (AD) patients both in the clinical and research settings has been represented by the validation of diagnostic biomarkers able to demonstrate the presence of pathological mechanisms of AD and to predict further cognitive decline and dementia onset since the stage of mild cognitive impairment (MCI) [1, 2]. Two main categories of biomarkers have been proposed to identify the prodromal stage of AD [2]. On the one side, amyloidosis biomarkers are able to identify the molecular/neuropathological feature of AD and include cerebrospinal fluid (CSF) amyloid-β_{1-42} reduction and brain amyloid accumulation as imaged through PET technology using radiopharmaceuticals that selectively bind to the fibrillar aggregates of amyloid-β plaques (AMY-PET) [2]. On the other side, neurodegeneration biomarkers reflect neuronal injury and downstream neurodegeneration which can be measured by the increase of tau protein in the CSF, regional atrophy on MRI, or

Robert Perneczky (ed.), *Biomarkers for Alzheimer's Disease Drug Development*, Methods in Molecular Biology, vol. 1750, https://doi.org/10.1007/978-1-4939-7704-8_13, © Springer Science+Business Media, LLC 2018

synaptic metabolic dysfunction on ^{18}F-Fluorodeoxyglucose PET (FDG-PET) [2]. In particular for AMY-PET imaging, while pathological validity and potential clinical usefulness have been proven in selected samples of patients, some methodological and clinical issues still need to be clarified to successfully implement the use of this tool in clinical routine care [3]. First, while qualitative findings has been consistent across a large number of centers, standardization is still an issue with respect the identification of both the optimal reading procedure (visual/binary versus semiquantitative) and a widely accepted and reproducible quantitative measures (i.e., method of analysis and universal cutoffs) [4]. Second, there's a need to clarify the prognostic value of AMY-PET in patients with borderline values with amyloid loads fallen just outside of the amyloid-negative [4]. Third, it is important to work for the integration of AMY-PET with other AD biomarkers and to include the tool in cost-effective clinical flowcharts able to impact on patients' management [3, 5].

2 Materials

Several radiotracers for amyloid PET have been investigated. In fact, the large body of evidence available on the usefulness of ^{11}C-Pittsburgh compound B (PiB) has been in the last few years followed by a growing number of publications on the ^{18}F-labeled compounds for amyloid PET imaging [6]. In fact in the last few years, three fluorinated tracers, ^{18}F-florbetaben (NeuraCeq), ^{18}F-florbetapir (Amyvid), and ^{18}F-flutemetamol (Vizamyl) have been approved by both the US and the European authorities [6]. Although these tracers share a common imaging target and similar imaging characteristics, Aβ radiopharmaceuticals differ in their tracer kinetics, target-to-background ratio, and specific binding ratios. These differences impact on recommended imaging parameters such as injected doses, uptake time after tracer administration, and scan durations (details are reported in Table 1).

Table 1
Recommended dose, uptake time, and scan duration for Amyloid PET tracers

Tracer	Recommended dose (MBq)	Uptake time (min)	Scan duration (min)
[18]F-florbetaben	300	90	20
[18]F-florbetapir	370	30–50	10
[18]F-flutemetamol	185	90	20

2.1 Patients' Preparation and Tracer Injection

1. There is no known evidence of drug interactions between amyloid radiotracers and common drugs prescribed for dementia patients.

2. No drug withdrawal is recommended, except for anti-Aβ antibodies administered in the context of experimental studies.

3. No rest condition is needed before the tracer injection. For patients requiring sedation, 18F-labeled radiopharmaceuticals should be injected before the administration of sedation to minimize any theoretic effects of sedatives on cerebral blood flow and radiotracer delivery.

4. The dose must be assayed in a suitable calibrator before administration. Tracers have to be injected using aseptic technique through a short intravenous catheter (approximately 4 cm/1.5 in. or less, to minimize the potential for adsorption of substantial amounts of the drug to the catheter) in a single intravenous bolus in a total volume of 10 mL or less, followed by the injection with an intravenous flush of 0.9% sterile sodium chloride solution. The injection site should be routinely inspected for dose infiltration.

2.2 Scan Acquisition

1. After a delay depending on the injected radiotracer, the scan acquisition time is usually 10–30 min (see Table 1).

2. Images should be acquired in three-dimensional mode with appropriate data corrections and reconstructed using attenuation correction with typical transaxial pixel sizes of 2–3 mm and a slice thickness of 2–4 mm. A dynamic scan can also be performed, lasting 60 or 90 min from the time of injection in order to calculate binding and to provide a distribution volume ratio.

3. The potential acquisition of early post-injection images has been reported as an aid for better image interpretation and improved accuracy [7]. In fact, it has been previously demonstrated that regional cerebral perfusion is usually coupled to cerebral metabolism which is coupled synaptic function [8]. Therefore, a "dual-phase brain PET" might be performed through the acquisition of a short image lasting 5 min, immediately after injection, mirroring perfusion imaging (potentially providing information on synaptic function/dysfunction). This acquisition will be followed by an interval of variable length depending on the kinetic properties of the specific tracer and by the late "standard" acquisition at equilibrium. Differently from the standard protocol, when dual-phase brain PET is performed, tracer injection should be performed under rest conditions. This approach is certainly of great interest and potentially cost-effective; however, large-scale validation studies are needed in order to validate and allow the introduction of this approach into the routine clinical practice.

2.3 Aβ Radiotracers

2.3.1 ^{11}C-PiB

PiB is a derivative of a fluorescent amyloid dye, thioflavin T, and has been shown to possess high affinity and high specificity for fibrillar Aβ in plaques and in other Aβ containing lesions. PiB also displays a much lower affinity toward other misfolded proteins with a similar-sheet secondary structure such as α-synuclein and tau [9]. However, the 20-min radioactive decay half-life of ^{11}C limits the use of ^{11}C-PiB to centers with an on-site cyclotron and ^{11}C radiochemistry expertise, making routine clinical use very expensive.

2.3.2 ^{18}F-Florbetaben

^{18}F-florbetaben (^{18}F-AV-1, ^{18}F-BAY-94-9172, Neuraceq®), developed by Bayer Healthcare and market by Piramal Imaging, binds with high affinity to Aβ in plaques and cerebral amyloid angiopathy in postmortem brain tissue sections with lack of binding to Lewy bodies or NFT at low nanomolar concentrations [10]. It received Food and Drug Administration (FDA) and European Medicines Agency (EMA) approval for clinical use in February and March 2014, respectively.

2.3.3 ^{18}F-Florbetapir

^{18}F-florbetapir (^{18}F-AV-45, Amyvid®) is a stilbene derivative, developed by Avid Radiopharmaceuticals (a wholly owned subsidiary of Lilly). Initial in vitro evaluation showed binding to Aβ plaques in AD brain sections [11]. ^{18}F-Florbetapir was the first radiotracer—and the first ^{18}F labeled radiotracer approved by FDG—approved by FDA in April 2012 and EMA in January 2013. Florbetapir is characterized by its rapid reversible binding characteristics allowing scanning at just 30–50 min after injection, similar to ^{11}C-PiB [11].

2.3.4 ^{18}F-Flutemetamol

^{18}F-flutemetamol (GE–067, Vizamyl®) is a fluoro derivative of ^{11}C-PiB developed by GE Healthcare. ^{18}F-flutemetamol brain retention is highly correlated with ^{11}C-PIB, and with Aβ burden as measured immunohistochemical assessment of brain biopsy tissue [12]. ^{18}F-flutemetamol received FDA approval in October 2013 and EMA approval in September 2014.

3   Methods

After the tracer is injected in the patient it rapidly enters the brain by passive diffusion through the blood–brain barrier and reaches the sites of interest in a time-interval mainly from the bloodstream. The lipophilic nature of the tracer, combined with a high lipid content in the white matter, leads to a nonspecific binding in brain white matter. By contrast, the high affinity binding to the amyloid fibrils results in a significantly slower clearance of the tracer bound to amyloid plaques in the gray matter [6]. Amyloid radiotracers have been compared ex vivo [9], finding that both the retention in the gray and white matter is slightly different for different ligands, whereas binding sites are substantially the same. This latter point ensures that all the radiopharmaceuticals may be used similarly and in reliable way to determine the density of cerebral amyloid plaques. In fact, the objective of AMY-PET image interpretation is to provide an estimate of the brain β-amyloid plaque density [6]. Accordingly a positive AMY-PET scan identifies the presence of brain amyloidosis and not necessarily the presence of AD (the results but must be considered in the context of the person's medical history, physical examination, and cognitive testing) [1, 2, 5, 6]. In fact, while all AMY-PET tracers have high affinity and selectively for β-amyloid plaques and not for other pathological proteins such us TAU pathology and alpha-synuclein deposits, the high affinity is paralleled by limited specificity for different amyloid type [1, 2, 5, 6, 13]. In fact, all AMY-PET tracers are able to bind classic ("AD-type") neuritic plaques, diffuse extracellular plaques (non-specific for AD) as well as vascular amyloid typical of Cerebral Amyloid Angiopathy [6]. By contrast given the repeatedly proven high negative predictive value of AMY-PET imaging, a negative amyloid PET scan is able to identify among cognitive impaired patients, subjects unlikely to be affected by AD.

3.1 Visual/ Qualitative Images Evaluation

1. Specific in vitro studies have demonstrated that all AMY-PET tracers share similar binding to a nanomolar high affinity site and thus these amyloid ligands can be used in a comparable and reliable manner to assess brain amyloid density [9].

2. The specific criteria for amyloid PET image visual interpretation differ among available radiotracers, and qualitative evaluation of images acquired with a given amyloid tracer should be performed using the instructions provided by the manufacturers. Some general principles should be considered when interpreting AMY-PET scans [6]. A suitable image scaling should be employed: a 16-bit scale is recommended for image display [6]. For 18F-Florbetaben and 18F-Florbetapir, PET images should be displayed using gray scale and inverse gray scale, respectively, while color scales (such as "cool" or "spectrum") are recommended for 18F-Flutemetamol. First evaluation should be in transversal orientation. Coronal and sagittal planes as well as PET/CT fused images can also be evaluated and can be of help especially to inspect specific brain regions (posterior cingulate in sagittal view) and to clarify doubtful cases in the presence of atrophy or noisy images. Image size should be optimized for a clear differentiation between nonspecific/physiologic white matter and pathologic gray matter uptake.

3. The cerebellar cortex is expected to be free of amyloid deposition even in subjects with cerebral cortical amyloid deposition. For this reason, white/gray matter contrast at cerebellar level is used as reference for 18F-Florbetapir scan evaluation. Conversely, the white matter maximum has been suggested as

a reference for AMY-PET scan when 18F-Florbetaben is used and for 18F-Flutemetamol it is recommended to set the scale intensity to a level of about 90% in the pons region [6].

4. The typical appearance of a negative AMY-PET scans is non-specific white matter uptake and little or no binding in the gray matter. Thus, negative scans have a clear gray/white matter contrast.

5. The evidence of radiotracer uptake extending to the edge of the cerebral cortex and forming a smooth, regular boundary reflects the presence of gray matter amyloidosis and thus a positive AMY-PET scan. Figure 1 shows the typical appearance of a negative (A) and a positive (B) AMY-PET scan.

3.2 Semiquantitative Approaches

Most amyloid-PET images are rather easily evaluated by a trained eye and the reliability of amyloid PET binary reads across different sites has been demonstrated to be high even in the multicenter settings [13]. However, as amyloid-PET becomes a widespread tool, uncertain instances are going to be met more frequently. Accordingly, more sophisticated approaches has been proposed and extensively evaluated with the aim of providing semiquantification of AMY-PET data.

1. Commercially semiquantification software are already available and they generally rely on the numerical estimation of the Standardized Uptake Value ratio (SUVr) [14]. SUVr procedure calculates the ratio of PET counts between a number of target regions of interest (ROI) versus a reference one. ROI number, placement, and size vary among implementations and they often require reader's feedback. SUVr was validated by histopathological studies of density of neuritic amyloid-β plaques and compared with CSF results with good agreement [15]. While a study comparing head-to-head SUVr results and correspondent cutoffs in the same patients with all the AMY-PET tracers has not been performed yet, cortical retention was strongly correlated in studies comparing pair of tracers regardless of reference region [16]. However SUVr values, and thus thresholds for discrimination between positive and negative scans, depend on the choice of the reference region (more often the cerebellum brainstem or cerebellar gray matter) and no standard or widely recognized cutoffs has been identified. In fact, the upper limit of normal binding varies per size and placement of cortical and reference regions of interest (generally between 1.3 and 1.6 for neocortical SUVr).

2. Other methods have been proposed to overcome the difficulties of image reading and the possible shortcomings of the SUVr methods. A SUVr-Independent Evaluation of Brain Amyloidosis named Evaluation of Brain Amyloidosis (ELBA)

A

B

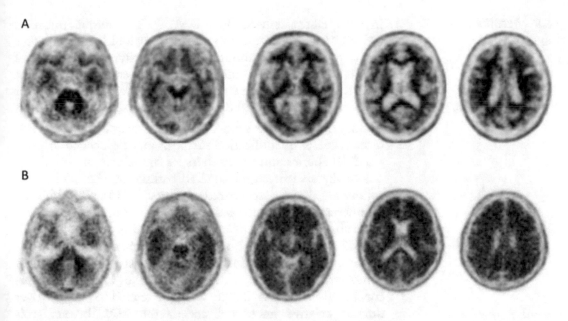

Fig. 1 Examples of positive and negative Amy PET scan. Panel (**a**) shows the typical appearance of a negative Amy PET scan in which the contrast between white and gray matter is represented in all brain areas, as in the cerebellum. Conversely, panel (**b**) represents a positive scan in which the radiotracer is widely distributed in all cortical areas

has been recently proposed [13]. ELBA does not rely on small, specific ROIs as it evaluates the whole brain and delivers a geometrical/intensity score to be used for ranking and dichotomic assessment. ELBA demonstrated to perform with area under the roc curve (AUC) = 0.997 versus the visual assessment. The longitudinal analysis estimated a test/retest error of 2.3% and longitudinal analysis suggests that the ELBA method accurately ranks the brain amyloid burden [13].

3. A working group has been formed within the Alzheimer's Imaging Consortium in 2012 with the aim of standardizing quantitative amyloid imaging measures by scaling the outcome of each particular analysis method or tracer to a 0 to 100 scale, anchored by young controls (≤45 years) and typical AD patients [4]. The units of this scale have been named "Centiloids." This approach aims to define "standard" method for analyzing PiB PET data and then a method for scaling any "nonstandard" method of Amy-PET analysis to the Centiloid scale. A key component of the optimal use of the Centiloid method is related to free access to all necessary data on a public database, and all of the scan data used in this initial report that has been deposited on the Global Alzheimer's Association Information Network (GAAIN; http://www.gaain.org) for free public access.

3.3 Quantification in Amyloid PET

1. In most clinical studies with AMY-PET, semiquantification with SUVr has been used to measure amyloid load [14]. This is due to a greater computational simplicity and the need of shorter scan duration (and thus less vulnerability to patient movement) with respect to the dynamic acquisition needed for absolute quantification and parametric analysis of tracer uptake.

2. Although SUVr may be acceptable for diagnostic purposes, more accurate quantification methods may be needed for longitudinal studies and/or to measure the effects of new drugs potentially able to target amyloid pathology. Van Berkel and colleagues directly compared changes in 11C-PiB binding parameters using different analytic methods and revealed that while absolute quantitative measures based on kinetic methods (RPM2 and reference Logan) showed relatively stable estimates of 11C-PiB binding in AD patients over time, SUVr demonstrated a decrease in 11C-PiB uptake [17]. The authors concluded that this variability could be related to changes over time in relative tracer delivery to the ROI, because this decreased over time in AD patients and that dynamic scanning protocols and fully quantitative data analysis methods are necessary as a solid baseline measurement to monitor their disease course and treatment response when only small changes in specific binding can be expected [17].

3.4 Integration Between Amyloid PET Data and Other AD Biomarkers

1. Different sets of criteria for diagnosis of AD at the stage of MCI have been proposed: the International Working Group (IWG)-1 [18] and IWG-2 [2], and National Institute of Ageing Alzheimer Association (NIA-AA) criteria [1]. Proposed criteria for diagnosis of AD at the stage of MCI partially differ from one another with respect to the combination of biomarker abnormalities needed to identify MCI at higher risk to convert to dementia [1, 2].

2. The IWG2 criteria, mainly developed for the research setting, propose to support the clinical suspicion of AD only by means of amyloidosis biomarkers (defined as diagnostic biomarkers) while neurodegeneration biomarkers such as Tau CSF levels, FDG PET, and MRI are considered as progression biomarkers due to their lower diagnostic specificity [2].

3. The use of AD biomarkers in routine clinical practice should take into account not only the diagnostic performances of a test but also cost-effectiveness estimates [3]. To guide clinicians on how best to apply amyloid PET in the clinical evaluation of people with cognitive decline, a working group convened by the Alzheimer's Association and the Society of Nuclear Medicine and Molecular Imaging (SNMMI) developed appropriate use criteria for brain amyloid PET scans [19]. According to this criteria amyloid PET should only be considered in

patients with clear, measurable cognitive deficits when there is substantial diagnostic uncertainty after a comprehensive evaluation by a dementia specialist.

4. The Amyloid Imaging Task force did not consider other proposed diagnostic biomarkers for AD and therefore did not draw any conclusions with regard to the relative value of amyloid PET compared with CFS, MRI, and FDG-PET. However, besides the clinical neuropsychological assessment, a comprehensive evaluation should certainly include an MRI scan while it is still to be clarified the cost-effectiveness of a flowchart proposing (or laying against) the use of FDG and/or CSF biomarkers before AMY-PET [5].

5. The conclusion of the Amyloid Imaging Task force [19] is that AMY-PET should have greatest value in patients with either: (1) progressive, unexplained mild cognitive impairment (MCI), or (2) dementia of uncertain cause due to atypical or mixed symptoms, or (3) unusually early age-of-onset.

References

1. Albert MS, DeKosky ST, Dickson D et al (2011) The diagnosis of mild cognitive impairment due to Alzheimer's disease: recommendations from the National Institute on Aging and Alzheimer's Association workgroup. Alzheimers Dement 7:270–279

2. Dubois B, Feldman HH, Jacova C et al (2014) Advancing research diagnostic criteria for Alzheimer's disease: the IWG-2 criteria. Lancet Neurol 13:614–629

3. Teipel S, Drzezga A, Grothe MJ et al (2015) Multimodal imaging in Alzheimer's disease: validity and usefulness for early detection. Lancet Neurol 14:1037–1353

4. Klunk WE, Koeppe RA, Price JC et al (2015) The Centiloid Project: standardizing quantitative amyloid plaque estimation by PET. Alzheimers Dement 11:11–15

5. Guerra UP, Nobili FM, Padovani A et al (2015) Recommendations from the Italian Interdisciplinary Working Group (AIMN, AIP, SINDEM) for the utilization of amyloid imaging in clinical practice. Neurol Sci 36:1075–1081

6. Minoshima S, Drzezga AE, Barthel H et al (2016) SNMMI procedure standard/EANM practice guideline for amyloid PET imaging of the brain 1.0. J Nucl Med 57:1316–1322

7. Garibotto V, Morbelli S, Pagani M (2016) Erratum to: dual-phase amyloid PET: hitting two birds with one stone. Eur J Nucl Med Mol Imaging 43:1747

8. Magistretti PJ (2000) Cellular bases of functional brain imaging: insights from neuron-glia metabolic coupling. Brain Res 886:108–112

9. Ni R, Gillberg PG, Bergfors A et al (2013) Amyloid tracers detect multiple binding sites in Alzheimer's disease brain tissue. Brain 136:2217–2227

10. Hsiao IT, Huang CC, Hsieh CJ et al (2012) Correlation of early-phase 18F-florbetapir (AV-45/Amyvid) PET images to FDG images: preliminary studies. Eur J Nucl Med Mol Imaging 39:613–620

11. Koole M, Lewis DM, Buckley C et al (2009) Whole-body biodistribution and radiation dosimetry of 18F-GE067: a radioligand for in vivo brain amyloid imaging. J Nucl Med 50:818–822

12. O'Keefe GJ, Saunder TH, Ng S et al (2009) Radiation dosimetry of beta-amyloid tracers 11C-PiB and 18F-BAY94-9172. J Nucl Med 50:309–315

13. Chincarini A, Sensi F, Rei L et al (2016) Alzheimer's Disease Neuroimaging Initiative. Standardized uptake value ratio-independent evaluation of brain amyloidosis. J Alzheimers Dis 54:1437–1457

14. Kinahan PE, Fletcher JW (2010) Positron emission tomography-computed tomography standardized uptake values in clinical practice and assessing response to therapy. Semin Ultrasound CT MR 31:496–505

15. Clark CM, Pontecorvo MJ, Beach TG et al (2012) Cerebral PET with florbetapir compared with neuropathology at autopsy for detection of neuritic amyloid-β plaques: a prospective cohort study. Lancet Neurol 11:669–678

16. Landau SM, Thomas BA, Thurfjell L et al (2014) Alzheimer's Disease Neuroimaging Initiative. Amyloid PET imaging in Alzheimer's disease: a comparison of three radiotracers. Eur J Nucl Med Mol Imaging 41:1398–1407

17. van Berckel BN, Ossenkoppele R, Tolboom N et al (2013) Longitudinal amyloid imaging using 11C-PiB: methodologic considerations. J Nucl Med 54:1570–1576

18. Dubois B, Feldman HH, Jacova C et al (2007) Research criteria for the diagnosis of Alzheimer's disease: revising the NINCDS-ADRDA criteria. Lancet Neurol 6:734–746

19. Johnson KA, Minoshima S, Bohnen NI et al (2013) Appropriate use criteria for amyloid PET: a report of the Amyloid Imaging Task Force, the Society of Nuclear Medicine and Molecular Imaging, and the Alzheimer's Association. Alzheimers Dement 9:e-1–e-16

Chapter 14

The Use of 18F-FDG PET in the Diagnostic Workup of Alzheimer's Dementia

Marion M. Ortner

Abstract

The diagnosis of dementia probably due to Alzheimer's disease is still primarily a clinical one. In cases that remain clinically unclear, however, biomarkers for amyloid deposition and neuronal injury can help to identify the underlying cause. One biomarker even for early neuronal injury in the stage of mild cognitive impairment is cerebral glucose hypometabolism measured by 18F-FDG PET. Distinct patterns of hypometabolism can be seen, for example, in dementia due to Alzheimer's disease, frontotemporal lobar degeneration, and dementia with Lewy bodies. This makes it possible to distinguish between different neurodegenerative diseases as well as major depressive disorder. While the sensitivity of 18F-FDG PET to detect Alzheimer's disease is high, specificity is low and the additional use of biomarkers for amyloid deposition might be beneficial in some cases. In conclusion, 18F-FDG PET is a useful tool when the cause for dementia remains unclear and different diagnosis would lead to different treatment approaches. Due to the lack of treatment options in pre-dementia stages, the use of 18F-FDG PET is currently not recommended for these cases in a purely clinical setting.

Key words Alzheimer's disease, Mild cognitive impairment (MCI), Alzheimer's disease dementia, Biomarker, 18F-FDG PET

1 Introduction

Alzheimer's disease (AD) is the most common cause of dementia [1]. It is neuropathologically defined by senile plaques containing β-Amyloid (Aβ) and neurofibrillary tangles with tau deposition in conjunction with loss of neurons and synapses [2, 3]. And while disease mechanisms are not fully comprehend yet, biomarkers for both amyloid pathology and neuronal loss helped to form hypotheses about the chronologic progression of pathologic changes occurring during the course of the disease. Biomarkers for Aβ deposition are low $A\beta_{42}$ in cerebrospinal fluid (CSF) and positive tracer uptake on amyloid positron emission tomography (PET) [4]. Biomarkers for neuronal injury and neuronal loss include elevated Tau protein in CSF, disproportionate atrophy on structural magnet resonance imaging (MRI) in medial, basal, lateral temporal lobe

Robert Perneczky (ed.), *Biomarkers for Alzheimer's Disease Drug Development*, Methods in Molecular Biology, vol. 1750, https://doi.org/10.1007/978-1-4939-7704-8_14, © Springer Science+Business Media, LLC 2018

and medial parietal cortex, and reduced ^{18}F-Fluordeoxyglucose (^{18}F-FDG) uptake on PET in temporoparietal cortex [4]. In research and clinical trials ^{18}F-FDG PET is commonly used to diagnose AD, even in pre-dementia stages, and to monitor disease progression. But what is its use in a purely clinical setting where the diagnosis of probable dementia due to AD is primarily a clinical one [4] and economic restrictions apply? This chapter aims to give an overview about the principle of ^{18}F-FDG PET and its application in diagnosing Alzheimer's dementia from a clinician's point of view.

2   Principles of ^{18}F-Fluordeoxyglucose Positron Emission Tomography

The most commonly used tracer for PET is FDG where basically a glucose analogue is labeled with the radioisotope fluorine-18 as a source of positrons. ^{18}F-FDG and glucose are both transported into cells by glucose transporters (GLUT) and become phosphorylated. In contrast to glucose, however, ^{18}F-FDG does not enter glycolysis after phosphorylation and is trapped inside the cell. When fluorine-18 decays, positrons are emitted. When these positrons collide with electrons two photons are emitted in a 180° angle. A ring-shaped detector which is positioned around the patient captures these photons and a computer calculates the point of origin of each photon pair. As cells with higher metabolism will take up more of the glucose analogue FDG while cells with lower metabolism will take up less FDG, measuring the radiation that is emitted over a certain time allows to indirectly assess metabolic activity for all points of origin. In the brain metabolic activity is mainly related to synaptic function. Compared to computed tomography (CT) or magnetic resonance imaging (MRI), the structural resolution of PET images is relatively poor. To be able to better relate the functional PET images to anatomic regions both modalities are usually combined in a PET-CT or PET-MRI scanner. 30 minutes after injection of ^{18}F-FDG PET imaging takes approximately 20 min.

2.1   High Blood Glucose Levels and Age Influence ^{18}F-FDG Uptake

Patients should be fasting for 4–6 h before the scan, and blood glucose levels need to be measured before the injection of ^{18}F-FDG. High blood glucose levels over 140 mg/dL or 7.8 mmol can interfere with ^{18}F-FDG uptake in the brain [5], in the worst case rendering the scan results useless by simulating a decreased cerebral glucose metabolism.

Although cerebral glucose metabolism decreases with age [6], not all brain regions are equally affected. Regions of hypometabolism typically associated with AD, such as the posterior cingulate cortex and the occipitotemporal cortex, show the least age-related changes [7]. For this reason, the diagnosis of AD based on results of F^{18}-FDG PET scans is vastly independent of the patients' age.

2.2 ¹⁸F-FDG-PET as a Tool in the Differential Diagnosis of Alzheimer's Disease

2.2.1 ¹⁸F-FDG-PET in the Differential Diagnosis Between Alzheimer's Dementia and Other Forms of Dementia

The use of ^{18}F-FDG PET is not generally recommended for the diagnostic workup of AD dementia by current guidelines [4, 8, 9]. However, it is an important tool when the cause of cognitive symptoms remains unclear, for example, in cases that could be either due to AD dementia, dementia with Lewy bodies (DLB), or frontotemporal lobar degeneration (FTLD) [8–10]. Different neurodegenerative diseases have unique patterns of hypometabolism. In AD dementia hypometabolism is primarily seen in the hippocampus, inferior parietal lobe, lateral temporal lobe, and posterior cingulate cortex. The prefrontal cortex can be affected as well, but typically to a lesser degree [11]. In the behavioral variant of FTLD the prefrontal cortex and lateral temporal lobe are primarily affected and to a lesser degree hypometabolism of the hippocampus and posterior cingulate cortex may occur [11, 12]. In dementia with Lewy bodies (DLB) the inferior parietal and occipital lobe are mainly affected [11]. In a study with neuropathologically confirmed cases Minoshima et al. found that ^{18}F-FDG PET was more sensitive in discriminating AD dementia from DLB than the clinical impression [13]. Specifics for sensitivity, specificity, and accuracy of ^{18}F-FDG PET in regard to different kinds of dementia are shown in Table 1.

^{18}F-FDG PET can also be used in the diagnostic workup of atypical presentations of AD such as posterior cortical atrophy (PCA) or logopenic variant of primary progressive aphasia (lvPPA) [14, 15]. PCA typically shows an occipito-parieto-temporal hypometabolism and lvPPA shows left inferior frontal and left temporo-parietal hypometabolism [16]. However, both PCA and lvPPA can also be caused by neurodegenerative diseases other than Alzheimer's disease, such as corticobasal degeneration, Creutzfeldt-Jakob disease, or FTLD [15, 17]. On the other hand, semantic variant of PPA, which is usually a variant of FTLD, can show typical neuropathologic changes of Alzheimer's disease [18, 19]. As the confirmation or exclusion of underlying Alzheimer's pathology will change therapeutic options, the additional use of a biomarker for Aβ pathology should be considered in these cases.

Table 1
Sensitivity, specificity, and accuracy of ^{18}F-FDG-PET to differentiate between AD dementia and other forms of dementia [10, 11, 13, 24, 31–34]

	Sensitivity [%]	Specificity [%]	Accuracy [%]
AD dementia vs. HC	86–100	73–100	88–100
AD dementia vs. bvFTLD	87–99	65–86	93–97
AD dementia vs. DLB	90–99	71–80	97

AD Alzheimer's disease, *HC* healthy control, *bvFTLD* behavioral variant of frontotemporal lobar degeneration, *DLB* dementia with Lewy bodies

^{18}F-FDG PET is also a useful tool to differentiate between Alzheimer's dementia and cognitive impairment caused by major depressive disorder where hypometabolism has been described mainly in the prefrontal cortex, insula, and the limbic system [20].

2.2.2 ^{18}F-FDG PET and MCI Due to Alzheimer's Disease

As AD is a progressive disease with gradual onset and increasing symptoms, there is a phase where cognitive impairment is evident; however, there is still independence in daily activities—the phase of mild cognitive impairment (MCI). Although many patients with MCI due to AD show already a similar pattern of hypometabolism as patients with AD dementia [11, 21], the use of ^{18}F-FDG PET in MCI is not recommended in a purely clinical setting [22, 23]. The Cochrane institute assesses the evidence insufficient to support routine use of ^{18}F-FDG PET for MCI in clinical practice as there is too much variability of specific values and lack of defined thresholds to determine scan positivity [23]. On the other hand, a negative ^{18}F-FDG PET scan, meaning normal cerebral glucose metabolism, is associated with a very low likelihood of developing Alzheimer's dementia over the next several years [24].

Should MCI patients seek out to know the underlying cause for their symptoms they should be referred to an expert to be counseled about possible tests such as ^{18}F-FDG PET, the value of the information gained by those tests, and possible therapeutic consequences [9]. Especially, as another factor to be considered in early diagnosis of Alzheimer's disease is the lack of treatment options in pre-dementia stages.

2.2.3 The Use of ^{18}F-FDG PET in Presymptomatic Alzheimer's Disease

The concept of preclinical AD is currently intended for research purposes only [25]. In a purely clinical setting the use of ^{18}F-FDG PET for the diagnosis of Alzheimer's disease in presymptomatic stages cannot be recommended and should not be offered, even if asked for by the patient. This is mainly due to ethical considerations. Up to this date there are no treatment options in presymptomatic Alzheimer's disease and the timeframe for an individual patient in which cognitive symptoms will develop cannot be predicted. Further information about the use of biomarkers in preclinical stages of AD can be found in the chapter "Patient benefit and ethical considerations: The ethics of biomarker-based preclinical diagnosis" by A. Kurz and N. Lautenschlager in this book.

2.3 ^{18}F-FDG PET in Combination with Other Biomarkers

While ^{18}F-FDG PET has a high sensitivity to detect AD the specificity is low [26]. For this reason a combination with other biomarkers, mainly those for amyloid pathology, such as amyloid PET with Pittsburgh compound B with high specificity and low sensitivity [26] may be useful in some cases. Although the combination of biomarkers for both Aβ pathology and neuronal injury can increase the probability of underlying AD pathology, they do not rule out a second underlying etiology [4]. Furthermore the results of biomarker testing are not always concordant within their group (e.g., total Tau and pTau181 in CSF and hypometabolism on FDG-PET as biomarkers for neuronal injury) or between groups (e.g., biomarkers for neuronal injury vs. Aβ deposition) [27, 28].

2.4 Limitations of ^{18}F-FDG PET (Cost, Availability, Radiation Exposure)

High costs compared to MRI scans or CSF analyses are a major disadvantage of ^{18}F-FDG PET. Beside the high cost PET scanners and tracer might not be ubiquitously available making it possibly difficult to obtain a ^{18}F-FDG PET scan within a reasonable travel distance for a patient. Although with 110 min relatively long, half life time might also be a factor to keep in mind when the tracer needs to be transported from manufacturing sites to remote sites of use.

Another factor that needs to be considered is radiation exposure. The exposure of the PET scan itself is about 7–10 mSv. For comparison, the mean effective dose of radiation exposure from natural sources in Germany is approximately 2.1 mSv/year [29], exposure during a transatlantic flight is about 0.08 mSv [30], and the average annual radon dose to people in Cornwall 6.9 mSv [30]. If combined with a CT scan additional radiation exposure will apply. This additional radiation can be avoided using PET-MRI scanners. However, PET-MRI scanners are far less common and might not be an option.

3   Conclusion

While the diagnosis of dementia due to probable AD is a clinical diagnosis, ^{18}F-FDG PET is a useful tool when the cause for dementia remains unclear. This is especially true if the correct diagnosis leads to different treatment approaches, e.g., if the differential diagnoses are AD, depression, and frontotemporal lobar degeneration. The use of ^{18}F-FDG PET in the pre-dementia state of MCI or cognitively normal should be limited to specialized settings and is not recommended in a purely clinical setting. This recommendation may change should treatment options for these early stages get available in the future.

References

1. Ferri CP, Prince M, Brayne C et al (2005) Global prevalence of dementia: a Delphi consensus study. Lancet 366(9503):2112–2117. https://doi.org/10.1016/S0140-6736(05)67889-0

2. Braak H, Braak E (1991) Neuropathological stageing of Alzheimer-related changes. Acta Neuropathol 82(4):239–259

3. Thal DR, Rub U, Orantes M et al (2002) Phases of A beta-deposition in the human brain and its relevance for the development of AD. Neurology 58(12):1791–1800

4. McKhann GM, Knopman DS, Chertkow H et al (2011) The diagnosis of dementia due to Alzheimer's disease: recommendations from the National Institute on Aging-Alzheimer's Association workgroups on diagnostic guidelines for Alzheimer's disease. Alzheimers Dement 7(3):263–269. https://doi.org/10.1016/j.jalz.2011.03.005

5. Kawasaki K, Ishii K, Saito Y et al (2008) Influence of mild hyperglycemia on cerebral FDG distribution patterns calculated by statistical parametric mapping. Ann Nucl Med 22(3):191–200. https://doi.org/10.1007/s12149-007-0099-7

6. Kuhl DE, Metter EJ, Riege WH et al (1982) Effects of human aging on patterns of local cerebral glucose utilization determined by the [18F]fluorodeoxyglucose method. J Cereb Blood Flow Metab 2(2):163–171. https://doi.org/10.1038/jcbfm.1982.15

7. Kalpouzos G, Chetelat G, Baron JC et al (2009) Voxel-based mapping of brain gray matter volume and glucose metabolism profiles in normal aging. Neurobiol Aging 30(1):112–124. https://doi.org/10.1016/j.neurobiolaging.2007.05.019

8. Soucy JP, Bartha R, Bocti C et al (2013) Clinical applications of neuroimaging in patients with Alzheimer's disease: a review from the fourth Canadian consensus conference on the diagnosis and treatment of dementia 2012. Alzheimers Res Ther 5(Suppl 1):S3. https://doi.org/10.1186/alzrt199

9. S3 Leitlinie "Demenz" (2015)

10. Foster NL, Heidebrink JL, Clark CM et al (2007) FDG-PET improves accuracy in distinguishing frontotemporal dementia and Alzheimer's disease. Brain 130(Pt 10):2616–2635. https://doi.org/10.1093/brain/awm177

11. Mosconi L, Tsui WH, Herholz K et al (2008) Multicenter standardized 18F-FDG PET diagnosis of mild cognitive impairment, Alzheimer's disease, and other dementias. J Nucl Med 49(3):390–398. https://doi.org/10.2967/jnumed.107.045385

12. Diehl-Schmid J, Grimmer T, Drzezga A et al (2007) Decline of cerebral glucose metabolism in frontotemporal dementia: a longitudinal 18F-FDG-PET-study. Neurobiol Aging 28(1):42–50. https://doi.org/10.1016/j.neurobiolaging.2005.11.002

13. Minoshima S, Foster NL, Sima AA et al (2001) Alzheimer's disease versus dementia with Lewy bodies: cerebral metabolic distinction with autopsy confirmation. Ann Neurol 50(3):358–365

14. Rabinovici GD, Jagust WJ, Furst AJ et al (2008) Abeta amyloid and glucose metabolism in three variants of primary progressive aphasia. Ann Neurol 64(4):388–401. https://doi.org/10.1002/ana.21451

15. Mesulam M, Wicklund A, Johnson N et al (2008) Alzheimer and frontotemporal pathology in subsets of primary progressive aphasia.

Ann Neurol 63(6):709–719. https://doi.org/10.1002/ana.21388

16. Laforce R Jr, Tosun D, Ghosh P et al (2014) Parallel ICA of FDG-PET and PiB-PET in three conditions with underlying Alzheimer's pathology. Neuroimage Clin 4:508–516. https://doi.org/10.1016/j.nicl.2014.03.005

17. Renner JA, Burns JM, Hou CE et al (2004) Progressive posterior cortical dysfunction: a clinicopathologic series. Neurology 63(7):1175–1180

18. Alladi S, Xuereb J, Bak T et al (2007) Focal cortical presentations of Alzheimer's disease. Brain 130(Pt 10):2636–2645. https://doi.org/10.1093/brain/awm213

19. Knibb JA, Xuereb JH, Patterson K et al (2006) Clinical and pathological characterization of progressive aphasia. Ann Neurol 59(1):156–165. https://doi.org/10.1002/ana.20700

20. Su L, Cai Y, Xu Y et al (2014) Cerebral metabolism in major depressive disorder: a voxel-based meta-analysis of positron emission tomography studies. BMC Psychiatry 14:321. https://doi.org/10.1186/s12888-014-0321-9

21. Drzezga A, Lautenschlager N, Siebner H et al (2003) Cerebral metabolic changes accompanying conversion of mild cognitive impairment into Alzheimer's disease: a PET follow-up study. Eur J Nucl Med Mol Imaging 30(8):1104–1113. https://doi.org/10.1007/s00259-003-1194-1

22. Albert MS, DeKosky ST, Dickson D et al (2011) The diagnosis of mild cognitive impairment due to Alzheimer's disease: recommendations from the National Institute on Aging-Alzheimer's Association workgroups on diagnostic guidelines for Alzheimer's disease. Alzheimers Dement 7(3):270–279. https://doi.org/10.1016/j.jalz.2011.03.008

23. Smailagic N, Vacante M, Hyde C et al (2015) (1)(8)F-FDG PET for the early diagnosis of Alzheimer's disease dementia and other dementias in people with mild cognitive impairment (MCI). Cochrane Database Syst Rev 1:CD010632. https://doi.org/10.1002/14651858.CD010632.pub2

24. Silverman DH, Small GW, Chang CY et al (2001) Positron emission tomography in evaluation of dementia: regional brain metabolism and long-term outcome. JAMA 286(17):2120–2127

25. Sperling RA, Aisen PS, Beckett LA et al (2011) Toward defining the preclinical stages of Alzheimer's disease: recommendations from the National Institute on Aging-

Alzheimer's Association workgroups on diagnostic guidelines for Alzheimer's disease. Alzheimers Dement 7(3):280–292. https://doi.org/10.1016/j.jalz.2011.03.003

26. Mosconi L, McHugh PF (2011) FDG- and amyloid-PET in Alzheimer's disease: is the whole greater than the sum of the parts? Q J Nucl Med Mol Imaging 55(3):250–264

27. Alexopoulos P, Kriett L, Haller B et al (2014) Limited agreement between biomarkers of neuronal injury at different stages of Alzheimer's disease. Alzheimers Dement 10(6):684–689. https://doi.org/10.1016/j.jalz.2014.03.006

28. Zwan MD, Rinne JO, Hasselbalch SG et al (2016) Use of amyloid-PET to determine cutpoints for CSF markers: a multicenter study. Neurology 86(1):50–58. https://doi.org/10.1212/WNL.0000000000002081

29. Federal Ministry for the Environment NC, Building and Nuclear Safety (2014) Umweltradioaktivität und Strahlenbelastung Jahresbericht 2014. http://www.bmub.bund.de/themen/atomenergie-strahlenschutz/strahlenschutz/atomenergie-strahlenschutz-download/artikel/umweltradioaktivitaet-und-strahlenbelastung-jahresbericht-2014-gesamtbericht/?tx_ttnews%5BbackPid%5D=347. Accessed 11 March 2017

30. England PH (2011) Guidance—ionising radiation: dose comparisons. https://www.gov.uk/government/publications/ionising-radiation-dose-comparisons/ionising-radiation-dose-comparisons. Accessed 22 Apr 2017

31. Mosconi L, Tsui WH, Pupi A et al (2007) (18) F-FDG PET database of longitudinally confirmed healthy elderly individuals improves detection of mild cognitive impairment and Alzheimer's disease. J Nucl Med 48(7):1129–1134. https://doi.org/10.2967/jnumed.107.040675

32. Chen WP, Samuraki M, Yanase D et al (2008) Effect of sample size for normal database on diagnostic performance of brain FDG PET for the detection of Alzheimer's disease using automated image analysis. Nucl Med Commun 29(3):270–276. https://doi.org/10.1097/MNM.0b013e3282f3fa76

33. Patwardhan MB, McCrory DC, Matchar DB et al (2004) Alzheimer disease: operating characteristics of PET—a meta-analysis. Radiology 231(1):73–80. https://doi.org/10.1148/radiol.2311021620

34. Bohnen NI, Djang DS, Herholz K et al (2012) Effectiveness and safety of 18F-FDG PET in the evaluation of dementia: a review of the recent literature. J Nucl Med 53(1):59–71. https://doi.org/10.2967/jnumed.111.096578

Chapter 15

Quantification of Tau Load in Alzheimer's Disease Clinical Trials Using Positron Emission Tomography

Tessa Timmers, Bart N.M. van Berckel, Adriaan A. Lammertsma, and Rik Ossenkoppele

Abstract

Alzheimer's disease is a neurodegenerative condition that is neuropathologically characterized by the presence of amyloid-β plaques and neurofibrillary tangles consisting of tau. Recently, several positron emission tomography (PET) tracers have been developed that yielded promising initial results. In this chapter, we discuss how tau PET can be used in the context in clinical trials. We argue that simplified reference tissue models based on dynamic data acquisition are most suitable for accurately measuring changes in tau pathology in trials tailored to reduce cerebral tau load. Therefore, we discuss the importance of tracer kinetic modeling and describe in detail how a reliable measurement of specific binding can be obtained.

Key words Tau, Positron emission tomography (PET), Alzheimer's disease (AD), AV1451, Clinical trial

1 Introduction

The core proteins involved in Alzheimer's disease (AD) pathogenesis are amyloid-β (Aβ) and hyperphosphorylated tau. Aβ deposits and tau tangles can be measured in the living human brain using positron emission tomography (PET) [1, 2]. The ability to probe both AD hallmarks in vivo offers great opportunities for AD research, clinical application (i.e., improving diagnosis and prognosis), and design, selection, and monitoring efficacy in clinical trials. This chapter will focus on how to perform quantitative tau PET scans optimally in the context of clinical trials.

Fundamental neuroscience studies have clearly pinpointed the central role of tau pathology as a driving force of neurodegeneration and cognitive decline in AD. Tau is a microtubule-associated protein that aggregates into intracellular neurofibrillary tangles (NFTs) and has a devastating effect on synaptic [3–5] and subsequent cognitive [6–8] function. The importance of mapping the

Robert Perneczky (ed.), *Biomarkers for Alzheimer's Disease Drug Development*, Methods in Molecular Biology, vol. 1750, https://doi.org/10.1007/978-1-4939-7704-8_15, © Springer Science+Business Media, LLC 2018

distribution of tau pathology in the living human brain is evident, but until recently this was not possible and tau pathology could only be examined in animal models, cell cultures, and cerebrospinal fluid. The advent of a series of PET tracers showing high in vitro affinity and selectivity for paired helical filament tau pathology [1, 9, 10], however, offers unique opportunities for in vivo assessment of regional tau load in AD. Due to differences in mRNA splicing of the microtubule-associated tau (MAPT) gene, distinct isoforms of tau exist in the human brain. The currently available tau PET ligands bind more strongly to the combination of 3-repeat (3R) and 4-repeat (4R) tau isoforms, a combination typically found in individuals with AD [9, 11, 12]. Therefore, tau imaging seems most useful across the spectrum of AD, and less in other tauopathies. Initial studies with these novel tau ligands are promising as they reveal retention patterns that closely resemble classical neuropathological Braak staging of NFTs [13, 14], clearly distinguish AD patients from individuals without dementia [13, 15], and show strong correlations with neurodegenerative markers and with cognition [16–19].

The selection of a specific PET method strongly depends on the research or clinical question at stake. For example, when the objective is to classify subjects into certain groups (for instance, $A\beta$ positive or negative), a visual read of a statically acquired PET scan could be sufficient [20]. However, when monitoring the effects of disease-modifying agents in AD clinical trials (which is the focus of this chapter), quantification methods are needed, since static scans cannot separate the confounding components of tracer delivery, uptake, retention, and clearance, which could all influence the net tracer uptake. Proper evaluation of the pharmacokinetic properties of the PET tracer is thus essential [21]. This provides knowledge about tracer delivery (i.e., tracer plasma concentration or blood flow), the amount of tracer binding sites, washout, and the presence of metabolites. This information is essential to determine the accuracy of the PET signal and can only be obtained following a procedure that includes dynamic scanning (i.e., monitoring the time course of radiotracer distribution during the entire scan after injection into the camera) and acquiring arterial blood samples during the scan. Only with these data, so-called plasma-input models can then serve as gold standard in tracer quantification. Using these plasma input models more simplified approaches can be validated, usually only possible when a reference region is available. A reference region is a brain region devoid of specific PET binding, for instance, cerebellar gray matter for tau pathology in AD. We propose that for clinical trials dynamic PET scans should be acquired, which should be analyzed with a validated reference tissue model [22, 23].

2   Materials

Various tau PET tracers are currently being used. In this chapter we focus on [^{18}F]AV1451 and describe the current PET acquisition and data analysis pipeline at VU University Medical Center for this specific tracer.

1. For the acquisition and analysis of dynamic [^{18}F]AV1451 PET scans, the following materials are needed:
   - Tau tracer.
   - PET scanner.
   - Atomic clock with hh:mm:ss notation.

2. For placement of the venous cannula:
   - Cannula for vein.
   - Gauzes.
   - Alcohol skin preparation solution.
   - 5 mL syringe with NaCl 0.9%.
   - Extension line with three-way stopcock.
   - Tape or adhesive plaster.

3. For injection of the tracer:
   - CT injection system (for instance, MEDRAD Stellant with workstation).
   - Extension lines.

4. To measure the injected dose:
   - Dose calibrator.
   - Atomic clock with hh:mm:ss notation.

5. For kinetic analysis:
   - PC with storage and software for analyses, such as
     (a) Vinci Software.
     (b) MatLab Software.
     (c) PVELab Software.
     (d) PPET Software.
     (e) Microsoft Excel.

3   Methods

For acquisition and analysis of dynamic tau PET scans, detailed planning and careful selection of equipment is essential. The ultimate goal is to derive regional or parametric outcome measures, reflecting tau burden. For this purpose, the following materials are needed.

3.1 Tau Tracer

While various tau PET tracers are currently being used, we focus in this chapter on [^{18}F]AV1451.

3.2 MRI Scan

For the purpose of co-registration, segmentation, and definition of volumes-of-interest (VOI), brain MRI including T1-weighted images are needed. Furthermore, MRI scans can be used for inclusion purposes, i.e., to rule out any anatomical abnormalities such as major stroke or mass that is likely to interfere with the interpretation of PET. Since dementia subjects are prone to progressive atrophy, time intervals between MRI and PET should ideally not exceed 6 months (particularly the case for clinical trials).

3.3 PET-CT and Scan Protocol

For longitudinal data and test–retest studies, it is preferred to perform all scans on the same PET-scanner, to obtain a homogenous dataset. Start the scanning protocol with a low dose CT for attenuation correction. After this, the dynamic scan should be started at the same time as the tracer is injected (*see* Subheading 3.5). For dynamic [^{18}F]AV1451 scans, different scan protocols are currently being used. Due to increased input function uncertainty and PET data noise at later time points, scanner protocols longer than 130 min are not recommended for this tracer. Perform short time frames in the first acquisition part to capture the bolus injection, and consider wider time frames in later parts of acquisition.

To reduce noise due to subject movement, the subject should be carefully instructed to lie still. Make sure the subject is as comfortable as possible for the duration of the PET scan, by using pillows or bindings. Using a head holder, foam, and band, head movement can be restricted. During the scan, head movements can be checked by projecting laser beams on set points projected on the head, and should be corrected immediately (*see* **Notes 1** and **2**).

3.4 Venous Cannula

Place a venous cannula in a superficial vein of the arm or hand using established procedures. This venous cannula will be used to inject the tracer (*see* **Note 3**).

3.5 Tracer Injection

Start the dynamic scanning protocol and inject the tracer simultaneously (*see* **Note 4**). For reproducibility purposes, it is preferred to inject the tracer with an CT injection system, for instance the MEDRAD Stellant CT injection system. Measure the radioactivity (MBq) in the syringe pre and post injection, as well as the extension lines. Tracer injection time should be noted as hh:mm:ss to calculate the net injected dose (*see* **Note 5**).

3.6 Storage and Reconstruction of PET Files

Code and store the PET files. The reconstruction for PET images is dependent on the type of PET-CT scanner and the software used. We use a Philips IngenuityTF PET/CT scanner with Astonish TF software for standard corrections for attenuation, scatter, and randoms: http://www.philips.nl/healthcare/product/HC459800473361/astonish-tf-timeofflight-technology.

3.7 Pre-processing PET-Images

The pre-processing for PET images is dependent on the type of PET-CT scanner and the software used. We use a Philips IngenuityTF PET/CT scanner with Astonish TF software for standard corrections of attenuation, scatter, and randoms.

First, convert Digital Imaging and Communications in Medicine (DICOM) files into ECAT files (an image format including a main header and at least one matrix list) to make them compatible for the software tool Vinci (i.e., Volume Imaging in Neurological Imaging). We have incorporated Vinci software into our pipeline because it has been shown to yield reliable results for image co-registration [24]. Open the files and check for errors in reconstruction. Next, check for head movements. This can be achieved by loading a range of non-attenuation corrected (NAC) frames (preferably a range in which sustainable uptake is seen), the CT image, and the average of CT-based attenuation correction (CTAC) frames. Using the contour tool and the fusion tool in Vinci, movement between CT and individual NAC frames and between CT and combined CTAC frames can be evaluated. Frame-by-frame motion correction can be applied using the NAC images [25] to increase the accuracy of PET quantification (*see* **Note 6**).

3.8 Generate Regional Time Activity Curves

By projecting regions of interest (ROI), delineated on T1-weighted MRI, on dynamic and motion corrected PET images, regional tissue time activity curves (TACs) can be generated. ROI delineation can be performed manually, or using "single-atlas" or "multi-atlas" approaches. In the context of clinical trials, manual ROI delineation is not preferable as it introduces additional noise caused by observer variability between baseline and follow-up scan(s). We prefer a probability-based multi-atlas approach, as this yields strong overlap between the ROI and its anatomical location on the PET image. First, co-register the MRI images to the PET frames using the MMM co-registration tool in Vinci [24] (*see* **Note 7**). Next, use the PVElab software to extract TACs (*see* **Note 8**). The program will load PET and MRI file, segment them in gray matter, white matter, and CSF, and warp them onto a multi-atlas brain template (in our case the Hammers template [26]). After generating the TACs for different ROIs, including TAC for the reference region (i.e., cerebellar gray matter), specific binding of the tracer can now be obtained. The following paragraphs describe how the most optimal method was selected.

3.9 Determine Optimal Tracer Kinetic Model

To determine the optimal tracer kinetic model, fit the regional TACs to different models, using standard nonlinear regression (NLR). Standard single tissue (1T2k), irreversible (2T3k) and reversible (2T4k) compartmental models with and without blood volume can be used. For selecting the optimal kinetics, Akaike criteria can be used. We have identified a reversible 2T4k model as the most optimal compartmental model for $[^{18}F]AV1451$ [23], but this procedure should be repeated for novel (tau) PET tracers.

3.10 Validate Simplified Reference Tissue Methods and Parametric Images

Full kinetic modeling is seen as the "gold standard," but once the optimal kinetic model has been selected, simplified reference tissue methods should be evaluated, since these methods are less invasive and reduce subject burden, improve computational simplicity, and reduce costs [27]. With the optimal tracer kinetic model, macroparameters such as binding potential (BP_{ND}) and distribution volume ratio (DVR) can be calculated, using simplified reference tissue methods such as reference Logan [28] or reference parametric mapping (RPM) [29, 30]. We have identified RPM as the most optimal reference tissue model for cross-sectional studies, but these validation steps should be repeated for next generation tau PET tracers. Figure 1 shows RPM-derived $[^{18}F]AV1451$ BP_{ND} images of three AD patients and three cognitively normal controls.

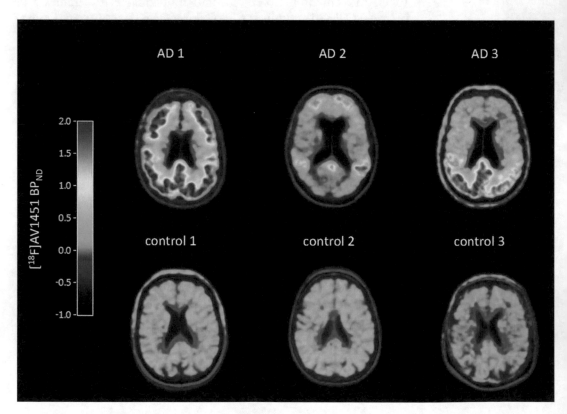

Fig. 1 $[^{18}F]AV1451$ BP_{ND} images of three AD patients and three cognitively normal controls

3.11 Test for Test–Retest Variability

Finally, the reliability of a PET-tracer can be tested using test–retest data. This is particularly important in studies monitoring disease progression over time. Difference between test and retest can be calculated for macroparameters obtained from the full kinetic modeling and for parameters obtained from simplified reference tissue methods. To date, no test–retest studies have been reported.

4 Notes

1. It is of great importance that head movement is restricted during scanning procedures. Therefore, instruct your subjects carefully and make sure they are lying comfortable before starting the scan procedures.

2. For subjects with severe cognitive decline, it can be challenging to complete the full procedure. Aim to select subjects who are likely able to lie still for a prolonged period of time.

3. When the amount of tracer is not fully submitted to subject's blood system, less tracer will be available to the binding sites. Therefore, check if the venous cannula is not placed subcutaneously, by flushing it with NaCl 0.9% before injection of the tracer. This can also be checked during tracer injection with the MEDRAD injection system, since it will provide an indication of the amount of pressure needed to inject the tracer.

4. To obtain reliable TACs, it is crucial to capture the first frames of the scan. Therefore, start the scanning procedures at exactly the same time as tracer injection. Use a clock with hh:mm:ss notation. This is especially important for longitudinal studies assessing changes with respect to the baseline condition.

5. Usually, a small amount of tracer is left behind in the syringe and extension lines. By measuring the syringe pre and post injection, you can measure the quantity of tracer that is left behind in the syringe, and correct for this by calculating the net injected dose.

6. When analyzing the scans, head movement can affect the reliability of your data. Carefully assess whether this is the case, and conduct a motion correction when appropriate.

7. To check gray and white matter segmentations, open the files and project them onto the MRI scan, using Vinci's MMM co-registration tool.

8. To test if PVElab software generated the time activity curves correctly, open the text-files and check if the start and ending times are correct.

References

1. Chien DT, Bahri S, Szardenings AK, Walsh JC, Mu F, Su MY, Shankle WR, Elizarov A, Kolb HC (2013) Early clinical PET imaging results with the novel PHF-tau radioligand [F-18]-T807. J Alzheimers Dis 34(2):457–468. https://doi.org/10.3233/JAD-122059

2. Klunk WE, Engler H, Nordberg A, Wang Y, Blomqvist G, Holt DP, Bergstrom M, Savitcheva I, Huang GF, Estrada S, Ausen B, Debnath ML, Barletta J, Price JC, Sandell J, Lopresti BJ, Wall A, Koivisto P, Antoni G, Mathis CA, Langstrom B (2004) Imaging brain amyloid in Alzheimer's disease with Pittsburgh Compound-B. Ann Neurol 55(3):306–319. https://doi.org/10.1002/ana.20009

3. Beharry C, Cohen LS, Di J, Ibrahim K, Briffa-Mirabella S, Alonso Adel C (2014) Tau-induced neurodegeneration: mechanisms and targets. Neurosci Bull 30(2):346–358. https://doi.org/10.1007/s12264-013-1414-z

4. Gomez-Isla T, Hollister R, West H, Mui S, Growdon JH, Petersen RC, Parisi JE, Hyman BT (1997) Neuronal loss correlates with but exceeds neurofibrillary tangles in Alzheimer's disease. Ann Neurol 41(1):17–24. https://doi.org/10.1002/ana.410410106

5. Spires-Jones TL, Hyman BT (2014) The intersection of amyloid beta and tau at synapses in Alzheimer's disease. Neuron 82(4):756–771. https://doi.org/10.1016/j.neuron.2014.05.004

6. Arriagada PV, Growdon JH, Hedley-Whyte ET, Hyman BT (1992) Neurofibrillary tangles but not senile plaques parallel duration and severity of Alzheimer's disease. Neurology 42(3 Pt 1):631–639

7. Nelson PT, Alafuzoff I, Bigio EH, Bouras C, Braak H, Cairns NJ, Castellani RJ, Crain BJ, Davies P, Del Tredici K, Duyckaerts C, Frosch MP, Haroutunian V, Hof PR, Hulette CM, Hyman BT, Iwatsubo T, Jellinger KA, Jicha GA, Kovari E, Kukull WA, Leverenz JB, Love S, Mackenzie IR, Mann DM, Masliah E, McKee AC, Montine TJ, Morris JC, Schneider JA, Sonnen JA, Thal DR, Trojanowski JQ, Troncoso JC, Wisniewski T, Woltjer RL, Beach TG (2012) Correlation of Alzheimer disease neuropathologic changes with cognitive status: a review of the literature. J Neuropathol Exp Neurol 71(5):362–381. https://doi.org/10.1097/NEN.0b013e31825018f7

8. Rolstad S, Berg AI, Bjerke M, Johansson B, Zetterberg H, Wallin A (2013) Cerebrospinal fluid biomarkers mirror rate of cognitive decline. J Alzheimers Dis 34(4):949–956. https://doi.org/10.3233/JAD-121960

9. Marquie M, Normandin MD, Vanderburg CR, Costantino IM, Bien EA, Rycyna LG, Klunk WE, Mathis CA, Ikonomovic MD, Debnath ML, Vasdev N, Dickerson BC, Gomperts SN, Growdon JH, Johnson KA, Frosch MP, Hyman BT, Gomez-Isla T (2015) Validating novel tau positron emission tomography tracer [F-18]-AV-1451 (T807) on postmortem brain tissue. Ann Neurol 78(5):787–800. https://doi.org/10.1002/ana.24517

10. Xia CF, Arteaga J, Chen G, Gangadharmath U, Gomez LF, Kasi D, Lam C, Liang Q, Liu C, Mocharla VP, Mu F, Sinha A, Su H, Szardenings AK, Walsh JC, Wang E, Yu C, Zhang W, Zhao T, Kolb HC (2013) [(18)F] T807, a novel tau positron emission tomography imaging agent for Alzheimer's disease. Alzheimers Dement 9(6):666–676. https://doi.org/10.1016/j.jalz.2012.11.008

11. Lowe VJ, Curran G, Fang P, Liesinger AM, Josephs KA, Parisi JE, Kantarci K, Boeve BF, Pandey MK, Bruinsma T, Knopman DS, Jones DT, Petrucelli L, Cook CN, Graff-Radford NR, Dickson DW, Petersen RC, Jack CR Jr, Murray ME (2016) An autoradiographic evaluation of AV-1451 Tau PET in dementia. Acta Neuropathol Commun 4(1):58. https://doi.org/10.1186/s40478-016-0315-6

12. Marquie M, Siao Tick Chong M, Anton-Fernandez A, Verwer EE, Saez-Calveras N, Meltzer AC, Ramanan P, Amaral AC, Gonzalez J, Normandin MD, Frosch MP, Gomez-Isla T (2017) [F-18]-AV-1451 binding correlates with postmortem neurofibrillary tangle Braak staging. Acta Neuropathol 134:619. https://doi.org/10.1007/s00401-017-1740-8

13. Scholl M, Lockhart SN, Schonhaut DR, O'Neil JP, Janabi M, Ossenkoppele R, Baker SL, Vogel JW, Faria J, Schwimmer HD, Rabinovici GD, Jagust WJ (2016) PET imaging of tau deposition in the aging human brain. Neuron 89(5):971–982. https://doi.org/10.1016/j.neuron.2016.01.028

14. Schwarz AJ, Yu P, Miller BB, Shcherbinin S, Dickson J, Navitsky M, Joshi AD, Devous MD Sr, Mintun MS (2016) Regional profiles of the candidate tau PET ligand 18F-AV-1451 recapitulate key features of Braak histopathological stages. Brain 139(Pt 5):1539–1550. https://doi.org/10.1093/brain/aww023

15. Johnson KA, Schultz A, Betensky RA, Becker JA, Sepulcre J, Rentz D, Mormino E, Chhatwal J, Amariglio R, Papp K, Marshall G, Albers M, Mauro S, Pepin L, Alverio J, Judge K, Philiossaint M, Shoup T, Yokell D, Dickerson B, Gomez-Isla T, Hyman B, Vasdev N, Sperling

R (2016) Tau positron emission tomographic imaging in aging and early Alzheimer disease. Ann Neurol 79(1):110–119. https://doi.org/10.1002/ana.24546

16. Cho H, Choi JY, Hwang MS, Kim YJ, Lee HM, Lee HS, Lee JH, Ryu YH, Lee MS, Lyoo CH (2016) In vivo cortical spreading pattern of tau and amyloid in the Alzheimer disease spectrum. Ann Neurol 80(2):247–258. https://doi.org/10.1002/ana.24711

17. Ossenkoppele R, Schonhaut DR, Baker SL, O'Neil JP, Janabi M, Ghosh PM, Santos M, Miller ZA, Bettcher BM, Gorno-Tempini ML, Miller BL, Jagust WJ, Rabinovici GD (2015) Tau, amyloid, and hypometabolism in a patient with posterior cortical atrophy. Ann Neurol 77(2):338–342. https://doi.org/10.1002/ana.24321

18. Ossenkoppele R, Schonhaut DR, Scholl M, Lockhart SN, Ayakta N, Baker SL, O'Neil JP, Janabi M, Lazaris A, Cantwell A, Vogel J, Santos M, Miller ZA, Bettcher BM, Vossel KA, Kramer JH, Gorno-Tempini ML, Miller BL, Jagust WJ, Rabinovici GD (2016) Tau PET patterns mirror clinical and neuroanatomical variability in Alzheimer's disease. Brain 139(Pt 5):1551–1567. https://doi.org/10.1093/brain/aww027

19. Sepulcre J, Schultz AP, Sabuncu M, Gomez-Isla T, Chhatwal J, Becker A, Sperling R, Johnson KA (2016) In vivo tau, amyloid, and gray matter profiles in the aging brain. J Neurosci 36(28):7364–7374. https://doi.org/10.1523/JNEUROSCI.0639-16.2016

20. Zwan MD, Ossenkoppele R, Tolboom N, Beunders AJ, Kloet RW, Adriaanse SM, Boellaard R, Windhorst AD, Raijmakers P, Adams H, Lammertsma AA, Scheltens P, van der Flier WM, van Berckel BN (2014) Comparison of simplified parametric methods for visual interpretation of 11C-Pittsburgh compound-B PET images. J Nucl Med 55(8):1305–1307. https://doi.org/10.2967/jnumed.114.139121

21. Lammertsma AA (2017) Forward to the past: the case for quantitative PET imaging. J Nucl Med 58:1019. https://doi.org/10.2967/jnumed.116.188029

22. van Berckel BN, Ossenkoppele R, Tolboom N, Yaqub M, Foster-Dingley JC, Windhorst AD, Scheltens P, Lammertsma AA, Boellaard R (2013) Longitudinal amyloid imaging using 11C-PiB: methodologic considerations. J Nucl Med 54(9):1570–1576. https://doi.org/10.2967/jnumed.112.113654

23. Golla SS, Timmers T, Ossenkoppele R, Groot C, Verfaillie S, Scheltens P, van der Flier WM, Schwarte L, Mintun MA, Devous M, Schuit RC, Windhorst AD, Lammertsma AA, Boellaard R, van Berckel BN, Yaqub M (2017) Quantification of tau load using [18F]AV1451 PET. Mol Imaging Biol 19:963. https://doi.org/10.1007/s11307-017-1080-z

24. Cizek J, Herholz K, Vollmar S, Schrader R, Klein J, Heiss WD (2004) Fast and robust registration of PET and MR images of human brain. Neuroimage 22(1):434–442. https://doi.org/10.1016/j.neuroimage.2004.01.016

25. Mourik JE, Lubberink M, van Velden FH, Lammertsma AA, Boellaard R (2009) Off-line motion correction methods for multi-frame PET data. Eur J Nucl Med Mol Imaging 36(12):2002–2013. https://doi.org/10.1007/s00259-009-1193-y

26. Hammers A, Allom R, Koepp MJ, Free SL, Myers R, Lemieux L, Mitchell TN, Brooks DJ, Duncan JS (2003) Three-dimensional maximum probability atlas of the human brain, with particular reference to the temporal lobe. Hum Brain Mapp 19(4):224–247. https://doi.org/10.1002/hbm.10123

27. Ossenkoppele R, Prins ND, van Berckel BN (2013) Amyloid imaging in clinical trials. Alzheimers Res Ther 5(4):36. https://doi.org/10.1186/alzrt195

28. Logan J, Fowler JS, Volkow ND, Wang GJ, Ding YS, Alexoff DL (1996) Distribution volume ratios without blood sampling from graphical analysis of PET data. J Cereb Blood Flow Metab 16(5):834–840. https://doi.org/10.1097/00004647-199609000-00008

29. Gunn RN, Lammertsma AA, Hume SP, Cunningham VJ (1997) Parametric imaging of ligand-receptor binding in PET using a simplified reference region model. Neuroimage 6(4):279–287. https://doi.org/10.1006/nimg.1997.0303

30. Lammertsma AA, Hume SP (1996) Simplified reference tissue model for PET receptor studies. Neuroimage 4(3 Pt 1):153–158. https://doi.org/10.1006/nimg.1996.0066

Chapter 16

Imaging Neuroinflammation: Quantification of Astrocytosis in a Multitracer PET Approach

Elena Rodriguez-Vieitez and Agneta Nordberg

Abstract

The recent progress in the development of in vivo biomarkers is rapidly changing how neurodegenerative diseases are conceptualized and diagnosed, and how clinical trials are designed today. Alzheimer's disease (AD)—the most common neurodegenerative disorder—is characterized by a complex neuropathology involving the deposition of extracellular amyloid-β (Aβ) plaques and intracellular neurofibrillary tangles (NFT) of hyperphosphorylated tau proteins, accompanied by the activation of glial cells—astrocytes and microglia—and neuroinflammatory responses, leading to neurodegeneration and cognitive dysfunction. An increasing diversity of positron emission tomography (PET) imaging radiotracers are available to selectively target the different pathophysiological processes of AD. Along with the success of Aβ PET and the more recent tau PET imaging, there is also a great interest to develop PET tracers to image glial activation and neuroinflammation. While most research to date has focused on imaging microgliosis, recent studies using ^{11}C-deuterium-L-deprenyl (^{11}C-DED) PET imaging suggest that astrocytosis may be present from very early stages of disease development in AD. This chapter provides a detailed description of the practical approach used for the analysis of ^{11}C-DED PET imaging data in a multitracer PET paradigm including ^{11}C-Pittsburgh compound B (^{11}C-PiB) and ^{18}F-fluorodeoxyglucose (^{18}F-FDG). The multitracer PET approach allows investigating the comparative regional and temporal patterns of in vivo brain astrocytosis, fibrillar Aβ deposition, and glucose metabolism in patients at different stages of disease progression. This chapter attempts to stimulate further research in the field, including the development of novel PET tracers that may allow visualizing different aspects of the complex astrocytic and microglial responses in neurodegenerative diseases. Progress in the field will contribute to the incorporation of PET imaging of glial activation and neuroinflammation as biomarkers with clinical application, and motivate further investigation on glial cells as therapeutic targets in AD and other neurodegenerative diseases.

Key words Alzheimer's disease, Amyloid, Astrocytosis, ^{11}C-deuterium-L-deprenyl (^{11}C-DED), ^{18}F-fluorodeoxyglucose (^{18}F-FDG), ^{11}C-Pittsburgh compound B (^{11}C-PiB), Neuroinflammation, Multitracer PET Imaging, Positron emission tomography

1 Introduction

Clinical practice in the field of neurodegenerative diseases is evolving toward an increasing reliance on in vivo biomarkers that will allow more accurate and differential diagnoses, and help provide individualized care. No disease-modifying treatment is yet

Robert Perneczky (ed.), *Biomarkers for Alzheimer's Disease Drug Development*, Methods in Molecular Biology, vol. 1750, https://doi.org/10.1007/978-1-4939-7704-8_16, © Springer Science+Business Media, LLC 2018

available for Alzheimer's disease (AD)—the most common neuro-degenerative and dementia disease—, but research on in vivo biomarkers is rapidly advancing our understanding of the disease pathology and progression. Biomarkers that can capture the earliest brain pathophysiological changes are needed for early diagnosis and as outcome measures in clinical trials of novel therapies at early stages [1], when treatments have the greatest chance to be efficacious.

Pathological hallmarks of AD include the abnormal deposition of extracellular amyloid-β (Aβ) plaques and intracellular aggregates of hyperphosphorylated tau proteins in the form of neurofibrillary tangles (NFTs) [2]. A commonly accepted model assumes that Aβ plaque deposition is an initiating event [3], followed by deposition of NFTs, neurodegeneration, and cognitive decline [4]. Alternatively, Aβ deposition and neurodegeneration may arise independently [5], and Aβ may interact with tau NFTs to accelerate downstream pathological changes leading to cognitive dysfunction [6]. Furthermore, there is increasing evidence that AD is complex and multifactorial including glial activation and neuroinflammation [7, 8] involving microglia and astrocytes, which may play beneficial and/or detrimental roles from early stages [9–11], and may even be drivers of synapse loss, synaptic dysfunction, and cognitive impairment [12]. There is also increasing evidence for heterogeneity in the clinical presentation and cognitive phenotypes of AD patients [13]. Thus, the availability of multiple in vivo biomarkers reflecting the diverse pathophysiological features of AD will help characterize patients, apply more individualized treatments, and stratify participants for enrichment of clinical trials.

Continuously evolving neuroimaging techniques allow investigating in vivo structural and molecular changes along disease progression. Positron emission tomography (PET) is a molecular imaging technique that allows visualization and absolute quantification of different brain pathophysiological changes at the molecular level [14]. Different modalities of PET imaging are currently used to track Aβ, tau NFTs, glucose metabolism, brain perfusion, glial activation, and neuroinflammatory changes in AD. The ongoing development of new PET modalities is greatly expanding the range of in vivo PET biomarkers that will become available in the near future.

PET imaging is based on the tracer concept. A tracer—labeled with a radioactive isotope and thus referred to as radiotracer—is injected into the subject's blood stream, eventually entering the brain and interacting selectively with a given target in a predictable way, without altering the brain system [15]. Table 1 lists the properties of a suitable radiotracer [15, 16]. As the radiotracer reaches the brain, the attached radioactive isotope—most frequently fluorine-18 (half-life of 110 min) or carbon-11 (half-life of 20 min)—decays by the emission of a positron. After traveling a distance of

Table 1
Properties of a suitable PET radiotracer

Properties
• Enters the brain: adequate lipophilicity, adequate ability to cross the blood–brain barrier
• High sensitivity: able to detect substances at the nanomolar concentration range
• High in vivo affinity and selectivity for a target
• Low nonspecific binding
• Suitable pharmacokinetic properties within the time interval of the PET scan
• Limited plasma binding and peripheral metabolism
• Low contamination from radioactive metabolites in brain: radioactive metabolites do not significantly cross the blood–brain barrier
• High specific activity that allows for reasonably low injected volumes

about 1–3 mm, the positron combines with an electron within the brain tissue, resulting in the emission of two oppositely directed (at approximately 180°) photons (511-keV γ-rays), which are detected in temporal coincidence by a ring of scintillator detectors in the PET scanner. The reconstruction of all such simultaneous γ-ray detection events, after correcting for attenuation and scatter of photons as well as for random coincidences, allows generating 3D brain images for visual assessment by clinicians. Brain PET images are also amenable to absolute quantification characterized by high sensitivity—typically able to quantify biochemical properties at the nanomolar concentration range. While the spatial resolution of PET (few mm) is lower than that of other brain imaging techniques such as magnetic resonance imaging (MRI), the strength of PET imaging is that it provides quantitative information on brain functional and biochemical changes at the molecular level.

The criteria for diagnosis of AD are continuously evolving toward a greater reliance on in vivo biomarkers including PET imaging [17, 18]. Recently, the Aβ PET tracers ^{18}F-florbetapir, ^{18}F-flutemetamol, and ^{18}F-florbetaben were approved by the European Medicines Agency and by the US Food and Drug Administration for assessing the presence of Aβ pathology in individuals with early memory disorders. Biomarkers are classified as either pathophysiological, indicating the presence of Aβ or tau pathology, or topographical, reflecting disease progression including dysfunction in glucose metabolism, or gray matter loss and atrophy [18].

Along with the success of Aβ PET, and the more recent tau PET imaging [19], there is also a great interest to develop PET tracers to image glial activation and neuroinflammation in AD and other neurodegenerative diseases [20–22]; Fig. 1 illustrates some

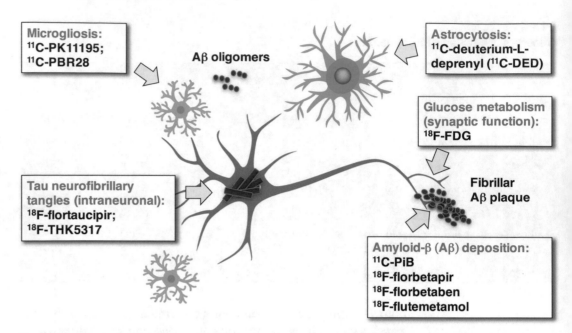

Fig. 1 Pathophysiological features of Alzheimer's disease and selected PET tracers that have been applied in human PET studies

of the most common PET tracers that have been applied in human studies to track different pathophysiological features of AD. Glial activation is meant to promote homeostasis, both in aging and neurodegenerative diseases, by surveying the brain environment for signs of harmful processes and then undergoing changes aimed at limiting the harm and repairing damage [23]. It is commonly accepted that a certain degree of activation is beneficial, but that chronic and excess activation may instigate neuroinflammatory responses that trigger further damage, and therefore may contribute to pathology. While it is not well known whether microglia or astrocytes are activated first, both undergo different stages of anti-inflammatory or pro-inflammatory activation, and they interact with each other to promote further activation and neuroinflammatory responses [7]. Today, PET imaging of neuroinflammation is not yet regarded as an in vivo biomarker for clinical diagnosis or to evaluate disease progression, but it may help in the future to diagnose neurodegenerative diseases and to test novel therapeutic agents targeting glial cells [24]; therefore, there is a significant interest to develop novel biomarkers for glial activation and neuroinflammation [1].

Most studies on PET imaging of neuroinflammation in AD have aimed at visualizing microglial activation, as measured by elevated expression of translocator protein 18 kDa (TSPO), a five transmembrane domain protein mainly located in the outer mitochondrial membrane of microglia; for comprehensive reviews on this topic, please *see* refs. 21, 22, 25–27. While a few studies claim that TSPO is also overexpressed in activated astrocytes [28, 29], the overall agreement is that TSPO is mostly a marker of microglial activation. ^{11}C-PK11195 is the most widely used TSPO PET tracer, although it has relatively low brain penetrance and high nonspecific binding [22, 30]. Second-generation TSPO PET tracers that have been already applied in human include ^{11}C-PBR28, ^{18}F-DPA-714, ^{18}F-FEPPA, ^{11}C-DAA1106, ^{18}F-PBR06, ^{18}F-PBR111, and ^{18}F-GE180 [22].

Very few PET tracers have been applied to investigate in vivo astrocyte activation, and the most common target has been monoamine oxidase B (MAO-B) as measured using ^{11}C-deuterium-L-deprenyl (^{11}C-DED) [22]. There is a current interest in developing other astrocyte tracers targeting, for example, Imidazoline$_2$ binding sites [31] or acetate metabolism [32]; however, no reports in human cases are yet available.

This chapter will focus on the practical procedures to investigate PET imaging of in vivo astrocyte activation, also known as astrocytosis, using the PET tracer ^{11}C-deuterium-L-deprenyl (^{11}C-DED). ^{11}C-DED binds specifically to MAO-B [33, 34], which is overexpressed in reactive astrocytes and serotonergic neurons [35–37]. Autoradiography studies using ^{3}H-L-deprenyl and glial fibrillary acidic protein (GFAP) immunohistochemistry have demonstrated that ^{3}H-L-deprenyl binding was co-localized with GFAP staining in brain tissue from patients with amyotrophic lateral sclerosis (ALS) [35, 36, 38] and AD [39–41], indicating a good level of specificity of MAO-B to activated astrocytes. An autoradiography study using ^{11}C-L-deprenyl in AD brain tissue showed the highest tracer binding in early Braak stages, thus suggesting an early involvement of astrocytes in the progression of the disease [42]. The laminar distribution of ^{3}H-L-deprenyl had a different pattern than that of Aβ deposition as measured by ^{3}H-PiB [40]; in contrast, the laminar pattern of ^{3}H-L-deprenyl was more similar to that of tau deposits as measured by ^{3}H-THK5117 [39].

In vivo PET investigations of MAO-B were initiated with a previously developed ^{11}C-L-deprenyl tracer (without deuterium in its formulation) [34], which showed too high affinity and irreversible binding to MAO-B. The deuterated version of the tracer (^{11}C-deuterium-L-deprenyl) had lower rate of radiotracer trapping in human brain compared to ^{11}C-L-deprenyl, showing improved pharmacokinetic properties, in particular a lower influence of brain perfusion on tracer binding [43, 44]. Thus, the deuterated formulation resulted in improved sensitivity to detect proliferation of glial cells in neurodegenerative disease [43].

[11]C-deuterium-L-deprenyl (^{11}C-DED) PET imaging has been used to investigate astrocytosis in neurodegenerative diseases including AD [45, 46], ALS [47] and Creutzfeldt–Jakob disease (CJD) [48, 49]. A multitracer PET imaging paradigm has been applied in recent studies, whereby each subject undergoes dynamic

PET imaging scans using three radiotracers: ^{11}C-DED, ^{11}C-Pittsburgh compound B (^{11}C-PiB), and ^{18}F-fluorodeoxyglucose (^{18}F-FDG). In these studies, significantly increased ^{11}C-DED binding was found in prodromal stages of AD in comparison to healthy controls or to patients with AD dementia [46], and ^{11}C-DED binding in prodromal AD patients was negatively correlated with gray matter density [50]. In addition, the early-phase uptake of ^{11}C-DED was demonstrated to be a surrogate marker for brain perfusion, allowing the tracer to have dual-use properties as a marker of both perfusion and astrocytosis [51]. The study of familial autosomal dominant AD (ADAD), for which mutation carriers develop clinical AD at a predictable age of onset, has allowed investigating brain pathophysiological and cognitive changes from early presymptomatic stages. By applying multitracer PET imaging in ADAD, the first in vivo observation of astrocytosis at early presymptomatic stages using the PET tracer ^{11}C-DED was reported [52], as well as diverging longitudinal trajectories showing increasing Aβ plaque deposition (^{11}C-PiB), while declining astrocytosis (^{11}C-DED) [53]. Early astrocytosis preceding Aβ plaque deposition was also observed in a transgenic mouse model of AD [54]. Thus, early elevation in astrocytosis suggested promising therapeutic potential [55].

In summary, the findings of very early astrocytosis using ^{11}C-DED PET imaging motivate further research on PET imaging of glial activation. This chapter provides a detailed description of the practical approach used for the analysis of ^{11}C-DED PET imaging data in a multitracer PET paradigm including ^{11}C-PiB and ^{18}F-FDG. The multitracer PET approach has shown great value to investigate the comparative regional and temporal patterns of in vivo brain astrocytosis, fibrillar Aβ deposition, and glucose metabolism in patients with sporadic or familial AD. In this chapter, the illustration of the multitracer PET imaging paradigm attempts to motivate further research in this field, including the development of novel PET tracers aimed at additional targets to visualize different stages of astrocytic and microglial activation. Progress in the field will promote the future incorporation of PET imaging of glial activation and neuroinflammation as biomarkers with clinical application in AD and other neurodegenerative diseases, and to further explore glial cells as promising therapeutic targets.

2 Materials

2.1 MRI Scanners   MRI scans are performed in a 3 Tesla (T) Siemens Trio scanner.

2.2 PET Scanners

PET imaging scans are performed at the Uppsala PET Centre (Uppsala, Sweden) on ECAT EXACT HR+ (Siemens/CTI) and GE discovery ST PET/CT scanners.

2.3 Image Analysis Software

1. The **Statistical Parametric Mapping (SPM)** software was developed by Friston and colleagues at University College London [56–58]. The SPM8 software version and its associated toolboxes can be freely downloaded (http://www.fil.ion.ucl.ac.uk/spm/), and it requires MATLAB (www.mathworks.com/products/matlab/).

2. **VINCI** ("Volume Imaging in Neurological Research, Co-Registration and ROIs included") is a software tool that was designed for the visualization and analysis of volume data generated by medical tomographical systems, with a special focus on the needs for data analysis in PET imaging (http://vinci.sf.mpg.de).

3. **VOIager** is an imaging software tool developed by GE Healthcare (https://www.ge.com/digital/industries/healthcare).

4. The **Hammers brain atlas** is a freely available adult brain maximum probability map in Montreal Neurological Institute (MNI) space (http://brain-development.org/brain-atlases/adult-brain-maximum-probability-map-hammers-mith-atlas-n30r83-in-mni-space/). In this study, a Hammers atlas version with 29 regions of interest (ROIs) is used.

5. **Imlook4d** (https://dicom-port.com/product/imlook4d/) is a free advanced medical imaging analysis software tool, which can be used for scripting and algorithm development, and is easily extended using MATLAB.

6. The **Biological Parametric Mapping (BPM)** software is a toolbox for multimodal image analysis based on a voxel-wise application of the general linear model (https://www.nitrc.org/projects/rbpm/). The BPM toolbox has been developed in MATLAB, it incorporates a user-friendly interface for performing voxel-wise correlation and regression analyses, and it relies on the SPM software for visualization and statistical inference [59].

3 Methods

This section illustrates the practical procedures for multitracer PET imaging, as applied in previously published studies by our group [46, 50–53, 60]. In summary, each participant receives, on the same day, three dynamic PET scans using the radiotracers ^{11}C-PiB, ^{11}C-DED, and ^{18}F-FDG. The description below includes the

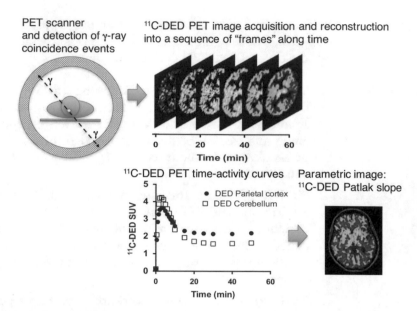

Fig. 2 Schematic diagram of PET imaging experimental setup for data acquisition, processing, and quantification. *DED* ^{11}C-deuterium-L-deprenyl, *PET* positron emission tomography, *SUV* standardized uptake value (PET radiotracer uptake normalized to injected dose and body weight)

procedures for the recruitment of participants, MRI image acquisition, PET radiotracer synthesis, PET image acquisition, reconstruction and analysis, and PET quantification. For ^{11}C-DED PET, fully quantitative analysis is performed using a graphical approach based on the modified reference Patlak model [47, 61], which was previously validated against a model using arterial sampling [62]. For ^{11}C-PiB and ^{18}F-FDG, semiquantitative analyses are performed by means of the standardized uptake value ratio (SUVr), using either the cerebellar gray matter or the pons as a reference region. Figure 2 presents an overview of the experimental setup for PET image scanning, image acquisition, processing, and quantification.

3.1 Participants

1. Patients, who were referred for memory problems to the Department of Geriatric Medicine, Karolinska University Hospital, Huddinge, Sweden, are recruited for the study.

2. Healthy elderly individuals, who may be recruited from advertising in the community, do not deviate from clinically normal in a physical examination and have normal MRI findings.

3. All participants sign a written informed consent to participate in the study, which is conducted according to the declaration of Helsinki and subsequent revisions. Prior to the study initiation, ethical approval is obtained from the regional Human Ethics Committee of Stockholm and the Faculty of Medicine and Radiation Hazard Ethics Committee of Uppsala University Hospital, Sweden.

4. Patients undergo a comprehensive clinical and imaging examination including medical history, neurological and psychiatric examination, MRI, apolipoprotein E (*APOE*) genotyping from blood, neuropsychological assessment, and cerebrospinal fluid (CSF) analysis.

5. Diagnoses are made during a consensus meeting where a geriatrician/neurologist, a neuropsychologist, and a nurse discuss the outcome of the assessment of the patients.

6. Patients are diagnosed as either mild cognitive impairment (MCI) or probable AD dementia.

7. The diagnosis of MCI is based on Petersen's criteria [63].

8. Probable AD dementia is diagnosed according to National Institute of Neurological and Communicative Disorders and Stroke, and the Alzheimer's Disease and Related Disorders Association (NINCDS-ADRDA) criteria [64].

9. MCI patients are further divided into PiB-positive and PiB-negative groups using a cutoff value of 1.41 neocortical SUVr with reference to the cerebellar gray matter, as previously described [65]. The subgroup of PiB-positive MCI patients fulfill the current diagnostic criteria for prodromal AD [18].

3.2   MRI

1. All participants undergo a structural 3D T_1 magnetization-prepared rapid-acquisition gradient-echo (MPRAGE) sequence on a 3 Tesla (T) Siemens Trio MRI scanner.

2. MRI images are acquired with a matrix size of $192 \times 256 \times 256$ and voxel size of $1.0 \times 0.98 \times 0.98$ mm, and are reconstructed to $1.0 \times 1.0 \times 1.0$ mm isometric voxels, with an echo time of 3.42 ms, repetition time of 1780 ms, inversion time of 900 ms, and flip angle of 9°.

3. To exclude patients with non-AD-related brain abnormalities and to examine possible brain abnormalities in healthy controls, fluid-attenuated inversion recovery T_2 and diffusion-weighted images are also acquired.

4. The structural T_1 MRI image for Subject 01 (as an example) is labeled: **01_T1_MRI.nii** (*see* **Note 1**).

3.3   Radiotracer Synthesis and Preparation

1. Production of ^{11}C-PiB, ^{11}C-DED, and ^{18}F-FDG is carried out according to the standard good manufacturing process at Uppsala University PET Centre.

2. Radiotracer synthesis procedures are reported elsewhere [44, 47, 62, 66, 67].

3.4   PET Image Acquisition

1. Each participant undergoes three PET scans on the same day, using three PET tracers in the following order: ^{11}C-PiB, ^{11}C-DED, and ^{18}F-FDG.

2. PET scans are acquired at the Uppsala PET Centre (Uppsala, Sweden) on either ECAT EXACT HR+ (Siemens/CTI) or GE discovery ST PET/CT scanners.

3. Participants are injected each radiotracer by intravenous injection. The mean injected doses for each tracer are 211 ± 65 MBq for ^{11}C-DED, 227 ± 76 MBq for ^{11}C-PiB, and 229 ± 42 MBq for ^{18}F-FDG, as previously reported [53].

4. Patients fast for 4 h preceding the ^{18}F-FDG scan.

5. The orbitomeatal line is used to center the head of the participants.

6. Image data are acquired as the patient lies in the scanner during 60 min for each of ^{11}C-PiB and ^{11}C-DED scans, and 45 min for the ^{18}F-FDG scan.

7. The PET data are acquired in three-dimensional mode, yielding a 155-mm field of view.

3.5 PET Image Reconstruction

1. All emission data are reconstructed with filtered back-projection using a 4-mm Hanning filter, resulting in a transaxial spatial resolution of 5 mm in the field of view. The matrix includes 128×128 pixels, and a zoom factor of 2.5 is used.

2. The ^{11}C-PiB acquisitions consist of 24 frames (4×30, 9×60, 3×180, and 8×300 s) over 60 min. The ^{11}C-DED reconstructed acquisitions consist of 19 time frames (4×30, 8×60, 4×300, and 3×600 s), with a total duration of 60 min. For each ^{18}F-FDG acquisition, 21 frames (4×30, 9×60, 3×180, and 5×300 s) are acquired over 45 min.

3.6 Within-Subject Realignment and Summation of PET Images

1. All reconstructed frames are realigned to correct for subject motion during each PET scan.

2. Using VOIager software, the dynamic PET data are processed to perform intra-subject realignment, by aligning each successive frame to the previous frame to correct for the mentioned possible motion of the subject during the scan.

3. For each of the tracers, the realigned dynamic series of each PET tracer is subsequently uploaded into VOIager, which is used to create average images of the late-frame PET tracer uptake, also called "summation images." More specifically, the following late-frame time-weighted averaged (or "summation") images are created: a 50-min static image for ^{11}C-DED, corresponding to 10- to 60-min; a 20-min static image for ^{11}C-PiB, corresponding to 40- to 60-min; and a 15-min static image for ^{18}F-FDG, corresponding to 30- to 45-min. These images are labeled as follows (for Subject 01): **01_DED_late_sum.nii; 01_PiB_late_sum.nii; 01_FDG_late_sum.nii.**

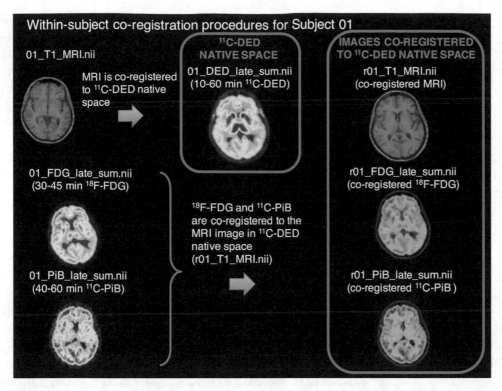

Fig. 3 Within-subject co-registration procedures for MRI and PET images, illustrated for an AD dementia patient

4. In addition, frames 3–6 of ^{11}C-DED, corresponding to 1- to 4-min tracer uptake, are summed to obtain a measure of brain perfusion: **01_DED_early_sum.nii**; this optimum early-phase time frame duration was previously reported to be a proxy for brain perfusion based on its close correlation with glucose metabolism as measured by ^{18}F-FDG in the same subjects [51].

3.7 Within-Subject Co-registration Procedures

1. Figure 3 illustrates the within-subject co-registration procedures for Subject 01, involving one structural MRI scan and three PET images using ^{11}C-DED, ^{11}C-PiB, and ^{18}F-FDG, respectively.

2. After the ^{11}C-DED PET data had been reconstructed, realigned, and the late frames summed, the ^{11}C-DED images are not transformed any further. Therefore, in this protocol, all the steps for the PET image analysis of one individual are performed in the subject's native ^{11}C-DED PET space.

3. For each participant, the T_1 MRI image **(01_T1_MRI.nii)** is co-registered onto the individual's ^{11}C-DED late-sum image in native ^{11}C-DED space **(01_DED_late_sum.nii)** using SPM8 (Functional Imaging Laboratory, Wellcome Department of Imaging Neuroscience, University College London) (*see* **Note 2**).

4. To perform this co-registration step, the function "Coregister (Estimate & Reslice)" is applied using the VBM/PET SPM8 module. The reference image (which remains static) is **01_DED_late_sum.nii**, the source image (the image that is moved onto the space of the reference image) is **01_T1_MRI.nii**. As a result of the procedure, the co-registered T_1 MRI image is automatically labeled with an r prefix, thus labeled: **r01_T1_MRI.nii** (*see* **Note 3**).

5. Also for each participant, the SPM8 function "Coregister (Estimate & Reslice)" is used to co-register the ^{11}C-PiB and ^{18}F-FDG late-sum images (**01_PiB_late_sum.nii** and **01_FDG_late_sum.nii**, used as source images) onto the individual T_1 MRI image (**r01_T1_MRI.nii**, used as reference image). As a result, the co-registered ^{11}C-PiB and ^{18}F-FDG late-sum images are labeled: **r01_PiB_late_sum.nii** and **r01_FDG_late_sum.nii** (*see* **Note 4**).

3.8 Subject-Specific Gray Matter Atlas for PET Image Quantification

1. Figure 4 illustrates the steps for within-subject PET image quantification (for Subject 01), which involves the creation of a subject-specific gray matter atlas, using the Hammers atlas as a basis.

2. After the individual T_1 MRI image was co-registered to native DED space (**r01_T1_MRI.nii,** described in Subheading 3.7, **step 4**), the MRI image is segmented into gray matter and white matter tissue classes using the unified segmentation algorithm of SPM8 [68]; the subject-specific probabilistic gray matter map for Subject 01 is saved as **r01_T1_MRI_GM_map.nii**. For this step, the "Segment" function of SPM8 is used with the default parameters. This segmentation step results in two matrices: a direct matrix **01_sn.mat** that transforms images from native ^{11}C-DED space into MNI space, and the corresponding inverse matrix **01_inv_sn.mat** that transforms images in the reverse direction: from MNI into native ^{11}C-DED space.

3. The inverse nonlinear transformation matrix from SPM8's segmentation algorithm (**01_inv_sn.mat**) is then used to warp the simplified digital probabilistic Hammers atlas (**Hammers_atlas.nii**) [69] consisting of 29 cortical and subcortical ROIs, as well as a hand-drawn whole pons region (**Pons_atlas.nii**)—both in MNI space—into the ^{11}C-DED native space of Subject 01 (**r01_Hammers_atlas.nii** and **r01_Pons_atlas.nii**, respectively). To perform this step, the "Normalise (write)" function from SPM8 is applied to the atlas and pons images in MNI space, using the **01_inv_sn.mat** matrix as the parameter file (*see* **Note 5**).

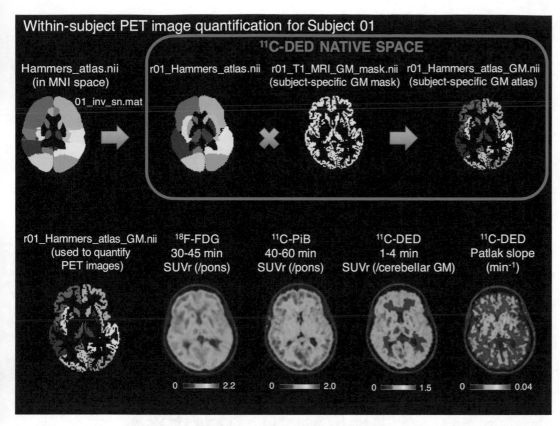

Fig. 4 Within-subject quantification of PET images, illustrated for an AD dementia patient. *GM* gray matter, *SUVr* standardized uptake value ratio

4. A threshold of 0.5 is applied to the subject-specific probabilistic gray matter map (**r01_T1_MRI_GM_map.nii**), whereby voxels with a probability greater than 50% of being gray matter are assigned a value of 1, and 0 otherwise. This step results in a subject-specific gray matter mask in native ^{11}C-DED space and is saved as **r01_T1_MRI_GM_mask.nii** (*see* **Note 6**).

5. The subject-specific Hammers atlas in ^{11}C-DED native space (**r01_Hammers_atlas.nii**) is multiplied by the corresponding binary gray matter mask (**r01_T1_MRI_GM_mask.nii**), which generates a gray-matter-specific digital atlas for Subject 01, saved as **r01_Hammers_atlas_GM.nii** (*see* **Note 7**).

3.9 Model for Quantification of ^{11}C-DED PET Image Data

1. For ^{11}C-DED quantification, a modified reference Patlak model [47, 61] is applied to the ^{11}C-DED dynamic PET data from 20 to 60 min, as previously described [46, 53] (*see* **Note 8**).

2. The modified reference Patlak model belongs to a group of graphical analysis techniques, and is based on the Patlak

linearization approach [61]. According to the Patlak approach, a scatter plot is created where the y axis is the measured PET activity in a target ROI divided by that in the reference tissue, and the x axis is a "normalized time" (integral of the reference time activity curve from the injection point to the current time point, and divided by the reference tissue PET activity at the current time point). The scatter plot is fitted by linear regression after an equilibration time t^*, and the slope of the regression line is the estimate of radiotracer binding in the target ROI (*see* **Note 9**).

3. The cerebellar gray matter is selected here as "modified reference," based on that it has the lowest specific binding of all brain regions, as reported in a previous autoradiography study using ^{11}C-DED in brain tissue from AD patients and healthy controls [42]. The cerebellar gray matter also showed the lowest ^{11}C-DED binding of all investigated regions in the present studies [46, 53].

4. The modified reference Patlak model assumes a cerebellar gray matter slope value of 0.01 min^{-1}, to take into account the fact that this region is not completely devoid of specific binding.

5. The graphical approach generates individual 3D parametric Patlak slope images, which are thus the estimates of ^{11}C-DED binding (units: min^{-1}). An individual Patlak slope parametric image for Subject 01 is illustrated in Fig. 4.

3.10 Semiquantitative Method for ^{11}C-PiB and ^{18}F-FDG PET Image Data

1. The previously co-registered and resliced ^{11}C-PiB and ^{18}F-FDG images for each participant, both in native ^{11}C-DED space (**r01_PiB_late_sum.nii** and **r01_FDG_late_sum.nii**), are sampled using the created individual gray matter atlas (**r01_Hammers_atlas_GM.nii**) and the individual pons atlas (**r01_Pons_atlas.nii**), both having been previously co-registered to native ^{11}C-DED space.

2. Either the whole pons or the cerebellar gray matter have been reported as suitable reference regions for both ^{11}C-PiB and ^{18}F-FDG PET quantification in sporadic AD. The whole pons is used as example in this protocol, because it was found to be preserved from pathology in both ADAD and sporadic AD [70, 71] (*see* **Note 10**).

3. Using the individual gray matter atlas, the average ^{11}C-PiB and ^{18}F-FDG uptake are calculated for each atlas ROI and then each are divided by the respective ^{11}C-PiB and ^{18}F-FDG average uptake in the reference region, which are called standardized uptake value ratios (SUVr) and are thus dimensionless. Images displaying PET quantification in SUVr units are illustrated in Fig. 4 (*see* **Note 11**).

3.11 Statistical Approaches for Comparison of PET Tracer Uptake Between Diagnostic Groups

1. A cross-sectional PET imaging study typically aims at comparing PET tracer uptake between a diagnostic group (for example, a group of prodromal AD or of AD dementia patients) and a healthy control group. A study will typically perform region-of-interest (ROI) and/or voxel-wise types of analyses, which may provide complementary information.

3.12 Region-of-Interest (ROI) Based Analyses

1. A number of brain ROIs are selected based on a hypothesis to be tested. Alternatively, an exploratory analysis over wide brain regions may be justified when investigating novel tracers, for which little previous information is available.

2. Parametric or nonparametric statistical tests are applied as appropriate to compare PET tracer uptake in the selected ROIs between a diagnostic and a control group (*see* **Note 12**).

3. Due to the multiple ROIs analyzed, appropriate methods for correction due to multiple comparisons are applied. For PET data analysis, a procedure controlling for false discovery rate as implemented in the Benjamini–Hochberg method [72] using pplot software [73] may be applied to correct for multiple regional tests.

3.13 Voxel-Wise Analyses

1. Voxel-wise analyses may be performed to compare the PET tracer uptake between a diagnostic and a control group.

2. Prior to voxel-wise analyses, individual PET images from different subjects need to be spatially normalized to MNI space, to allow for comparisons across individuals. The normalization step is performed using SPM8 "Normalise (write)" and applying the previously obtained transformation matrix (**01_sn.mat**) as parameter file for conversion of the individual PET images from native ^{11}C-DED space to MNI space.

3. Normalized images are smoothed by an 8-mm full width at half maximum (FWHM) Gaussian filter using the VBM/PET SPM8 "Smooth" function, and masked using a gray matter mask to allow for sampling of only gray matter regions.

4. A voxel-wise comparison between PET tracer uptake in a diagnostic vs. a control group is performed using SPM8 two-sample t-test function for group comparisons.

5. A voxel-wise correlation analysis between two PET imaging modalities across subjects within a given diagnostic group is performed using Biological Parametric Mapping (BPM, v3.3) [59].

6. BPM correlation maps and SPM8 T-maps are thresholded at $p < 0.001$ (uncorrected, $\geq$20-voxel cluster extent) and projected onto a template cortical surface using FreeSurfer

(v5.3, https://surfer.nmr.mgh.harvard.edu) or BrainNet Viewer (a toolbox for SPM8; https://www.nitrc.org/projects/bnv/). Clusters that remain significant after family-wise error (FWE, $p < 0.05$) correction for multiple comparisons are tabulated.

4 Notes

1. Brain images are typically in NIftI (Neuroimaging InFormatics Technology Initiative) format and have an extension .nii. Other widely used formats for medical images include DICOM (Digital Imaging and Communications in Medicine), Analyze, ECAT, and Interfile.

2. Alternatively, a subject's static MRI scan may be used as template (native space), and the individual's PET image (or images) are co-registered to the MRI template. In the protocol described in this chapter, the intention was to preserve the ^{11}C-DED image quality as closely as possible to the original image data to allow for accurate modeling and quantification of this tracer.

3. Given that this co-registration step is a within-subject registration procedure, a 6-parameter rigid-body transformation is applied using the "Coregistration (Estimate & Reslice)" option in SPM8, and Normalised Mutual Information as Objective Function. Reslice options are trilinear interpolation, no wrapping, and no masking of images.

4. When performing multiple image processing steps in SPM8 for a cohort of participants, it is useful to develop MATLAB scripts that allow for automatization of the processes (https://en.wikibooks.org/wiki/SPM/Programming_intro).

5. The SPM8 "Normalise (write)" function is applied using the Nearest Neighbour Interpolation option, no wrapping, and preserving concentrations (all parameters for bounding box and voxel sizes are entered as NaN).

6. This thresholding step can be performed using the Image Calculator ("ImCalc") option in SPM8, or other imaging software tools such as VINCI, using the Threshold Tool, and Image Volume Arithmetics.

7. The segmented gray matter from the MRI is used to restrict the sampling to gray matter areas within each region of interest in the Hammers atlas. This multiplication step can be performed using "ImCalc" option in SPM8.

8. Ideally, a reference region has virtually no specific binding of the tracer. A "modified reference" is a region with a relatively low specific binding of the tracer, substantially lower than that in target brain regions.

9. The modified reference Patlak graphical approach can be applied in two ways: to fit time-activity curves extracted from each of the ROIs of the atlas, or by fitting the dynamic ^{11}C-DED PET data pixel-by-pixel and thus obtaining parametric images of the ^{11}C-DED binding. Both approaches are implemented in MATLAB scripts using Imlook4d.

10. If the study involves familial ADAD participants, it is important to note that the cerebellar gray matter has been found to contain Aβ plaque deposits, and it is thus typically not used as a reference region in ADAD [71]; the pons may be used instead. The pons has been used as reference for both ^{11}C-PiB and ^{18}F-FDG in sporadic or familial forms of AD [53, 74].

11. The semiquantification of ^{11}C-PiB and ^{18}F-FDG in terms of SUVr is very common in the literature, and has the advantage of simplicity and thus ease of application in the clinic. Previous studies have validated the SUVr semiquantitative approach for ^{11}C-PiB and ^{18}F-FDG PET against other available fully quantitative modeling approaches [75, 76].

12. Statistical analyses are performed using SPSS (IBM SPSS Statistics, version 22.0) and R (v. 3.1.2, R Foundation for Statistical Computing, Vienna, Austria).

Acknowledgements

We are grateful to the staff at the Uppsala PET Centre. This work was financially supported by grants from the Swedish Research Council (project 05817), the Swedish Foundation for Strategic Research (SSF), the Strategic Research Programme in Neuroscience at Karolinska Institutet, Neuroscience program, the Stockholm County Council-Karolinska Institutet regional agreement on medical training and clinical research (ALF grant), the Swedish Brain Foundation, the Swedish Alzheimer Foundation (Alzheimerfonden), Demensfonden, the EU FP7 large-scale integrating project INMiND (http://www.uni-muenster.de/INMiND), the Foundation for Old Servants, Karolinska Institutet's Foundation for Aging Research, Gun and Bertil Stohne's Foundation, Loo and Hans Osterman's Foundation, and Åke Wiberg's Foundation.

References

1. Mattsson N, Carrillo MC, Dean RA, Devous MD Sr, Nikolcheva T, Pesini P, Salter H, Potter WZ, Sperling RS, Bateman RJ, Bain LJ, Liu E (2015) Revolutionizing Alzheimer's disease and clinical trials through biomarkers. Alzheimers Dement (Amst) 1(4):412–419. https://doi.org/10.1016/j.dadm.2015.09.001

2. Braak H, Braak E (1991) Neuropathological stageing of Alzheimer-related changes. Acta Neuropathol 82(4):239–259

3. Hardy J, Selkoe DJ (2002) The amyloid hypothesis of Alzheimer's disease: progress and problems on the road to therapeutics. Science 297(5580):353–356. https://doi.org/10.1126/science.1072994

4. Jack CR Jr, Knopman DS, Jagust WJ, Petersen RC, Weiner MW, Aisen PS, Shaw LM, Vemuri P, Wiste HJ, Weigand SD, Lesnick TG, Pankratz VS, Donohue MC, Trojanowski JQ (2013) Tracking pathophysiological processes in Alzheimer's disease: an updated hypothetical model of dynamic biomarkers. Lancet Neurol 12(2):207–216. https://doi.org/10.1016/S1474-4422(12)70291-0

5. Jack CR Jr, Wiste HJ, Weigand SD, Knopman DS, Lowe V, Vemuri P, Mielke MM, Jones DT, Senjem ML, Gunter JL, Gregg BE, Pankratz VS, Petersen RC (2013) Amyloid-first and neurodegeneration-first profiles characterize incident amyloid PET positivity. Neurology 81(20):1732–1740. https://doi.org/10.1212/01.wnl.0000435556.21319.e4

6. Sperling R, Mormino E, Johnson K (2014) The evolution of preclinical Alzheimer's disease: implications for prevention trials. Neuron 84(3):608–622. https://doi.org/10.1016/j.neuron.2014.10.038

7. Heneka MT, Carson MJ, El Khoury J, Landreth GE, Brosseron F, Feinstein DL, Jacobs AH, Wyss-Coray T, Vitorica J, Ransohoff RM, Herrup K, Frautschy SA, Finsen B, Brown GC, Verkhratsky A, Yamanaka K, Koistinaho J, Latz E, Halle A, Petzold GC, Town T, Morgan D, Shinohara ML, Perry VH, Holmes C, Bazan NG, Brooks DJ, Hunot S, Joseph B, Deigendesch N, Garaschuk O, Boddeke E, Dinarello CA, Breitner JC, Cole GM, Golenbock DT, Kummer MP (2015) Neuroinflammation in Alzheimer's disease. Lancet Neurol 14(4):388–405. https://doi.org/10.1016/S1474-4422(15)70016-5

8. De Strooper B, Karran E (2016) The cellular phase of Alzheimer's disease. Cell 164(4):603–615. https://doi.org/10.1016/j.cell.2015.12.056

9. Acosta C, Anderson HD, Anderson CM (2017) Astrocyte dysfunction in Alzheimer disease. J Neurosci Res 95:2430. https://doi.org/10.1002/jnr.24075

10. Verkhratsky A, Marutle A, Rodriguez-Arellano JJ, Nordberg A (2015) Glial asthenia and functional paralysis: a new perspective on neurodegeneration and Alzheimer's disease. The Neuroscientist 21(5):552–568. https://doi.org/10.1177/1073858414547132

11. Thal DR (2012) The role of astrocytes in amyloid beta-protein toxicity and clearance. Exp Neurol 236(1):1–5. https://doi.org/10.1016/j.expneurol.2012.04.021

12. Chung WS, Welsh CA, Barres BA, Stevens B (2015) Do glia drive synaptic and cognitive impairment in disease? Nat Neurosci 18(11):1539–1545. https://doi.org/10.1038/nn.4142

13. Murray ME, Graff-Radford NR, Ross OA, Petersen RC, Duara R, Dickson DW (2011) Neuropathologically defined subtypes of Alzheimer's disease with distinct clinical characteristics: a retrospective study. Lancet Neurol 10(9):785–796. https://doi.org/10.1016/S1474-4422(11)70156-9

14. Jones T, Townsend D (2017) History and future technical innovation in positron emission tomography. J Med Imaging (Bellingham) 4(1):011013. https://doi.org/10.1117/1.JMI.4.1.011013

15. Turkheimer FE, Veronese M, Dunn J (2014) Experimental design and practical data analysis in positron emission tomography. King's College, London

16. Pike VW (2009) PET radiotracers: crossing the blood-brain barrier and surviving metabolism. Trends Pharmacol Sci 30(8):431–440. https://doi.org/10.1016/j.tips.2009.05.005

17. McKhann GM, Knopman DS, Chertkow H, Hyman BT, Jack CR Jr, Kawas CH, Klunk WE, Koroshetz WJ, Manly JJ, Mayeux R, Mohs RC, Morris JC, Rossor MN, Scheltens P, Carrillo MC, Thies B, Weintraub S, Phelps CH (2011) The diagnosis of dementia due to Alzheimer's disease: recommendations from the National Institute on Aging-Alzheimer's association workgroups on diagnostic guidelines for Alzheimer's disease. Alzheimers Dement 7(3):263–269. https://doi.org/10.1016/j.jalz.2011.03.005

18. Dubois B, Feldman HH, Jacova C, Hampel H, Molinuevo JL, Blennow K, DeKosky ST, Gauthier S, Selkoe D, Bateman R, Cappa S, Crutch S, Engelborghs S, Frisoni GB, Fox NC, Galasko D, Habert MO, Jicha GA, Nordberg A, Pasquier F, Rabinovici G, Robert P, Rowe C, Salloway S, Sarazin M, Epelbaum S, de Souza LC, Vellas B, Visser PJ, Schneider L, Stern Y, Scheltens P, Cummings JL (2014) Advancing research diagnostic criteria for Alzheimer's disease: the IWG-2 criteria. Lancet Neurol 13(6):614–629. https://doi.org/10.1016/S1474-4422(14)70090-0

19. Saint-Aubert L, Lemoine L, Chiotis K, Leuzy A, Rodriguez-Vieitez E, Nordberg A (2017) Tau PET imaging: present and future directions. Mol Neurodegener 12(1):19. https://doi.org/10.1186/s13024-017-0162-3

20. Jacobs AH, Tavitian B, INMiND Consortium (2012) Noninvasive molecular imaging of neuroinflammation. J Cereb Blood Flow Metab 32(7):1393–1415. https://doi.org/10.1038/jcbfm.2012.53

21. Albrecht DS, Granziera C, Hooker JM, Loggia ML (2016) In vivo imaging of human neuroinflammation. ACS Chem Neurosci 7(4):470–483. https://doi.org/10.1021/acschemneuro.6b00056

22. Varrone A, Nordberg A. (2015) Molecular imaging of neuroinflammation in Alzheimer's disease. Clin Transl Imaging 3:437–447

23. Burda JE, Sofroniew MV (2014) Reactive gliosis and the multicellular response to CNS damage and disease. Neuron 81(2):229–248. https://doi.org/10.1016/j.neuron.2013.12.034

24. Hamby ME, Sofroniew MV (2010) Reactive astrocytes as therapeutic targets for CNS disorders. Neurotherapeutics 7(4):494–506. https://doi.org/10.1016/j.nurt.2010.07.003

25. Stefaniak J, O'Brien J (2016) Imaging of neuroinflammation in dementia: a review. J Neurol Neurosurg Psychiatry 87(1):21–28. https://doi.org/10.1136/jnnp-2015-311336

26. Varley J, Brooks DJ, Edison P (2015) Imaging neuroinflammation in Alzheimer's disease and other dementias: recent advances and future directions. Alzheimers Dement 11(9):1110–1120. https://doi.org/10.1016/j.jalz.2014.08.105

27. Lagarde J, Sarazin M, Bottlaender M (2017) In vivo PET imaging of neuroinflammation in Alzheimer's disease. J Neural Transm (Vienna). https://doi.org/10.1007/s00702-017-1731-x

28. Lavisse S, Guillermier M, Herard AS, Petit F, Delahaye M, Van Camp N, Ben Haim L, Lebon V, Remy P, Dolle F, Delzescaux T, Bonvento G, Hantraye P, Escartin C (2012) Reactive astrocytes overexpress TSPO and are detected by TSPO positron emission tomography imaging. J Neurosci 32(32):10809–10818. https://doi.org/10.1523/JNEUROSCI.1487-12.2012

29. Cosenza-Nashat M, Zhao ML, Suh HS, Morgan J, Natividad R, Morgello S, Lee SC (2009) Expression of the translocator protein of 18 kDa by microglia, macrophages and astrocytes based on immunohistochemical localization in abnormal human brain. Neuropathol Appl Neurobiol 35(3):306–328. https://doi.org/10.1111/j.1365-2990.2008.01006.x

30. Turkheimer FE, Rizzo G, Bloomfield PS, Howes O, Zanotti-Fregonara P, Bertoldo A, Veronese M (2015) The methodology of TSPO imaging with positron emission tomography. Biochem Soc Trans 43(4):586–592. https://doi.org/10.1042/BST20150058

31. Parker CA, Nabulsi N, Holden D, Lin SF, Cass T, Labaree D, Kealey S, Gee AD, Husbands SM, Quelch D, Carson RE, Nutt DJ, Huang Y, Tyacke RJ (2014) Evaluation of 11C-BU99008, a PET ligand for the imidazoline2 binding sites in rhesus brain. J Nucl Med 55(5):838–844. https://doi.org/10.2967/jnumed.113.131854

32. Wyss MT, Magistretti PJ, Buck A, Weber B (2011) Labeled acetate as a marker of astrocytic metabolism. J Cereb Blood Flow Metab 31(8):1668–1674. https://doi.org/10.1038/jcbfm.2011.84

33. Fowler JS, Logan J, Volkow ND, Wang GJ (2005) Translational neuroimaging: positron emission tomography studies of monoamine oxidase. Mol Imaging Biol 7(6):377–387. https://doi.org/10.1007/s11307-005-0016-1

34. Fowler JS, MacGregor RR, Wolf AP, Arnett CD, Dewey SL, Schlyer D, Christman D, Logan J, Smith M, Sachs H et al (1987) Mapping human brain monoamine oxidase A and B with 11C-labeled suicide inactivators and PET. Science 235(4787):481–485

35. Ekblom J, Jossan SS, Bergstrom M, Oreland L, Walum E, Aquilonius SM (1993) Monoamine oxidase-B in astrocytes. Glia 8(2):122–132. https://doi.org/10.1002/glia.440080208

36. Ekblom J, Jossan SS, Oreland L, Walum E, Aquilonius SM (1994) Reactive gliosis and monoamine oxidase B. J Neural Transm Suppl 41:253–258

37. Levitt P, Pintar JE, Breakefield XO (1982) Immunocytochemical demonstration of monoamine oxidase B in brain astrocytes and serotonergic neurons. Proc Natl Acad Sci U S A 79(20):6385–6389

38. Jossan SS, Ekblom J, Aquilonius SM, Oreland L (1994) Monoamine oxidase-B in motor cortex and spinal cord in amyotrophic lateral sclerosis studied by quantitative autoradiography. J Neural Transm Suppl 41:243–248

39. Lemoine L, Saint-Aubert L, Nennesmo I, Gillberg PG, Nordberg A (2017) Cortical laminar tau deposits and activated astrocytes in Alzheimer's disease visualised by 3H-THK5117 and 3H-deprenyl autoradiography. Sci Rep 7:45496. https://doi.org/10.1038/srep45496

40. Marutle A, Gillberg PG, Bergfors A, Yu W, Ni R, Nennesmo I, Voytenko L, Nordberg A (2013) (3)H-deprenyl and (3)H-PIB autoradiography show different laminar distributions of astroglia and fibrillar beta-amyloid in Alzheimer brain. J Neuroinflammation 10:90. https://doi.org/10.1186/1742-2094-10-90

41. Saura J, Luque JM, Cesura AM, Da Prada M, Chan-Palay V, Huber G, Loffler J, Richards JG (1994) Increased monoamine oxidase B activity in plaque-associated astrocytes of Alzheimer brains revealed by quantitative enzyme radioautography. Neuroscience 62(1):15–30

42. Gulyas B, Pavlova E, Kasa P, Gulya K, Bakota L, Varszegi S, Keller E, Horvath MC, Nag S, Hermecz I, Magyar K, Halldin C (2011) Activated MAO-B in the brain of Alzheimer patients, demonstrated by [11C]-L-deprenyl

using whole hemisphere autoradiography. Neurochem Int 58(1):60–68. https://doi.org/10.1016/j.neuint.2010.10.013

43. Fowler JS, Wang GJ, Logan J, Xie S, Volkow ND, MacGregor RR, Schlyer DJ, Pappas N, Alexoff DL, Patlak C et al (1995) Selective reduction of radiotracer trapping by deuterium substitution: comparison of carbon-11-L-deprenyl and carbon-11-deprenyl-D2 for MAO B mapping. J Nucl Med 36(7):1255–1262

44. Fowler JS, Wolf AP, MacGregor RR, Dewey SL, Logan J, Schlyer DJ, Langstrom B (1988) Mechanistic positron emission tomography studies: demonstration of a deuterium isotope effect in the monoamine oxidase-catalyzed binding of [11C]L-deprenyl in living baboon brain. J Neurochem 51(5):1524–1534

45. Santillo AF, Gambini JP, Lannfelt L, Langstrom B, Ulla-Marja L, Kilander L, Engler H (2011) In vivo imaging of astrocytosis in Alzheimer's disease: an (1)(1)C-L-deuteriodeprenyl and PIB PET study. Eur J Nucl Med Mol Imaging 38(12):2202–2208. https://doi.org/10.1007/s00259-011-1895-9

46. Carter SF, Scholl M, Almkvist O, Wall A, Engler H, Langstrom B, Nordberg A (2012) Evidence for astrocytosis in prodromal Alzheimer disease provided by 11C-deuterium-L-deprenyl: a multitracer PET paradigm combining 11C-Pittsburgh compound B and 18F-FDG. J Nucl Med 53(1):37–46. https://doi.org/10.2967/jnumed.110.087031

47. Johansson A, Engler H, Blomquist G, Scott B, Wall A, Aquilonius SM, Langstrom B, Askmark H (2007) Evidence for astrocytosis in ALS demonstrated by [11C](L)-deprenyl-D2 PET. J Neurol Sci 255(1–2):17–22. https://doi.org/10.1016/j.jns.2007.01.057

48. Engler H, Lundberg PO, Ekbom K, Nennesmo I, Nilsson A, Bergstrom M, Tsukada H, Hartvig P, Langstrom B (2003) Multitracer study with positron emission tomography in Creutzfeldt-Jakob disease. Eur J Nucl Med Mol Imaging 30(1):85–95. https://doi.org/10.1007/s00259-002-1008-x

49. Engler H, Nennesmo I, Kumlien E, Gambini JP, Lundberg P, Savitcheva I, Langstrom B (2012) Imaging astrocytosis with PET in Creutzfeldt-Jakob disease: case report with histopathological findings. Int J Clin Exp Med 5(2):201–207

50. Choo IL, Carter SF, Scholl ML, Nordberg A (2014) Astrocytosis measured by (1)(1)C-deprenyl PET correlates with decrease in gray matter density in the parahippocampus of prodromal Alzheimer's patients. Eur J Nucl Med Mol Imaging 41(11):2120–2126. https://doi.org/10.1007/s00259-014-2859-7

51. Rodriguez-Vieitez E, Carter SF, Chiotis K, Saint-Aubert L, Leuzy A, Scholl M, Almkvist O, Wall A, Langstrom B, Nordberg A (2016) Comparison of early-phase 11C-deuterium-l-Deprenyl and 11C-Pittsburgh compound B PET for assessing brain perfusion in Alzheimer disease. J Nucl Med 57(7):1071–1077. https://doi.org/10.2967/jnumed.115.168732

52. Scholl M, Carter SF, Westman E, Rodriguez-Vieitez E, Almkvist O, Thordardottir S, Wall A, Graff C, Langstrom B, Nordberg A (2015) Early astrocytosis in autosomal dominant Alzheimer's disease measured in vivo by multi-tracer positron emission tomography. Sci Rep 5:16404. https://doi.org/10.1038/srep16404

53. Rodriguez-Vieitez E, Saint-Aubert L, Carter SF, Almkvist O, Farid K, Scholl M, Chiotis K, Thordardottir S, Graff C, Wall A, Langstrom B, Nordberg A (2016) Diverging longitudinal changes in astrocytosis and amyloid PET in autosomal dominant Alzheimer's disease. Brain 139(Pt 3):922–936. https://doi.org/10.1093/brain/awv404

54. Rodriguez-Vieitez E, Ni R, Gulyas B, Toth M, Haggkvist J, Halldin C, Voytenko L, Marutle A, Nordberg A (2015) Astrocytosis precedes amyloid plaque deposition in Alzheimer APPswe transgenic mouse brain: a correlative positron emission tomography and in vitro imaging study. Eur J Nucl Med Mol Imaging 42(7):1119–1132. https://doi.org/10.1007/s00259-015-3047-0

55. Schott JM, Fox NC (2016) Inflammatory changes in very early Alzheimer's disease: friend, foe, or don't know? Brain 139(Pt 3):647–650. https://doi.org/10.1093/brain/awv405

56. Acton PD, Friston KJ (1998) Statistical parametric mapping in functional neuroimaging: beyond PET and fMRI activation studies. Eur J Nucl Med 25(7):663–667

57. Friston KJ (1995) Commentary and opinion: II. Statistical parametric mapping: ontology and current issues. J Cereb Blood Flow Metab 15(3):361–370. https://doi.org/10.1038/jcbfm.1995.45

58. Kiebel SJ, Ashburner J, Poline JB, Friston KJ (1997) MRI and PET coregistration—a cross validation of statistical parametric mapping and automated image registration. NeuroImage 5(4 Pt 1):271–279. https://doi.org/10.1006/nimg.1997.0265

59. Casanova R, Srikanth R, Baer A, Laurienti PJ, Burdette JH, Hayasaka S, Flowers L, Wood F, Maldjian JA (2007) Biological parametric mapping: a statistical toolbox for multimodality brain image analysis. NeuroImage 34(1):137–143. https://doi.org/10.1016/j.neuroimage.2006.09.011

60. Farid K, Carter SF, Rodriguez-Vieitez E, Almkvist O, Andersen P, Wall A, Blennow K, Portelius E, Zetterberg H, Nordberg A (2015) Case report of complex amyotrophic lateral sclerosis with cognitive impairment and cortical amyloid deposition. J Alzheimers Dis 47(3):661–667. https://doi.org/10.3233/JAD-141965

61. Patlak CS, Blasberg RG (1985) Graphical evaluation of blood-to-brain transfer constants from multiple-time uptake data. Generalizations. J Cereb Blood Flow Metab 5(4):584–590. https://doi.org/10.1038/jcbfm.1985.87

62. Bergstrom M, Kumlien E, Lilja A, Tyrefors N, Westerberg G, Langstrom B (1998) Temporal lobe epilepsy visualized with PET with 11C-L-deuterium-deprenyl—analysis of kinetic data. Acta Neurol Scand 98(4):224–231

63. Petersen RC (2004) Mild cognitive impairment as a diagnostic entity. J Intern Med 256(3):183–194. https://doi.org/10.1111/j.1365-2796.2004.01388.x

64. McKhann G, Drachman D, Folstein M, Katzman R, Price D, Stadlan EM (1984) Clinical diagnosis of Alzheimer's disease: report of the NINCDS-ADRDA Work Group under the auspices of Department of Health and Human Services Task Force on Alzheimer's disease. Neurology 34(7):939–944

65. Nordberg A, Carter SF, Rinne J, Drzezga A, Brooks DJ, Vandenberghe R, Perani D, Forsberg A, Langstrom B, Scheinin N, Karrasch M, Nagren K, Grimmer T, Miederer I, Edison P, Okello A, Van Laere K, Nelissen N, Vandenbulcke M, Garibotto V, Almkvist O, Kalbe E, Hinz R, Herholz K (2013) A European multicentre PET study of fibrillar amyloid in Alzheimer's disease. Eur J Nucl Med Mol Imaging 40(1):104–114. https://doi.org/10.1007/s00259-012-2237-2

66. Klunk WE, Engler H, Nordberg A, Wang Y, Blomqvist G, Holt DP, Bergstrom M, Savitcheva I, Huang GF, Estrada S, Ausen B, Debnath ML, Barletta J, Price JC, Sandell J, Lopresti BJ, Wall A, Koivisto P, Antoni G, Mathis CA, Langstrom B (2004) Imaging brain amyloid in Alzheimer's disease with Pittsburgh Compound-B. Ann Neurol 55(3):306–319. https://doi.org/10.1002/ana.20009

67. Mathis CA, Wang Y, Holt DP, Huang GF, Debnath ML, Klunk WE (2003) Synthesis and evaluation of 11C-labeled 6-substituted 2-arylbenzothiazoles as amyloid imaging agents. J Med Chem 46(13):2740–2754. https://doi.org/10.1021/jm030026b

68. Ashburner J, Friston KJ (2005) Unified segmentation. NeuroImage 26(3):839–851. https://doi.org/10.1016/j.neuroimage.2005.02.018

69. Hammers A, Allom R, Koepp MJ, Free SL, Myers R, Lemieux L, Mitchell TN, Brooks DJ, Duncan JS (2003) Three-dimensional maximum probability atlas of the human brain, with particular reference to the temporal lobe. Hum Brain Mapp 19(4):224–247. https://doi.org/10.1002/hbm.10123

70. Minoshima S, Frey KA, Foster NL, Kuhl DE (1995) Preserved pontine glucose metabolism in Alzheimer disease: a reference region for functional brain image (PET) analysis. J Comput Assist Tomogr 19(4):541–547

71. Lippa CF, Saunders AM, Smith TW, Swearer JM, Drachman DA, Ghetti B, Nee L, Pulaski-Salo D, Dickson D, Robitaille Y, Bergeron C, Crain B, Benson MD, Farlow M, Hyman BT, George-Hyslop SP, Roses AD, Pollen DA (1996) Familial and sporadic Alzheimer's disease: neuropathology cannot exclude a final common pathway. Neurology 46(2):406–412

72. Benjamini Y, Hochberg Y. (1995) Controlling the false discovery rate—a practical and powerful approach to multiple testing. J Roy Stat Soc B Met 57:289–300

73. Turkheimer FE, Smith CB, Schmidt K (2001) Estimation of the number of "true" null hypotheses in multivariate analysis of neuroimaging data. NeuroImage 13(5):920–930. https://doi.org/10.1006/nimg.2001.0764

74. Edison P, Hinz R, Ramlackhansingh A, Thomas J, Gelosa G, Archer HA, Turkheimer FE, Brooks DJ (2012) Can target-to-pons ratio be used as a reliable method for the analysis of [11C]PIB brain scans? NeuroImage 60(3):1716–1723. https://doi.org/10.1016/j.neuroimage.2012.01.099

75. Herholz K (2010) Cerebral glucose metabolism in preclinical and prodromal Alzheimer's disease. Expert Rev. Neurother 10(11):1667–1673. https://doi.org/10.1586/ern.10.136

76. Lopresti BJ, Klunk WE, Mathis CA, Hoge JA, Ziolko SK, Lu X, Meltzer CC, Schimmel K, Tsopelas ND, DeKosky ST, Price JC (2005) Simplified quantification of Pittsburgh compound B amyloid imaging PET studies: a comparative analysis. J Nucl Med 46(12):1959–1972

Part VI

Neuropathology

Chapter 17

Unbiased Lipidomics and Metabolomics of Human Brain Samples

Giuseppe Astarita, Matteo Stocchero, and Giuseppe Paglia

Abstract

Mass spectrometry (MS)-based lipidomics and metabolomics approaches have been used to discover new diagnostic and therapeutic targets of neurodegenerative disorders. Here, we describe a protocol to conduct an integrated metabolomics and lipidomics profiling of postmortem brains of frozen tissue samples from clinically characterized patients and age-matched controls. Metabolites and lipids can be extracted from each brain tissue sample, using a biphasic liquid/liquid extraction method. An unbiased liquid chromatography MS-based lipidomics and metabolomics workflows allows to screen for the content and composition of lipids and polar metabolites for each brain tissue. Data processing and statistical analysis are then used to compare the molecular content of all the samples, grouping them into cluster based on molecular similarities. The final results highlight classes of metabolites and biochemical pathways that are altered in brain samples from diseased brains compared to those from healthy subjects, helping to generate novel hypotheses on their mechanistic and functional significance.

Key words Lipidomics, Lipids, Metabolomics, Metabolites, Liquid chromatography mass spectrometry, Brain, Metabolic pathways

1 Introduction

Metabolites and lipids play essential roles in energy metabolism, membrane structure, and signaling. Thus, alterations in metabolites and lipid metabolism have been linked to the development of many diseases, including neurodegenerative disorders [1]. By profiling the overall content of lipids and metabolites, lipidomic and metabolomics approaches provide a snapshot of the physiological and pathological status of a biological system [2–4]. Such a bird's-eye view of the metabolism might help to determine the biochemical pathways that are altered in diseased compared to healthy brains and generate novel hypotheses on molecular targets for diagnostics and therapeutics [1].

Liquid chromatography combined with mass spectrometry (MS) is the method of choice for metabolomics and lipidomics due to the sensitivity and selectivity of analysis. Advancement in analytical technology and data processing allows to profile thousands

Robert Perneczky (ed.), *Biomarkers for Alzheimer's Disease Drug Development*, Methods in Molecular Biology, vol. 1750, https://doi.org/10.1007/978-1-4939-7704-8_17, © Springer Science+Business Media, LLC 2018

of molecular species and compare their composition between healthy and diseased samples. A growing number of clinical research laboratories use MS-based metabolomics and lipidomics to study neurodegenerative disorders for translational research and biomarker discovery [5–7].

In this chapter, we describe a protocol for conducting integrated lipidomics and metabolomics analyses of frozen brain tissue samples from diseased and control subjects (Fig. 1). First, we describe a procedure for the simultaneous extraction of lipids and polar metabolites from the same tissue using a biphasic, liquid-liquid extraction procedure. Next, we describe a workflow for conducting an unbiased analysis using liquid chromatography-mass spectrometry (MS). Lipids are separated using a reversed-phase chromatography, whereas polar metabolites are separated using a

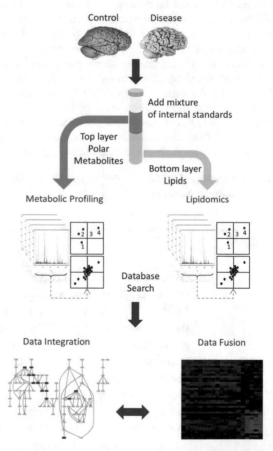

Fig. 1 Representative lipidomics and metabolomics experimental workflow. Brain samples from diseased subjects and healthy control cohorts are extracted via a biphasic method. After centrifugation, top layer is analyzed by a metabolomics approach for polar metabolites; bottom layer is analyzed by a lipidomics approach for lipids. The results can then be fused and integrated within known biochemical pathways

hydrophobic interaction liquid chromatography. Accurate mass and fragmentation MS/MS data are used in combination with retention time to increase confidence of lipid and metabolite identification. Finally, we present a workflow to process lipidomic and metabolomic data and identify specific metabolites of interest mapping them into known biochemical pathways (Fig. 2).

2 Materials

2.1 Equipment

1. Analytical balance.
2. Chemical fume-hood.
3. Homogenizer, such as TissueLyser (QIAGEN).
4. Vortex.
5. Centrifuge.
6. UHPLC such as Acquity UPLC (Waters).
7. Time of Flight mass spectrometer, such as a Synapt G2 mass spectrometer (Waters).
8. Vacuum evaporator.

2.2 Solvents and Chemicals

1. Water (MS grade).
2. Methanol (MS grade).
3. Chloroform (HPLC grade).
4. Formic acid (MS grade).
5. Ammonium formate (MS grade).
6. Isopropanol (MS grade).
7. Acetonitrile (MS grade).
8. Internal Standards: d8 arachidonic acid (Cayman Chemicals); cholesterol-d7 (Avanti), C17:0-cholesteryl ester (Avanti); 1,2-dimyristoyl-sn-glycero-3-phosphoethanolamine (Avanti), 1,2-dimyristoyl-sn-glycero-3-phosphocholine (Avanti), 1-heptadecanoyl-2-hydroxy-sn-glycero-3-phosphocholine (Avanti), SPLASH™ Lipidomix® Mass Spec Standard (Avanti), phenylalanine d2, [Sigma Aldrich], succinate d4, [Sigma Aldrich], glucose 13C6, [Sigma Aldrich]; carnitine d9, [Sigma Aldrich]: glutamic acid d5, [Sigma Aldrich]; lysine d4 [Sigma Aldrich]; alanine d4 [Sigma Aldrich].
9. Leukine enkephalin [Sigma Aldrich].
10. System-suitability standard solution for polar metabolites. Nicotinamide, 5-oxoproline, phenylalanine, succinic acid, hypoxanthine, arginine, inosine, S-Adenosyl-L-homocysteine (SAH), and raffinose [Sigma Aldrich].
11. System-suitability standard solution for lipids: Differential Ion Mobility System Suitability Lipidomix® Kit (Avanti).

258   Giuseppe Astarita et al.

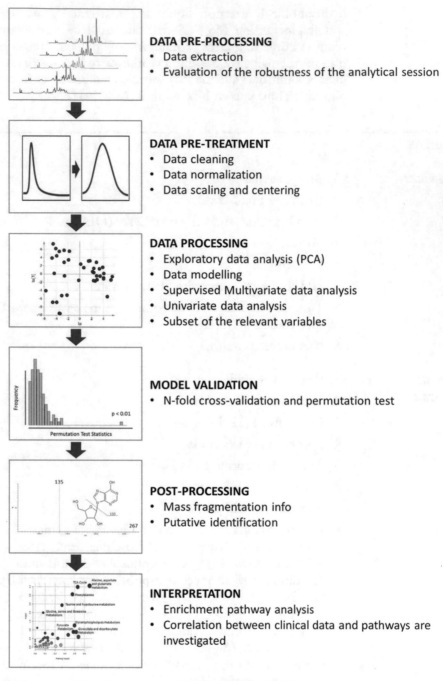

Fig. 2 Workflow for the analysis of lipidomics and metabolomics data

2.3 Supplies	1. ACQUITY CSH C18 column (2.1 × 100 mm ID, 1.7 μm).
	2. ACQUITY UPLC BEH Amide column (2.1 × 150 mm ID, 1.7 μm).
	3. Glass Vials 1.5-mL for autosampler and LC/MS analysis.

3   Methods

3.1   Considerations on the Experiment Design

During the experimental design it is important to include criteria for subject selection. For instance, based on previously published studies, cohort sizes for metabolomics and lipidomics analysis of human brain should be at least of 20 subjects per group. Sample groups should be matched by age, sex, and postmortem interval. The selection of a particular brain region or subregion should be carefully evaluated before the analysis; considerations on white and gray matter should be taken into account (*see* **Note 1**).

3.2   Sample Preparation for Lipidomics and Metabolomics Analysis

A biphasic liquid/liquid extraction method can be used to extract polar metabolites in the aqueous phase and lipids in the organic phase. The solvent mixture allows the precipitation of proteins, which after centrifugation appear as a disk at the interface of the upper and lower phase. To allow normalization for both extraction efficiency and instrument response, a mixture of internal standards is added before the extraction process (*see* Reagents). Generally, internal standards are non-endogenous or isotopically labeled compounds that have chemical similarity with the class of metabolites or lipids to be analyzed. After extraction, both the upper and lower phases are dried down and resuspended for further LC/MS analyses (Fig. 1).

1. Label tubes according to the number of tissue samples to analyze.

2. Prepare an ice-cold methanol solution containing a mixture of the following internal standards: d8 arachidonic acid (0.1 μg/mL), cholesterol-d7 (50 μg/mL), C17:0-cholesteryl ester (1 μg/mL), 1,2-dimyristoyl-sn-glycero-3-phosphoethanolamine (10 μg/mL), 1,2-dimyristoyl-sn-glycero-3-phosphocholine (10 μg/mL), 1-heptadecanoyl-2-hydroxy-sn-glycero-3-phosphocholine (1 μg/mL), phenylalanine d2 (1.5 μg/mL), succinate d4 (1.5 μg/mL), glucose 13C6 (60 μg/mL), carnitine d9 (0.15 μg/mL), glutamic acid d5 (1.2 μg/mL), lysine d4 (1.5 μg/mL), and alanine d4 (3 μg/mL).

3. Add 0.2 mL of methanol containing the internal standards in each tube.

4. Weigh the frozen tissues (20 mg) (*see* **Note 2**) and transfer them in the previously prepared tubes containing methanol with internal standards.

5. Homogenize the tissues keeping the tubes in cold (*see* **Note 3**).

6. Add 0.4-mL of chloroform and vortex for 10 s (*see* **Note 4**).

7. Add 0.15 mL of water and vortex for 10 s.

8. Centrifuge at $4000 \times g$ for 10 min at 4 °C to the mixture into two phases with a protein interface.

9. Recover the upper phase (polar metabolome) and the bottom phase (lipidome) and transfer them into two separate vials.

10. Dry lipids extracts (bottom phase) using a vacuum evaporator for 30 min at 35 °C and reconstitute in 2-propanol/acetonitrile/water (4:3:1 v/v/v, 0.1 mL) (*see* **Note 5**).

11. Create a QC pool sample by collecting and pooling together a small amount (5–10 μL) from each lipid extract sample. Use this QC pool sample as quality control during the LC–MS analyses.

12. Dry polar metabolites extracts using a vacuum evaporator for 3 h at 35 °C and reconstitute in acetonitrile/water (1:1 v/v, 0.2 mL).

13. Create a QC pool sample by collecting and pooling together a small amount (5–10 μL) from each polar metabolite extract sample. Use this QC pool sample as quality control during the LC–MS analyses.

3.3 LC/MS Analysis of Polar Metabolites

Metabolic profiling of the polar metabolome is achieved by using HILIC coupled with high-resolution mass spectrometry to obtain both retention time and accurate mass information (Fig. 3). In addition, fragmentation experiments on the pooled sample allow to increase the confidence in metabolite identification.

1. System-suitability standard solution for polar metabolites. Prepare 100 μL of a solution in acetonitrile:water (50:50 v:v) containing the following metabolites at the concentration of 10 μg/mL: nicotinamide, 5-oxoproline, phenylalanine, succinic acid, hypoxanthine, arginine, inosine, SAH, and raffinose.

2. Prepare mobile phase A by adding 1 mL of formic acid in 1 L of ACN.

3. Prepare mobile phase B by adding 1 mL of formic acid in 1 L of water.

4. Weak wash solvent for polar metabolites analysis. Prepare 500 mL of a solution of acetonitrile/water (10:90, vol/vol).

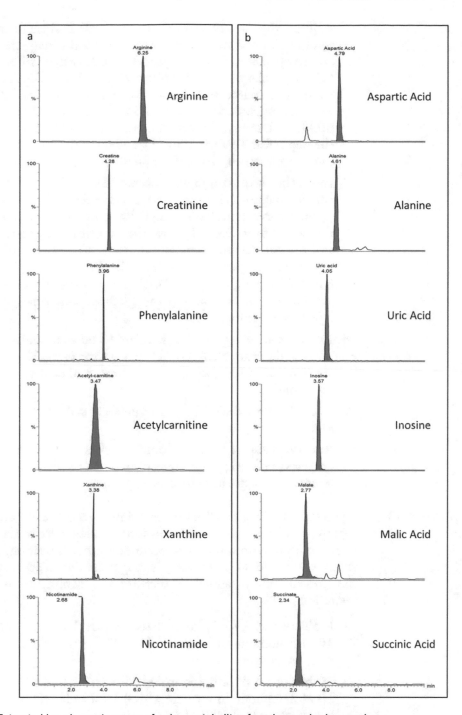

Fig. 3 Extracted ion chromatograms of polar metabolites from human brain samples

5. Strong wash solvent for polar metabolites analysis. Prepare 500 mL of a solution of acetonitrile/water (40:60, vol/vol).

6. Prepare the mass spectrometer. For untargeted metabolomics, use high-resolution mass spectrometry, such as a Q-TOF mass spectrometer. For example, for a Synapt G2 instrument,

calibrate the mass spectrometer using sodium formate in both positive and negative ionization mode. Set the mass spectrometer to operate in data-independent mode (MS^E) (*see* **Note 6**). Set the capillary and cone voltage at 1.5 kV and 30 V, respectively. The source and desolvation temperatures at 120 and 500 °C, respectively, and the flow rate of desolvation gas at 800 L/h. During MS^E experiments, set the collision energy in the trap cell at 4 eV (function 1), and ramp the collision energy in the transfer cell, from 15 to 30 eV (function 2).

7. Insert the chromatographic column (ACQUITY UPLC BEH Amide column, 2.1 × 150 mm, particle size 1.7 μm) into the column compartment. Set the column temperature to 45 °C, the flow rate to 0.4 mL/min, the injection volume to 5 μL, and the autosampler temperature to 4 °C. Use the following linear elution gradient: 0 min, 99% of A; 6 min, 40% of A; 8 min, 99% of A; 10 min, 99% of A. Equilibrate the chromatographic system by running the gradient four times without injecting any sample.

8. Inject the system-suitability standard solution for polar metabolites and ensure that the LC–MS system is working fine by checking mass accuracy, retention time, and area of the polar metabolites.

9. Inject 15 times the QC pooled sample to stabilize the LC–MS system.

10. Run the samples in a randomized order and include a QC pooled sample every eight injections or at least five times within your sample sequence (*see* **Note 7**).

3.4 LC/MS Analysis of Lipids

Lipidomic profiling is achieved by using reversed-phase chromatography coupled with high-resolution mass spectrometry to obtain both retention time and accurate mass information. As for the metabolomics LC/MS analysis, fragmentation experiments on the pooled sample allow to increase the confidence in lipid identification.

1. Mobile phase A for lipids analysis. Prepare 1 L of a solution of 10 mM ammonium formate with 0.1% formic acid in acetonitrile/water 40:60 (vol/vol).

2. Mobile phase B for lipids analysis. Prepare 1 L of a solution of 10 mM ammonium formate with 0.1% formic acid in acetonitrile/isopropanol 10:90 (vol/vol).

3. Weak wash solvent for lipids analysis. Prepare 500 mL of a solution of acetonitrile/water/isopropanol (30:30:40, vol/vol/vol).

4. Strong wash solvent for lipids analysis. Prepare 500 mL of a solution of isopropanol/water/formic acid/dichloromethane (95:5:2:1, vol/vol/vol/vol).

5. Prepare the mass spectrometer. For untargeted lipidomics, use high-resolution mass spectrometry, such as a Q-TOF mass spectrometer. For example, for a Synapt G2 instrument, calibrate the mass spectrometer using sodium formate in both positive and negative ionization mode. Set the mass spectrometer to operate in data-independent mode (MS^E) (*see* **Note 6**). Set the capillary and cone voltage at 2.5 kV and 35 V, respectively. The source and desolvation temperatures at 120 and 500 °C, respectively, and the flow rate of desolvation gas at 1000 L/h. During MS^E experiments, set the collision energy in the trap cell at 4 eV (function 1), and ramp the collision energy in the transfer cell, from 15 to 30 eV (function 2).

6. Insert the chromatographic column (ACQUITY UPLC CSH C18 column, 2.1 × 100 mm, particle size 1.7 μm) into the column compartment. Set the column temperature to 45 °C, the flow rate to 0.4 mL/min, the injection volume to 5 μL, and the autosampler temperature to 4 °C. Use the following linear elution gradient: 0 min, 99% of A; 6 min, 40% of A; 8 min, 99% of A; 10 min, 99% of A. Equilibrate the chromatographic system by running the gradient four times without injecting any sample.

7. Inject the system-suitability standard solution for lipids and ensure that the LC–MS system is working fine by checking mass accuracy, retention time, and area of the polar metabolites.

8. Inject five times the QC pooled sample to stabilize the LC–MS system.

9. Run the samples in a randomized order and include a QC pooled sample every eight injections or at least five times within your sample sequence (*see* **Note 7**).

3.5 Data Processing and Analysis

Lipidomics and metabolomics dataset are processed using an identical workflow involving the following steps.

3.5.1 Data Pre-processing

Raw data are characterized by a data structure with three dimensions for each sample: retention time, m/z, and intensity. Commonly used univariate and multivariate data analysis tools work on data tables, which are data structures with two dimensions for each sample. Thus, raw data must be transformed into suitable data structures where variables are well defined and quantified (i.e., peak area) prior to perform data analysis.

1. *Data extraction*. A data table where each sample is described by the so-called m/z_time variables is obtained for each analytical

session. The main steps of data extraction are the following (*see* **Note 8**):

- Baseline correction.

- Peak detection; for each sample, a mass list (detected ions) is generated for each time scan.

- Chromatogram building; for each detected peak, a chromatogram is generated continuously over the time scans.

- Chromatogram deconvolution; for each sample, chromatograms are deconvoluted and the obtained peaks are integrated and identified as m/z_time variable (m/z is the mass-to-charge ratio whereas time is the retention time of the peak); as a result, each sample is described by a peak list of m/z_time variables.

- Time alignment; the time of the m/z_time variable is corrected for a suitable function in order to take into account the retention time variability of the same compound in different runs; the deviation of retention times between the m/z_time lists is reduced.

- Peak list matching; the m/z_time variables are matched over the samples to obtain a data table.

- Gap filling. The raw data are re-processed to impute the missing values present in the data table (*see* **Note 9**).

2. *Evaluation of the robustness of the analytical session.* A preliminary data analysis is performed to check the robustness of the analytical session.

   - The coefficient of variation is estimated for each variable of the QC.

   - The trend of the total sum of the variable intensity is monitored as a function of the run order.

   - Principal Component Analysis (PCA) is applied to evaluate the reproducibility of the QCs against the variability of the analytical samples; outliers are identified and excluded if necessary.

3.5.2 Data Pretreatment

1. *Data cleaning.* Variables with more than a pre-defined number of imputed missing or zeroes values (e.g., 50%) and/or with an unsatisfactory coefficient of variation (e.g., CV > 30%) are excluded.

2. *Data normalization.* Normalization is applied in order to remove systematic sources of variation. We suggest to apply median fold change normalization for data obtained by mass spectrometry.

3. *Data scaling and centering.* Variables are log-transformed and mean centered.

3.5.3 Data Processing

1. Exploratory data analysis. PCA is applied to detect specific patterns in the data.

2. Data modeling.

   - Multivariate data analysis. Supervised multivariate data analysis is applied to distinguish the groups of samples under investigation. Specifically, Projection to Latent Structures-Discriminant Analysis (PLS-DA) is used to obtain reliable discriminant models. A subset of relevant variables characterizing each group is selected by variable influence analysis (*see* **Note 10**).

   - Univariate data analysis. *t*-Test with false discovery rate is performed to complete the results of multivariate data analysis. Variables with q-values less than a defined threshold are selected (see **Note 11**).

   - Subset of the relevant variables. The results of multivariate and univariate data analysis are merged to obtain the subset of relevant variables able to characterize the investigated groups of samples.

3.5.4 Model Validation

N-fold cross-validation with different values of N, permutation test on the response, and stability test are applied to evaluate the reliability of the multivariate models (*see* **Note 12**).

3.5.5 Post-processing. Relevant Variables Are Confirmed to Be Chemical Compounds

1. *Mass fragmentation info.* Raw data are re-processed for extracting the traces corresponding to the relevant m/z_time variables. The fragmentation pattern is extracted for each variable. Once the variables are confirmed, putative identification is performed.

2. *Putative identification.* Metabolites and lipids of interest are identified by searching in various publicly available databases (e.g., METLIN [8], the Human Metabolome Database (HMDB) [9], and LipidMaps [10]) or in-house databases filtering by a defined tolerance for Delta ppm of precursors and fragments, retention time range and isotope similarities.

3.5.6 Interpretation

Enrichment pathway analysis is performed on the relevant identified metabolites to highlight the pathways perturbed by the disease. The relationships between clinical data and pathways are investigated by Projection to Latent Structures regression (PLS) (*see* **Note 13**).

3.6 Maintenance and System Suitability Test for LC/MS Analysis

In the following sections we report general procedures for the maintenance and system suitability testing used to validate the LC/MS lipidomic and metabolomics analysis.

3.6.1 LC/MS
Maintenance

To avoid contaminations routinely preventive maintenance is performed.

1. Replacing the spray needle and cleaning ionization spray chamber or other accessible MS components.

2. Replacing inline filters and frits, the injector needle and capillaries or other accessible LC components; flushing the system with a mixture of cyclohexane/acetonitrile/isopropanol (1/1/2, v/v/v).

3.6.2 Quality Assurance

1. To assure equilibration of the LC column, 15 pooled samples are run before sequence.

2. As quality control, pooled samples are run before, between, and after biological samples.

3.6.3 Storage of Lipid
and Metabolite Extracts

Lipid and metabolites extracts are usually stored in a freezer at −80 °C. It was shown that after storage up to 4 years at −80 °C, the blood lipid composition is practically unchanged [11].

4 Notes

1. In order to limit artifacts due to sample degradation, in the experimental design consider to perform sampling using a postmortem interval average of less than 4 h.

2. Both lipid and metabolite composition are altered during thawing at room temperature. To limit artifacts due to enzymatic reactions and oxidation, brain samples should be weighed while still frozen and then quenched with ice-cold methanol.

3. We suggest to normalize lipids and metabolites levels by using tissue weight or volumes in case of biofluids. In cases when working with small amount of tissues, a small aliquot from the homogenate solution can be used to quantify proteins for normalization.

4. Methanol/chloroform mixture is irritating to skin and eyes, and toxic. Alternative extraction procedures that use less toxic organic solvents have been proposed for a wide range of tissues [12, 13]. Handle any organic solvents with gloves in a chemical fume-hood, avoiding health hazard by accidental spills, skin contact, and breathing of vapors.

5. Alternative extraction protocol could be used for the analysis of acidic phospholipids, such as gangliosides and phosphoinositides [14, 15].

6. In order to identify lipids and metabolites, it is necessary to collect fragmentation information for metabolites of interest.

Using data-dependent and data-independent acquisition modes on the pooled sample, you can generate fragmentation spectra that can be used after statistical analyses to confirm the analyte identification [16].

7. In untargeted metabolomics/lipidomics, blank samples are normally used to remove background noise during data pretreatment. However, blank samples analyzed during the analytical batch might affect the metabolic profile of the first real sample analyzed after the blank sample. We suggest to run blank samples at the very beginning or at the end of the analytical batch.

8. Several workflows are discussed in literature and implemented in freeware software; here, we report the workflow implemented in the freeware software MZmine 2 [17], that is very similar to the workflow implemented in the freeware R-package XCMS [18]; the main differences between MZmine 2 and XCMS are in the algorithms used for peak alignment; we remark that different software produce different data tables; we suggest to use the same software for all the analytical sessions (with suitable protocols).

9. Missing values and zeroes values might cause difficulties for downstream statistical analysis. Most missing or zeroes values are caused by low abundance lipids and metabolites, which cannot be detected. Various methods may be applied to deal with zeroes or missing values, including replacing them with a small values (for example, using the half of the minimum positive values in the original data) or mean/median values, or using Probabilistic or Bayesian PCA method or Singular Value Decomposition method [19].

10. Several solution can be adopted for implementing PLS-DA. It is possible to use the commercial software SIMCA from Umetrics, or PLS-DA can be performed by R-package "pls" or by R-package "BioMark") or by using Metaboanalyst [19].

11. Univariate data analysis can be performed by Metaboanalyst [19] as well as R (e.g., t-test with false discovery rate is available in the R-package "qvalue").

12. Metaboanalyst [19] and SIMCA from Umetrics performs only N-fold cross-validation and permutation test; for a full model validation is required to implement suitable R-functions based on R-package "pls" and/or R-package "BioMark".

13. Targeted lipidomics and metabolomics approaches (i.e., using internal standards to quantify) are used to confirm and validate any potential biomarkers in larger patient cohorts.

References

1. Toledo JB, Arnold M, Kastenmuller G, Chang R, Baillie RA, Han X, Thambisetty M, Tenenbaum JD, Suhre K, Thompson JW, John-Williams LS, MahmoudianDehkordi S, Rotroff DM, Jack JR, Motsinger-Reif A, Risacher SL, Blach C, Lucas JE, Massaro T, Louie G, Zhu H, Dallmann G, Klavins K, Koal T, Kim S, Nho K, Shen L, Casanova R, Varma S, Legido-Quigley C, Moseley MA, Zhu K, Henrion MY, van der Lee SJ, Harms AC, Demirkan A, Hankemeier T, van Duijn CM, Trojanowski JQ, Shaw LM, Saykin AJ, Weiner MW, Doraiswamy PM, Kaddurah-Daouk R, Alzheimer's Disease Neuroimaging I, the Alzheimer Disease Metabolomics C (2017) Metabolic network failures in Alzheimer's disease-A biochemical road map. Alzheimer's Dement 13:965. https://doi.org/10.1016/j.jalz.2017.01.020

2. Paglia G, Stocchero M, Cacciatore S, Lai S, Angel P, Alam MT, Keller M, Ralser M, Astarita G (2016) Unbiased metabolomic investigation of Alzheimer's disease brain points to dysregulation of mitochondrial aspartate metabolism. J Proteome Res 15(2):608–618. https://doi.org/10.1021/acs.jproteome.5b01020

3. Fonteh AN, Harrington RJ, Huhmer AF, Biringer RG, Riggins JN, Harrington MG (2006) Identification of disease markers in human cerebrospinal fluid using lipidomic and proteomic methods. Dis Markers 22(1–2):39–64

4. Astarita G, Jung KM, Vasilevko V, Dipatrizio NV, Martin SK, Cribbs DH, Head E, Cotman CW, Piomelli D (2011) Elevated stearoyl-CoA desaturase in brains of patients with Alzheimer's disease. PLoS One 6(10):e24777. https://doi.org/10.1371/journal.pone.0024777

5. Astarita G, Jung KM, Berchtold NC, Nguyen VQ, Gillen DL, Head E, Cotman CW, Piomelli D (2010) Deficient liver biosynthesis of docosahexaenoic acid correlates with cognitive impairment in Alzheimer's disease. PLoS One 5(9):e12538. https://doi.org/10.1371/journal.pone.0012538

6. Inoue K, Tsutsui H, Akatsu H, Hashizume Y, Matsukawa N, Yamamoto T, Toyo'oka T (2013) Metabolic profiling of Alzheimer's disease brains. Sci Rep 3:2364. https://doi.org/10.1038/srep02364

7. Graham SF, Chevallier OP, Roberts D, Holscher C, Elliott CT, Green BD (2013) Investigation of the human brain metabolome to identify potential markers for early diagnosis and therapeutic targets of Alzheimer's disease. Anal Chem 85(3):1803–1811. https://doi.org/10.1021/ac303163f

8. Zhu ZJ, Schultz AW, Wang J, Johnson CH, Yannone SM, Patti GJ, Siuzdak G (2013) Liquid chromatography quadrupole time-of-flight mass spectrometry characterization of metabolites guided by the METLIN database. Nat Protoc 8(3):451–460. https://doi.org/10.1038/nprot.2013.004

9. Wishart DS, Jewison T, Guo AC, Wilson M, Knox C, Liu Y, Djoumbou Y, Mandal R, Aziat F, Dong E, Bouatra S, Sinelnikov I, Arndt D, Xia J, Liu P, Yallou F, Bjorndahl T, Perez-Pineiro R, Eisner R, Allen F, Neveu V, Greiner R, Scalbert A (2013) HMDB 3.0—the human metabolome database in 2013. Nucleic Acids Res 41(Database issue):D801–D807. https://doi.org/10.1093/nar/gks1065

10. Fahy E, Subramaniam S, Murphy RC, Nishijima M, Raetz CR, Shimizu T, Spener F, van Meer G, Wakelam MJ, Dennis EA (2009) Update of the LIPID MAPS comprehensive classification system for lipids. J Lipid Res 50(Suppl):S9–14. https://doi.org/10.1194/jlr.R800095-JLR200

11. Lau OW, Wong SK (2000) Contamination in food from packaging material. J Chromatogr A 882(1–2):255–270

12. Lin JH, Liu LY, Yang MH, Lee MH (2004) Ethyl acetate/ethyl alcohol mixtures as an alternative to folch reagent for extracting animal lipids. J Agric Food Chem 52(16):4984–4986. https://doi.org/10.1021/jf049360m

13. Hara A, Radin NS (1978) Lipid extraction of tissues with a low-toxicity solvent. Anal Biochem 90(1):420–426

14. Bian L, Yang J, Sun Y (2015) Isolation and purification of monosialotetrahexosylgangliosides from pig brain by extraction and liquid chromatography. Biomed Chromatogr 29(10):1604–1611. https://doi.org/10.1002/bmc.3467

15. Garcia AD, Chavez JL, Mechref Y (2014) Rapid and sensitive LC-ESI-MS of gangliosides. J Chromatogr B Anal Technol Biomed Life Sci 947-948:1–7. https://doi.org/10.1016/j.jchromb.2013.11.025

16. Fu W, Magnusdottir M, Brynjolfson S, Palsson BO, Paglia G (2012) UPLC-UV-MS(E) analysis for quantification and identification of major carotenoid and chlorophyll species in algae. Anal Bioanal Chem 404(10):3145–3154. https://doi.org/10.1007/s00216-012-6434-4

17. Pluskal T, Castillo S, Villar-Briones A, Oresic M (2010) MZmine 2: modular framework for processing, visualizing, and analyzing mass spectrometry-based molecular profile data. BMC Bioinformatics 11:395. https://doi.org/10.1186/1471-2105-11-395

18. Huan T, Forsberg EM, Rinehart D, Johnson CH, Ivanisevic J, Benton HP, Fang M, Aisporna A, Hilmers B, Poole FL, Thorgersen MP, Adams MWW, Krantz G, Fields MW, Robbins PD, Niedernhofer LJ, Ideker T, Majumder EL, Wall JD, Rattray NJW, Goodacre R, Lairson LL, Siuzdak G (2017) Systems biology guided by XCMS online metabolomics. Nat Methods 14(5):461–462. https://doi.org/10.1038/nmeth.4260

19. Xia J, Wishart DS (2016) Using MetaboAnalyst 3.0 for comprehensive metabolomics data analysis. Curr Protoc Bioinformatics 55:14.10.11–14.10.91. https://doi.org/10.1002/cpbi.11

Chapter 18

Neuropathological Assessment as an Endpoint in Clinical Trial Design

Steve Gentleman and Alan King Lun Liu

Abstract

Different neurodegenerative conditions can have complex, overlapping clinical presentations that make accurate diagnosis during life very challenging. For this reason, confirmation of the clinical diagnosis still requires postmortem verification. This is particularly relevant for clinical trials of novel therapeutics where it is important to ascertain what disease and/or pathology modifying effects the therapeutics have had. Furthermore, it is important to confirm that patients in the trial actually had the correct clinical diagnosis as this will have a major bearing on the interpretation of trial results. Here we present a simple protocol for pathological assessment of neurodegenerative changes.

Key words Clinical trial, Neurodegeneration, Postmortem, Diagnosis, Neuropathology

1 Introduction

Examination of postmortem human brain tissue has been key to many of the major advances in our understanding of neurodegenerative disorders over the past 30 years. The detection of the new variant Creutzfeldt–Jakob disease in the 1990s [1], the identification of the multiple molecular mechanisms underlying different frontotemporal dementias [2], and the emergence of new disease entities, such as chronic traumatic encephalopathy [3], have all been due to observations made on examination of autopsy brains. Postmortem examination is also crucial for clinical audit when the clinical diagnosis is not straightforward. For example, the most common cause of parkinsonism is Parkinson's disease but there are a number of other disorders, such as multiple system atrophy (MSA) and progressive supranuclear palsy (PSP), which can also present in this way. These disorders have different cellular and molecular mechanisms of pathogenesis and it is sometimes only by postmortem examination that the correct diagnosis can be confirmed. With increasing life expectancy, a further complication is the fact that many elderly patients may have more than one disease

Robert Perneczky (ed.), *Biomarkers for Alzheimer's Disease Drug Development*, Methods in Molecular Biology, vol. 1750,
https://doi.org/10.1007/978-1-4939-7704-8_18, © Springer Science+Business Media, LLC 2018

pathology which may make their clinical presentation very difficult to interpret [4]. These problems with clinical diagnostic accuracy have been highlighted recently in relation to immunotherapy trials for Alzheimer's disease. Autopsy studies revealed that a proportion of people enrolled on the trial, which was specifically based on removal of Aβ peptide, did not actually have Alzheimer's disease [5]. For all of these reasons we feel that postmortem follow-up is essential for clinical trials and we present here a protocol for assessment of neurodegenerative changes which is based on what we routinely use in the Parkinson's UK tissue bank (The Parkinson's UK Brain Bank, https://www.parkinsons.org.uk/content/parkinsons-uk-brain-bank).

2 Materials

Brain donations can be made in a number of different ways. A hospital postmortem can be requested by a physician after the death of an inpatient, particularly if there is uncertainty over diagnosis. However, for research purposes, many brain tissue banks will prospectively consent patients who have expressed a wish to donate their brain (UK Brain Banks Network, https://www.mrc.ac.uk/research/facilities-and-resources-for-researchers/brain-banks/; The Parkinson's UK Brain Bank). The prospective nature of this consenting process usually facilitates a more rapid retrieval of tissue when the patient dies because the next of kin and/or the attending health care professionals are aware of the patient's wishes and will inform the tissue banks soon after death. Ideally, a similar premortem prospective consent procedure should be included in clinical trial designs.

3 Methods

When a brain donation is received, the protocol for neuropathological assessment entails tissue dissection, sampling, preparation, sectioning, staining, and examination. In some cases donations will be of whole fixed brains but, if possible, fresh brains should be bisected and frozen tissue should be retained from one half of the brain. This tissue is not only useful for research purposes but will also aid in the biochemical and genetic workup of the case.

3.1 Macroscopic Dissection (Fresh Tissue)

1. Weigh the whole brain.

2. Aliquot cerebrospinal fluid, measure pH, and store at −80 °C.

3. Separate the brainstem and cerebellum from the cerebrum by cutting though the midbrain at the level of the oculomotor nerve (CNIII).

4. Bisect the cerebrum along the longitudinal fissure. Place one hemisphere into 4% formalin solution for subsequent diagnostic examination.

5. Bisect the brainstem in the mid-sagittal plane and fix the half contralateral to the fixed cerebral hemisphere.

6. Coronally slice the unfixed hemisphere at 1 cm intervals with the first cut made at the level of the mammillary body. Dissect each slice into 2 cm² blocks using a grid system, photograph the dissected slice with each block having a unique grid coordinate, flash freeze, and store at −80 °C.

7. Separate the cerebellum from the brainstem by cutting the three cerebellar peduncles. Slice the cerebellum in the sagittal plane. Slice the brainstem in the horizontal plane. Photograph, flash freeze, and store at −80 °C.

3.2 Macroscopic Dissection (Fixed Tissue)

Tissue should be fixed in the 4% formalin solution for 4–5 weeks before dissection (Fig. 1).

1. Examine the meninges for evidence of infection and fibrosis.

2. Examine the cortical gyration pattern and determine if there is a global or any regional atrophy.

3. Examine the basal blood vessels.

4. Determine if there is any uncal indentation or tonsillar prominence suggestive of raised intracranial pressure in vivo.

5. Coronally slice the cerebral hemisphere at the level of the mammillary body.

6. Make coronal slices of the anterior and posterior cerebrum using a 1 cm cut guide.

7. Separate the cerebellum from the brainstem by cutting the three cerebellar peduncles.

8. Slice the cerebellum at 0.5 cm intervals in the sagittal plane.

9. Slice the brainstem at 0.5 cm intervals in the horizontal plane.

3.3 Tissue Sampling and Preparation

The following anatomical areas are sampled for diagnostic assessment:

1. Superior and middle frontal gyrus at level of genu of corpus callosum.

2. Cingulate gyrus at level of nucleus accumbens.

3. Nucleus accumbens.

4. Superior temporal gyrus at level of mammillary body.

5. Basal ganglia at level of anterior commissure (containing the nucleus basalis of Meynert).

6. Hypothalamus at level of mammillary body.

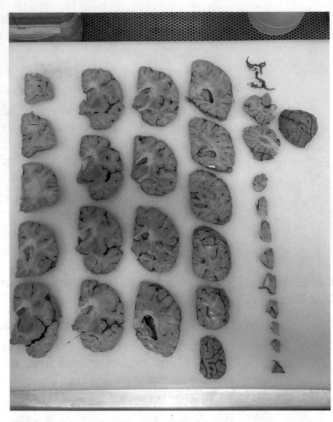

Fig. 1 Completed dissection of a single hemisphere and contralateral hemi-brainstem/cerebellum prior to tissue sampling

7. Amygdala.

8. Thalamus to include subthalamic nucleus.

9. Anterior hippocampus.

10. Posterior hippocampus at level of lateral geniculate nucleus.

11. Precentral gyrus (Primary motor cortex).

12. Occipital cortex to include calcarine fissure.

13. Inferior parietal lobule.

14. Cerebellum to include folia and dentate nucleus.

15. Midbrain at level of oculomotor nerve (containing substantia nigra).

16. Pons to include locus coeruleus.

17. Medulla to include inferior olive and dorsal motor nucleus of the vagus.

The selected blocks of tissue are placed in processing cassettes for paraffin wax embedding. Following embedding 6–8 μm sections are cut for staining.

3.4 Histological Staining

A section from each block is stained with hematoxylin and eosin (H&E).

1. Deparaffinize and rehydrate sections by immersing in: (a) xylene [3 × 5 min] (in a fume hood), (b) 100% industrial methylated spirit (IMS) [2 × 5 min], (c) 90% IMS [5 min], (d) 70% IMS [5 min], and (e) distilled water [5 min].

2. Immerse in filtered Mayer's Hematoxylin [5 min].

3. Wash in running tap water (or Scott's Tap Water Substitute) for blueing of sections.

4. Check sections under the microscope and briefly differentiate in 1% acid-alcohol if necessary.

5. Nuclei should be a deep blue color with the vesicular nuclei showing a well-marked chromatin pattern. The background should show only weak residual hematoxylin coloration.

6. If the staining is too pale or too dark, immerse in hematoxylin or acid-alcohol again, respectively, for as long as necessary.

7. Immerse in filtered 1% eosin [5 min].

8. Wash briefly (as this will bleach the eosin stain) in running tap water.

9. If the stain is too dark, it can be bleached by washing for longer. If too pale, immerse the sections in 1% eosin again for as long as necessary.

10. Dehydrate by immersing briefly (as this also will bleach the eosin stain) in: (a) 70% IMS, (b) 90% IMS, and finally wash in 100% IMS (2 × 5 min).

11. Clear by immersing in xylene [3 × 5 min] (in fume hood).

12. Mount sections in distrene–plasticizer–xylene (DPX; a xylene-based mountant), in the fume hood.

The result of this protocol is that the nuclei are stained blue, cytoplasmic constituents are stained red to pink, and red blood cells are stained red to orange.

3.5 Immuno-cytochemistry

In order for the pathological changes in the brain to be staged, immunocytochemical staining is required. The key antibodies for this assessment are against hyperphosphorylated tau, Aβ peptide, α-synuclein (αSN, Fig. 2), and TDP-43. There are a variety of commercial antibodies available and each will require individual staining protocol optimization. The anatomical areas that require immunostaining for each of these antibodies are detailed in Table 1.

1. Dewax and rehydrate tissue sections as described above.

2. Immerse in 1% hydrogen peroxide (H_2O_2)/phosphate-buffered saline (PBS, pH 7.4) for 30 min at room temperature for quenching of endogenous peroxidase activity.

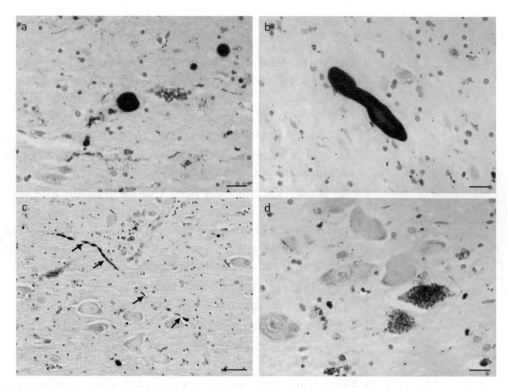

Fig. 2 Examples of αSN-immunopositive pathological structures. **(a)** and **(b)** extracellular Lewy body-like inclusions. **(c)** αSN-immunopositive Lewy neurites (arrows). **(d)** Granular cytoplasmic staining within magnocellular neurons. Scale bars = 20 μm **(a, b, d)**; 50 μm (c)

3. Wash in distilled water (5 min).

4. Carry out antigen retrieval procedures (if necessary):

   - **Heat-induced antigen retrieval:** e.g., Place sections in pressure cooker in 0.01 M sodium citrate buffer (pH 6) (25 min) or microwave in 1 mM EDTA buffer (pH 8) (20 min) or steamer in 0.01 M sodium citrate buffer (20 min).

   - Place in 80% formic acid (10 min) [essential for anti-αSN and anti-Aβ antibodies].

5. Wash in distilled water (5 min).

6. Wash in PBS (3 × 5 min).

7. Incubation with primary antibodies (diluted in 0.3% TritonX-100 in PBS) at 4 °C overnight (example of antibodies used is listed in Table 2).

8. Wash in PBS (3 × 5 min).

9. Incubation with biotinylated secondary antibodies (diluted in 0.3% Triton-X 100/PBS) (1 h).

10. Signal amplification with avidin–biotin complex (ABC) (as per manufacturer's protocol).

Table 1
H&E and immunocytochemistry to be carried out on sections from the different anatomical blocks

Block #	Anatomical area	H&E	Tau	Aβ	αSN	TDP-43
1	Frontal cortex	x	x	x	x	x
2	Cingulate cortex	x			x	
3	Ant basal ganglia	x				
4	Sup temporal gyrus	x	x	x	x	
5	Basal ganglia	x	x	x	x	
6	Hypothalamus	x				
7	Amygdala	x	x	x	x	x
8	Thalamus	x				
9	Ant hippocampus	x	x	x	x	
10	Post hippocampus	x	x	x	x	x
11	Precentral gyrus	x				
12	Occipital cortex	x	x	x		
13	Parietal cortex	x	x	x		
14	Cerebellum	x		x	x	
15	Midbrain	x	x	x	x	
16	Pons	x	x	x	x	
17	Medulla	x	x	x	x	

11. Wash in PBS (3 × 5 min).

12. Visualization with 3′3-diaminobenzidine (DAB) (5 min)

13. Wash in distilled water (2 × 5 min).

14. Counterstaining with Meyer's hematoxylin (30 s).

15. Rinsing in running tap water.

16. Dehydration and clearing as described above and sections coverslipped with DPX.

3.6 Pathology Staging

The standard protocol for the reporting of microscopic neurodegenerative pathology is constantly evolving but the current protocol most widely used is that of the National Institute on Aging-Alzheimer's Association [6]. This is reported in the ABC format with the A relating to assessment of Aβ spread [7], B relating to tau pathology (Braak tau staging) [8], and C the assessment of neuritic plaques (CERAD score). For Lewy body related αSN pathology the staging of the BrainNet Europe Consortium and McKeith criteria are used to classify pathology into brainstem, limbic or neocortical subtypes [9, 10]. TDP-43 is used to screen for other rarer neurodegenerative disorders.

Table 2
Examples of antibodies used for neuropathological assessment

Antibody	Host	Clonality	Immunogen	Company	Catalogue number	Pretreatment
Alpha-synuclein (Clone 42)	Mouse	Monoclonal (IgG$_1$)/Clone 42	Rat Synuclein-1 aa. 15–123	BD Transduction Laboratories	610787	10 min 80% formic acid
Amyloid-beta	Mouse	Monoclonal (IgG$_{2b}$)/Clone 4G8	β amyloid aa 17–24	Covance (Signet)	800704/800705/ 800706	10 min 80% formic acid
Tau (Phospho-PHF-tau pSer202 + Thr205)	Mouse	Monoclonal (IgG$_1$)/Clone AT8	Partially purified human PHF-Tau	Pierce Thermo Scientific	MN1020	Nil

Acknowledgments

The authors would like to thank Parkinson's UK, registered charity 258197, for their continued support as well as the donors and family for their invaluable donation of brain tissue to the Parkinson's UK Tissue Bank.

References

1. Will RG, Ironside JW, Zeidler M et al (1996) A new variant of Creutzfeldt-Jakob disease in the UK. Lancet 347(9006):921–925

2. Lashley T, Rohrer JD, Mead S et al (2015) Review: an update on clinical, genetic and pathological aspects of frontotemporal lobar degenerations. Neuropathol Appl Neurobiol 41(7):858–881

3. McKee AC, Stein TD, Kiernan PT et al (2015) The neuropathology of chronic traumatic encephalopathy. Brain Pathol 25(3):350–364. https://doi.org/10.1111/bpa.12248

4. Attems J (2017) The multi-morbid old brain. Acta Neuropathol 134(2):169–170

5. Buckland GR, Harrison CH, Love S et al (2016) Topographical distribution of A-beta resulting from A-beta immunotherapy in Alzheimer's disease. Neuropathol Appl Neurobiol 42 (Supp 1) 16

6. Montine TJ, Phelps CH, Beach TG et al (2012) National Institute on Aging-Alzheimer's Association guidelines for the neuropathologic assessment of Alzheimer's disease: a practical approach. Acta Neuropathol 123(1):1–11

7. Thal DR, Rub U, Orantes M et al (2002) Phases of A beta-deposition in the human brain and its relevance for the development of AD. Neurology 58(12):1791–1800

8. Braak H, Alafuzoff I, Arzberger T et al (2006) Staging of Alzheimer disease-associated neuro-fibrillary pathology using paraffin sections and immunocytochemistry. Acta Neuropathol 112(4):389–404

9. Alafuzoff I, Ince PG, Arzberger T et al (2009) Staging/typing of Lewy body related alpha-synuclein pathology: a study of the BrainNet Europe Consortium. Acta Neuropathol 117(6):635–652

10. McKeith IG, Dickson DW, Lowe J et al (2005) Diagnosis and management of dementia with Lewy bodies: third report of the DLB Consortium. Neurology 65(12):1863–1872

Part VII

Genomic Methods

Chapter 19

Analysis of Micro-RNA Expression by qPCR on a Microfluidics Platform for Alzheimer's Disease Biomarker Discovery

Petros Takousis

Abstract

Changes associated with neurodegeneration at the cellular level are manifestations of deregulated biochemical pathways, and typically precede neuronal loss. Incorporation of molecular markers in the diagnostic process could aid detection of early changes, prior to extensive neuronal loss, as early as the presymptomatic stages of the disorder, thus enabling improved patient stratification for targeted drug development. Such biomarkers should be sufficiently sensitive and specific to distinguish AD from other disorders with overlapping symptoms. Easily accessible biosamples, simple methodology, and low overall cost would enable population screening, which would not be feasible with other modalities. Non-coding (nc)RNAs have a crucial role in the entire spectrum of cellular processes, from development and differentiation to homeostatic maintenance, and have been implicated in different diseases; micro-RNAs (miRNAs) are a family of ncRNA molecules with an important role in posttranscriptional gene silencing. The early advances in the study of miRNAs as noninvasive biomarkers in cancer inspired their study for other conditions, including AD. Several deregulated miRNAs in brain, CSF, and blood have been associated with AD and other brain disorders. Their high stability makes miRNAs attractive for biomarker development, and a number of platforms are currently available for their analysis. qPCR is a technology characterized by high sensitivity and is suitable for focused analysis of specific candidates (assays) in a large number of samples. Microfluidic-based qPCR platforms have minimal RNA requirements and can yield thousands of datapoints in one qPCR experiment. Here, I present the use of miScript qPCR miRNA assays with the Fluidigm BioMark HD System.

Key words Micro-RNA (miRNA), qPCR, miScript, Microfluidics, Fluidigm BioMark

1 Introduction

The gradual and progressive loss of neuronal structure and function, and ultimately neuronal death, is a common characteristic of neurodegenerative disorders, and eventually leads to nervous system dysfunction. Distinct cognitive, behavioral, and motor symptoms, characteristic of a specific disorder, become manifest as neurodegeneration progresses, reflecting the brain region and neuronal type affected and the extent of damage. Changes associ-

Robert Perneczky (ed.), *Biomarkers for Alzheimer's Disease Drug Development*, Methods in Molecular Biology, vol. 1750,
https://doi.org/10.1007/978-1-4939-7704-8_19, © Springer Science+Business Media, LLC 2018

ated with neurodegeneration at the cellular level, such as neurite retraction, synaptic dysfunction, and axonal transport defects, typically precede neuronal loss [1]. These changes are manifestations of deregulated biochemical pathways, and may result in imbalanced metabolite levels and biomolecule leakage in intercellular space or unconventional secretions, including shedding vesicles (or ectosomes) [2].

Incorporation of molecular markers in the diagnostic process could aid detection of early changes, prior to extensive neuronal loss, as early as the presymptomatic stages of the disorder, thus enabling improved patient stratification for targeted drug development. Such biomarkers should be sufficiently sensitive and specific to distinguish AD from other disorders with overlapping symptoms, especially at early disease stages, and thus provide window of opportunity for therapeutic intervention and contribute to improved patient outcomes. They could also serve as a tool to assess disease stage and monitor disease progression. Easily accessible biosamples collected by non- or minimally invasive procedures, simple methodology with short processing time to generate results, and low overall cost would avail such tool to population screening, which would not be feasible with other modalities, like novel neuroimaging approaches.

Non-coding (nc)RNAs have a crucial role in the entire spectrum of cellular processes, from development and differentiation to homeostatic maintenance, and have been implicated in different diseases. Micro-RNAs (miRNAs) are a family of ncRNA molecules that were first described in 1993. Long miRNA transcripts, known as pri-miRNA, are enzymatically processed into the mature form (~22 nucleotides); these short RNA molecules accomplish post-transcriptional gene silencing by binding complementary sequences at the 3'UTR of target mRNAs, leading to mRNA degradation or translation inhibition (reviewed in [3]). Multiple mRNAs may be targets of a specific miRNA and several miRNAs may target a specific mRNA. Around 2600 human mature miRNAs have been characterized (miRBase release 21) [4].

The majority of miRNA profiling studies focus on solid tissues, but due to their high stability, miRNAs released by peripheral tissues are detectable in blood and blood components, like serum and plasma. MiRNAs are also detectable in other biofluids, such as cerebrospinal fluid (CSF), urine, and saliva [5–7]. The potential of circulating miRNAs as biomarkers in blood or blood components was indicated by studies examining patients with various malignancies [8, 9]. Boeri and colleagues demonstrated that circulating miRNAs could be used to predict disease in samples taken from lung cancer patients, several years before the onset of disease [10]. Another study reported lower expression of two miRNAs in saliva from oral squamous cell carcinoma patients compared to healthy individuals [11]. Keller et al. analyzed blood samples from patients diagnosed with one of 14 diseases, which included different cancers and autoimmune conditions, and found that over 100 miRNAs were deregulated for each disease; they were able to predict the disease in nearly 7 out of 10 patients being studied [12].

The early advances in the study of miRNA as noninvasive biomarkers in cancer inspired their study for other conditions, including AD. Several deregulated miRNAs in brain, CSF, and blood have been associated with AD and other brain disorders (reviewed in [13] and [1]).

Interestingly, changes in miRNA concentrations in a bodily fluid and in an organ involved in pathology are not always concordant and sometimes change in opposite directions. For instance, serum hsa-miR-501-3p levels were downregulated in AD patients, its lower levels significantly correlating with lower Mini-Mental State Examination scores, but it was upregulated in the postmortem brains of the same donors [14]. Although miRNA expression may be discordant between biofluid and affected tissue, and irrespective of whether changes in expression are causal or consequential to the pathological process, discovery of novel miRNA biomarkers would improve patient stratification and targeted drug development.

Several measurement platforms have been developed to determine relative miRNA abundance in biological samples using different technologies, such as narrow-assay-focus and high-sample-throughput (e.g., reverse transcription-quantitative PCR; RT-qPCR), and broad-assay-focus and low-sample-throughput techniques (e.g., sequencing and microarrays). In a recent study, 12 commercially available platforms for analysis of miRNA expression were systematically compared, and platform performance was assessed for reproducibility, sensitivity, accuracy, specificity, and concordance of differential expression. Two miRNA sequencing platforms, three miRNA hybridization platforms, and seven RT-qPCR platforms were included in the assessment. Each method had its strengths and weaknesses, and researchers can refer to those findings to guide their selection according to the aims of their project.[15] While broad assay focus techniques are useful in identifying promising candidates in a small number of samples, focused analysis of specific candidates (assays) in a large number of samples is better served by a technology such as RT-qPCR. RT-qPCR is characterized by an overall high sensitivity, especially prominent when working with samples with low RNA quantity, which is of particular importance when miRNA expression is studied in body fluids. The advent of microfluidic-based qPCR platforms, such as the Fluidigm BioMark HD System, can yield as many as 9216 datapoints in one qPCR experiment (e.g., if using a 96×96 chip); it has the capacity for high-sample-throughput but minimal RNA requirements.

The miScript qPCR System has more than 2400 validated human miRNA assays and allows the flexibility to study any subset of these. It uses a poly-A universal reverse transcription (RT) step, followed by oligo-dT priming. Universal RT is less complicated and quicker than target-specific RT alternatives, and allows greater flexibility for downstream analysis of the whole miRNome as compared to a multiplex reaction which is confined to the number of assays included in the RT step. Internal controls such as the miRNA reverse transcription control (miRTC), which is added in the RT Mix, and the positive PCR control (PPC), which is dispensed on pre-spotted PCR Arrays, are typical of this platform and allow evaluation of important stages of the procedure.

A detailed account of a three-step workflow for multi-well plates pre-spotted with qPCR primer assays, which includes quality checkpoints after each step: (1) RT and quality control of the RT product by evaluation of miRTC levels, (2) preamplification and evaluation of the preamplified miRTC product, and (3) qPCR assessment of spike-in controls miRTC and PPC, together with miRNAs of interest; a discussion of important considerations regarding RNA quantity; as well as explanations of the most suitable normalization procedure have previously been covered in another volume of this series [16]. Here, I present the protocol for users of the Fluidigm BioMark HD System [17].

2   Materials

The following materials and reagents are required for this protocol:

- 96-well plate containing assays in solution.
- 20× DNA Binding Dye Sample Loading Reagent.
- 8-strip PCR tubes.
- Low EDTA-TE buffer (0.1 mM EDTA).
- RT^2 Microfluidics qPCR Reagent System.

3   Method

3.1   Protocol Overview

In this protocol, cDNA synthesis is performed using the RT^2 Microfluidics qPCR Reagent System. Next, preamplification is performed using the RT^2 PreAMP Pathway Primer Mix Format H. Finally, real-time PCR is performed using RT^2 Profiler PCR Array Format H in combination with Microfluidics qPCR Master Mix (contains EvaGreen).

3.2 Considerations of RNA Amount to Be Used

The RT^2 Microfluidics qPCR System yields results with as little as 10 ng or as much as 1 μg total RNA per well reaction. However, the optimal amount of starting material depends on the relative abundance of the transcripts of interest. Lower abundance transcripts require more RNA; higher abundance transcripts require less RNA. Greater amounts of input RNA yield greater number of positive calls; that is, genes expressed in the linear dynamic range of the method.

Important: Use a consistent amount of total RNA for all samples in a single experiment to be characterized and compared.

3.3 Procedure

3.3.1 cDNA Synthesis Using the RT^2 Microfluidics qPCR Reagent System

1. Thaw Buffer GE2 and BC4 Solution (RT master mix). Mix each solution by flicking the tubes. Centrifuge briefly to collect residual liquid from the sides of the tubes and then store on ice.

2. Prepare the genomic DNA elimination mix for each RNA sample in one well of a 96-well plate according to Table 1.

3. Incubate the genomic DNA elimination mix for 5 min at 37 °C, then place immediately on ice for at least 1 min.

4. Add 6 μL BC4 Solution to each well, mix by carefully pipetting up and down (can be done with a multi-channel pipette). Centrifuge briefly to collect residual liquid from the sides of the tubes.

5. Program a thermal cycler for a single cycle as follows: 42 °C for 60 min, 95 °C for 5 min, 4 °C hold. Place the 96-well plate in the cycler and run the program (*see* **Note 1**).

6. Place the reactions on ice and proceed with the preamplification protocol (*see* **Note 2**).

3.3.2 Preamplification Using RT^2 PreAMP Primer Mix Format H

1. Thaw RT^2 PreAMP Primer Mix and RT^2 PreAMP PCR Mastermix (PA-30) on ice. Mix each solution by flicking the tubes. Centrifuge briefly to collect residual liquid from the sides of the tubes and then store on ice.

Table 1
Genomic DNA elimination mix

Component	Amount for each well
RNA	10 ng–1 μg[a]
Buffer GE2	6 μL
RNase-free water	Variable
Total volume	**14 μL**

[a]If performing the experiment for the first time, we recommend 1 μg RNA

Table 2
Preamplification mix

Component	Amount for one sample (µL)	Amount for 96 wells[a] (µL)
RT² PreAMP Primer Mix	3	330
RT² PreAMP PCR Mastermix (PA-30)	5	550
Total volume	**8**	**880**

[a]These volumes provide 15% more mix than is required to allow for pipetting errors

Table 3
Cycling conditions for preamplification

Cycles	Duration	Temperature (°C)	Comments
1	10 min	95	HotStart DNA *Taq* Polymerase is activated by this heating step
14	15 s	95	
	2 min	60	
Hold		4	

2. Prepare preamplification mix according to Table 2.

3. Pipet 8 µL preamplification mix into each well of an empty 96-well plate.

4. Add 2 µL of first-strand cDNA from each well of the 96-well plate in **step 6** to each well of the 96-well plate in **step 9** using an 8-channel pipette (*see* **Note 3**).

5. Mix by carefully pipetting up and down and spin briefly.

6. Program the real-time cycler according to Table 3. Place the 96-well plate in the real-time cycler and start the program.

7. When cycling is finished, take the plate from the real-time cycler and place on ice.

8. Add 1 µL Side Reaction Reducer to each well. Mix gently by pipetting up and down and spin briefly.

9. Incubate at 37 °C for 15 min followed by heat inactivation at 95 °C for 5 min.

10. Add 44 µL low EDTA–TE buffer (0.1 mM EDTA) to each well (*see* **Note 4**).

11. Place on ice prior to real-time PCR, or store at −15 to −30 °C.

Table 4
Sample mix

Component	Volume for one reaction (µL)	Volume for a BioMark 96.96/48.48 Dynamic Array™[a] (µL)
2× Microfluidics qPCR Master Mix	3	330/165
20× DNA Binding Dye Sample Loading Reagent (Fluidigm, cat. no. 100-0388)	0.3	33/16.5
1× Low EDTA-TE buffer (0.1 mM EDTA)	0.7	77/38.5
Total volume	4.0	440/220

[a]These volumes provide 15% more mix than is required to allow for pipetting errors

3.3.3 Sample Mix Preparation

1. Prepare a sample mix according to Table 4.

2. Pipette 53 µL (96.96 Dynamic Array) or 26 µL (48.48 Dynamic Array) sample mix into each tube of an 8-strip PCR tube.

3. Using an 8-channel pipette, transfer 4 µL sample mix into each well of an empty 96-well plate (for the 48.48 Dynamic Array, use only half of the 96-well plate).

4. Add 2 µL of each preamplified sample from **step 17** to a well of the 96-well plate containing the sample mix (*see* **Note 5**).

5. Cover the plate with plate sealer. Mix and spin briefly.

6. Label the plate as "sample."

3.3.4 Assay Mix Preparation

1. Remove the RT² Profiler PCR Array Format H from −15 to −30 °C. Thaw for 10 min at room temperature (15–25 °C). Briefly vortex and spin the plate to bring the contents to the bottom of the wells.

2. Mark the caps of the RT² Profiler PCR Array so that they can be replaced in the original order. Remove the caps.

3. Pipet 45 µL 2× Assay Loading Reagent (provided by Fluidigm) into each tube of an 8-strip PCR tube.

4. Transfer 3 µL 2× Assay Loading Reagent from the 8-strip tube into each well of an empty 96-well plate (*see* **Notes 6** and **7**).

5. Transfer 3 µL from each well of the RT² Profiler PCR Array to the corresponding well of the 96-well plate from **step 27**.

6. Cover the plate with a plate sealer. Mix by vortexing and spin briefly.

7. Label this plate as "assay."

*3.3.5 Priming
and Loading the Fluidigm
BioMark HD Dynamic Array*

1. Peel the blue protective film from the underside of the BioMark Chip. Place the BioMark Dynamic Array into the IFC Controller.

2. Prime the Dynamic Array using standard Fluidigm protocols.

3. Using an 8-channel pipette, aliquot 5 μL from each well of the "sample" plate into appropriate sample inlets on the BioMark Dynamic Array (loading wells on the right side of the chip).

4. Using an 8-channel pipette, aliquot 5 μL from each well of the "assay" plate into appropriate assay inlets on the BioMark Dynamic Array (loading wells on the left side of the chip).

5. Using the IFC Controller HX (96.96 Dynamic Arrays) or the IFC Controller MX (48.48 Dynamic Arrays), run the Load Mix (136×) Script for 96.96 IFCs or the Load Mix (113×) Script for 48.48 IFCs.

6. Remove the BioMark Dynamic Array from the IFC Controller.

7. Remove any dust particles from the BioMark Chip surface.

*3.3.6 Running
the BioMark Dynamic Array
IFC*

1. Double-click the "Data Collection Software" icon to launch the software.

2. Click "Start a New Run," place the chip into the reader, and click "Load."

3. Verify chip barcode and chip type, choose project settings (if applicable), and click "Next."

4. Chip run file: Select "New" or "Predefined," browse to a file location for data storage, and click "Next."

5. For "Application, Reference, Probes," select the following: (a) "Application Type: Gene Expression," (b) "Passive Reference: ROX," (c) "Select Assay: single probe," (d) "Select probe type: EvaGreen." Click "Next."

6. Click "Browse" to find thermal protocol file "GE 96×96 Standard v1.pcl." or "GE 48x48 Standard v1.pcl" (*see* **Note 8**).

7. Change the thermal protocol file to the conditions in Table 5.

Table 5
Cycling conditions for Fluidigm BioMark 96.96 Dynamic Array IFCs

Cycles	Duration (s)	Temperature (°C)	Comments
1	120	50	Thermal Mix[a] (only for 96.96 Dynamic Array IFC,
1	1800	70	Thermal Mix not needed for 48.48 Dynamic Array IFC)
1	600	25	HotStart DNA *Taq* Polymerase is activated by this
1	600	95	heating step
40	15	94	
40	60	60	Perform fluorescence data collection

Ramp rate: slow 1 °C/s
[a]If you are using a 96.96 Dynamic Array IFC, add a Thermal Mix segment by checking the box. The Thermal Mix is a step that helps the assay and sample chambers diffuse better on the small chambers on the 96.96 Dynamic Array. You do not need a Thermal Mix if you are using any kind of chip other than the 96.96 Dynamic Array IFC

8. Confirm that "Auto Exposure" is selected and click "Next."

9. Verify the Dynamic Array run information and click "Start Run."

4 Notes

1. This is the reverse transcription step.

2. Reactions can be stored in a -15 to -30 °C freezer at this point.

3. The remaining first-strand cDNA can be stored for use in future experiments.

4. This is a fivefold dilution (11 µL preamplification mix +44 µL buffer). This dilution can be optimized if desired. (Undiluted cDNA can be used for qPCR if needed.)

5. Preamplified sample can be transferred using an 8-channel pipette.

6. This step can be performed using an 8-channel pipette.

7. For a 96.96 Dynamic Array, all 96 assays can be used at one time. When using a 48.48 Dynamic Array, only 48 assays can be used at once. A second 48.48 Dynamic Array must be run to utilize all 96 assays.

8. A 96.96-specific protocol or 48.48-specific protocol must be used depending on the Dynamic Array type.

References

1. Grasso M, Piscopo P, Confaloni A, Denti MA (2014) Circulating miRNAs as biomarkers for neurodegenerative disorders. Molecules 19(5):6891–6910. https://doi.org/10.3390/molecules19056891

2. Schneider A, Simons M (2013) Exosomes: vesicular carriers for intercellular communication in neurodegenerative disorders. Cell Tissue Res 352(1):33–47. https://doi.org/10.1007/s00441-012-1428-2

3. He L, Hannon GJ (2004) MicroRNAs: small RNAs with a big role in gene regulation. Nat Rev Genet 5(7):522–531. https://doi.org/10.1038/nrg1379

4. Kozomara A, Griffiths-Jones S (2014) miR-Base: annotating high confidence microRNAs using deep sequencing data. Nucleic Acids Res 42(Database issue):D68–D73. https://doi.org/10.1093/nar/gkt1181

5. Cogswell JP, Ward J, Taylor IA, Waters M, Shi Y, Cannon B, Kelnar K, Kemppainen J, Brown D, Chen C, Prinjha RK, Richardson JC, Saunders AM, Roses AD, Richards CA (2008) Identification of miRNA changes in Alzheimer's disease brain and CSF yields putative biomarkers and insights into disease pathways. J Alzheimers Dis 14(1):27–41

6. Hanke M, Hoefig K, Merz H, Feller AC, Kausch I, Jocham D, Warnecke JM, Sczakiel G (2010) A robust methodology to study urine microRNA as tumor marker: microRNA-126 and microRNA-182 are related to urinary bladder cancer. Urol Oncol 28(6):655–661. https://doi.org/10.1016/j.urolonc.2009.01.027

7. Michael A, Bajracharya SD, Yuen PS, Zhou H, Star RA, Illei GG, Alevizos I (2010) Exosomes from human saliva as a source of microRNA biomarkers. Oral Dis 16(1):34–38. https://doi.org/10.1111/j.1601-0825.2009.01604.x

8. Xing L, Todd NW, Yu L, Fang H, Jiang F (2010) Early detection of squamous cell lung cancer

in sputum by a panel of microRNA markers. Mod Pathol 23(8):1157–1164. https://doi.org/10.1038/modpathol.2010.111

9. Huang Z, Huang D, Ni S, Peng Z, Sheng W, Du X (2010) Plasma microRNAs are promising novel biomarkers for early detection of colorectal cancer. Int J Cancer 127(1):118–126. https://doi.org/10.1002/ijc.25007

10. Boeri M, Verri C, Conte D, Roz L, Modena P, Facchinetti F, Calabro E, Croce CM, Pastorino U, Sozzi G (2011) MicroRNA signatures in tissues and plasma predict development and prognosis of computed tomography detected lung cancer. Proc Natl Acad Sci U S A 108(9):3713–3718. https://doi.org/10.1073/pnas.1100048108

11. Park NJ, Zhou H, Elashoff D, Henson BS, Kastratovic DA, Abemayor E, Wong DT (2009) Salivary microRNA: discovery, characterization, and clinical utility for oral cancer detection. Clin Cancer Res 15(17):5473–5477. https://doi.org/10.1158/1078-0432.CCR-09-0736

12. Keller A, Leidinger P, Bauer A, Elsharawy A, Haas J, Backes C, Wendschlag A, Giese N, Tjaden C, Ott K, Werner J, Hackert T, Ruprecht K, Huwer H, Huebers J, Jacobs G, Rosenstiel P, Dommisch H, Schaefer A, Muller-Quernheim J, Wullich B, Keck B, Graf N, Reichrath J, Vogel B, Nebel A, Jager SU, Staehler P, Amarantos I, Boisguerin V, Staehler C, Beier M, Scheffler M, Buchler MW, Wischhusen J, Haeusler SF, Dietl J, Hofmann S, Lenhof HP, Schreiber S, Katus HA, Rottbauer W, Meder B, Hoheisel JD, Franke A, Meese E (2011) Toward the blood-borne miRNome of human diseases. Nat Methods 8(10):841–843. https://doi.org/10.1038/nmeth.1682

13. Kumar S, Reddy PH (2016) Are circulating microRNAs peripheral biomarkers for Alzheimer's disease? Biochim Biophys Acta 1862(9):1617–1627. https://doi.org/10.1016/j.bbadis.2016.06.001

14. Hara N, Kikuchi M, Miyashita A, Hatsuta H, Saito Y, Kasuga K, Murayama S, Ikeuchi T, Kuwano R (2017) Serum microRNA miR-501-3p as a potential biomarker related to the progression of Alzheimer's disease. Acta Neuropathol Commun 5(1):10. https://doi.org/10.1186/s40478-017-0414-z

15. Mestdagh P, Hartmann N, Baeriswyl L, Andreasen D, Bernard N, Chen C, Cheo D, D'Andrade P, DeMayo M, Dennis L, Derveaux S, Feng Y, Fulmer-Smentek S, Gerstmayer B, Gouffon J, Grimley C, Lader E, Lee KY, Luo S, Mouritzen P, Narayanan A, Patel S, Peiffer S, Ruberg S, Schroth G, Schuster D, Shaffer JM, Shelton EJ, Silveria S, Ulmanella U, Veeramachaneni V, Staedtler F, Peters T, Guettouche T, Wong L, Vandesompele J (2014) Evaluation of quantitative miRNA expression platforms in the microRNA quality control (miRQC) study. Nat Methods 11(8):809–815. https://doi.org/10.1038/nmeth.3014

16. Zeka F, Mestdagh P, Vandesompele J (2015) RT-qPCR-based quantification of small non-coding RNAs. Methods Mol Biol 1296:85–102. https://doi.org/10.1007/978-1-4939-2547-6_9

17. Qiagen-GmbH (2014) RT² Profiler PCR array handbook. QIAGEN. https://www.qiagen.com/at/resources/download.aspx?id=6161ebc1-f60f-4487-8c9e-9ce0c5bc3070&lang=en. Accessed 3 July 2017

Chapter 20

Telomere Length Shortening in Alzheimer's Disease: Procedures for a Causal Investigation Using Single Nucleotide Polymorphisms in a Mendelian Randomization Study

Yiqiang Zhan and Sara Hägg

Abstract

Measuring the length of telomeres, repetitive nucleotide sequences capping the chromosomes which shortens by each cell division, has become a popular way of attaining a marker of biological aging processes. Several observational studies have investigated the associations between telomere length and Alzheimer's disease (AD) with the overall conclusion being shorter telomeres provide an increased risk for AD development. Here we present an alternative approach for addressing the topic where additional evidence on causality can be drawn. To do so, we include information on single nucleotide polymorphisms (SNPs) using nature's own experiment with random segregation of alleles at conception. The protocol describes the full process of the so-called *Mendelian Randomization* by selecting appropriate SNPs for the analysis, discussing different data sources that can be used and inform about methods, assumptions and suitable software packages including Stata code.

Key words Telomere length, Alzheimer's disease, Single nucleotide polymorphisms, Causality, Mendelian randomization

1 Introduction

Telomeres are short repetitive nucleotide sequences $(TTAGGG)_n$ found at the chromosomal ends. Telomeres protect the chromosomes from degradation during cell division when the end replication problem arises. Instead, the enzyme telomerase extends the unreplicated DNA allowing for DNA polymerase to complete replication of the lagging strand [1]. However, insufficient telomerase and oxidative stress throughout the life course makes the telomeres shorten by about 20–30 bases per year. When critically short, the cell will enter a senescent state. Hence, telomere shortening is ongoing all life, but at old ages, when telomeres become critically short, individuals will experience decline in

Robert Perneczky (ed.), *Biomarkers for Alzheimer's Disease Drug Development*, Methods in Molecular Biology, vol. 1750, https://doi.org/10.1007/978-1-4939-7704-8_20, © Springer Science+Business Media, LLC 2018

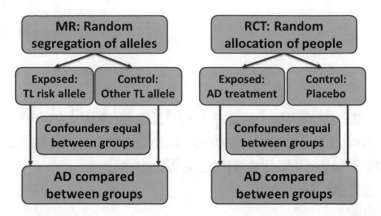

Fig. 1 Mendelian Randomization in comparison to a Randomized Clinical Trial. A Mendelian Randomization (MR) study can be considered as nature's own version of a Randomized Clinical Trial (RCT). In the MR approach, random segregation of risk alleles for having shorter telomere length (TL) at conception is mimicking the randomization of treatment or placebo in an RCT. Thus, because of the randomization, confounders are expected to be equal between the groups and conclusions about the risk of developing Alzheimer's disease (AD) can be compared between the groups

body function and increased susceptibility to age-related diseases such as Alzheimer's disease (AD). Several studies showed associations between short telomere lengths (TL), as measured from leukocytes in blood, and increased risk of AD [2–4]. Leukocyte TL is shown to reflect TL in the cerebellum [5], and may thus act as a proxy for brain deterioration, although more studies are needed to confirm this correlation. Furthermore, it is not well understood how the link from TL to AD works, though inflammation and increased oxidative stress are suggested pathways [1, 6], and, moreover, whether the association is cause or consequence of disease.

In epidemiology, a rising trend to investigate causality is by the use of genetic information in a so-called *Mendelian Randomization* (MR) study [7]. By taking advantage of Mendel's second law—the random assortment of alleles at conception—a randomized clinical trial can be mimicked using disease affecting alleles from single nucleotide polymorphisms (SNPs) as treatments (Fig. 1). In the end, conclusions can be drawn on disease risk in individuals carrying the effect allele compared to those without the effect allele. Here we provide a detailed tutorial for how to carry out a causal investigation in your data by using the MR design. We describe the data needed for analysis, what models to run, and how to address model assumptions and draw conclusions. Throughout the protocol, examples are given from simulated data, as well as from a recent MR study on TL and AD [8], using Stata software.

2   Materials

To conduct an MR study, investigators need to have access to epidemiological data collected in a prospective or case-control study setting, well suited for the topic of choice. At least three variables need to be available in the data: (1) genotypes (e.g., SNPs associated with TL), (2) exposure (e.g., TL), and (3) outcome (e.g., AD). Depending on the data sources where these variables come from, MR studies can be performed using two different approaches: (1) the one-sample approach where all variables are measured in the same study sample, and (2) the two-sample approach where genetic variants and exposure come from one study sample while the same genetic variants and outcome come from another study sample (Fig. 2) [9].

2.1   The One-Sample Approach

In the one-sample approach, all measurements and analyses are to be performed on the same study participants. This approach is straightforward and intuitive; individual level data should be available for all participants. However, an MR study usually requires a large sample size to achieve sufficient power [10]. When it is unfeasible to carry out all analyses on the same study participants, the two-sample approach should be considered.

2.2   The Two-Sample Approach

For a two-sample approach, genetic variants and exposure are assessed in one sample while the same genetic variants and outcome are measured in another sample. This approach is extremely appealing when measuring the exposure variable is expensive, as it thus can be measured in a subset of samples. When a case-control study design is used, it is recommended to assess the genetic association with exposure only in controls. Control samples represent the general population where the genetic association with the exposure should be tested. In addition, existing genome-wide association

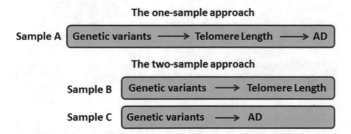

Fig. 2 Conceptual overview of the one-sample vs. the two-sample approach. The one-sample approach in Mendelian Randomization studies performs all analyses within the same sample (Sample A). All data are available on individual level with genetic variants, telomere length, and Alzheimer's disease (AD) assessed in the same study participants. In the two-sample approach, data on genetic variants and telomere length come from one sample (Sample B), whereas data on genetic variants and AD come from another sample (Sample C). However, sample B and C are assumed to be representations of the same underlying population. The two-sample approach can be performed using group level data, preferably summary statistics from genome-wide association studies

study (GWAS) summary statistics, which are widely available from different consortia, can also be used. As such, only group level data are used in the MR analysis. However, the two-sample approach comes with a caveat: it should be assumed that the genetic association with the exposure (outcome) in one sample is the same as in the other sample. Hence, the two samples should be drawn from the same underlying population. In reality, the exposure in one sample cannot affect the outcome in another sample, but biologically we have to assume it would if they were the same sample. A greater discussion and comparison of the one-sample and the two-sample approaches can be found elsewhere [9].

We are now ready to describe how to analyze these data, using either the one-sample or the two-sample approach, where discussions around the assumptions will be included.

3 Methods

An MR analysis is a form of instrumental variable (IV) analysis which uses genetic variants to infer causality. Three assumptions essential for performing an IV analysis also apply to the MR analysis. The directed acyclic graph in Fig. 3 describes the three assumptions: (1) the genetic variants should be strongly associated with the exposure (e.g., TL), (2) the genetic variants should not be associated with measured or unmeasured confounders of exposure and outcome, and (3) the effect of the genetic variants on the outcome should only go through the exposure [11]. These assumptions are sufficient for testing if there is a causal effect from the exposure on the outcome. Additional assumptions are needed if a point estimate of the causal effect should be obtained.

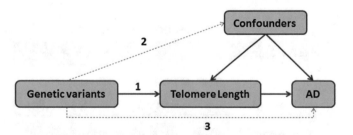

Fig. 3 Mendelian Randomization framework. In the directed acyclic diagram (DAG) used to illustrate causal inference methods, each line with single-headed arrow represents a direct link from a causal factor to an intermediate factor or outcome. Three main assumptions have to be fulfilled: (1) the genetic variants used need to have a strong association with the exposure, here telomere length, hence, there is direct causal effect from genetic variants to telomere length indicated by a solid line, (2) the genetic variants cannot be associated with confounders important to the exposure or outcome, the dashed line indicates that this link should not be present, and (3) the effect from the genetic variants on the outcome, here Alzheimer's disease (AD), has to go through the exposure (telomere length), hence, the dashed line from telomere length to AD should not exist

We start by simulating a cohort of 400,000 participants for illustrative purposes. In the following text, the genotype for each genetic variant (coded as 0, 1, and 2), the continuous exposure TL, the binary outcome AD (coded as 0 or 1), and the continuous unmeasured confounder are denoted by G, X, Y, and U, respectively. The effect allele frequency is assumed to be 25%, and the other variables are simulated as follows: U ~ uniform(−1, 1), X ~ normal(−0.1G − U, 1), p = exp(−3.5−0.4X + U), Y ~ bernoulli(p). By using this setup, the causal risk ratio for AD is exp(0.4) = 1.5 for one unit decrease in TL. The following code will implement the simulation in Stata 14.1:

```
version 14
clear
set seed 20170101
set obs 400000
gen g1 = runiform() < 0.25
gen g2 = runiform() < 0.25
gen g = g1 + g2
gen u = runiform(-1,1)
gen x = -0.1 *g - u + rnormal()
gen plog = exp(-3.5-0.4*x+u)
gen y = rbinomial(1, plog)
```

3.1 Selection of Appropriate SNPs

Selecting appropriate SNPs as IV is not an easy task. Priority should be given to the SNPs where the potential biological function on the exposure is known. In other words, the closer the SNP is to the exposure, the better. As an example, rs10936599, located within the telomerase RNA component gene (*TERC*), is tightly connected to the function of telomeres. Insufficient biological knowledge of a genetic variant requires more analyses to out rule pleiotropy (alternative pathways, other than through the exposure, from the genetic variant on the outcome). In order to increase power, a genetic risk score (GRS) can be constructed by summing multiple individual genetic variants (Table 1, *see* **Note 1**).

Table 1

Example of calculating a non-weighted genetic risk score

ID	Genotype	*TERC* (risk allele = T)	Genotype	*TERT* (risk allele = A)	Non-weighted genetic risk score
1	TT	2	AC	1	2 + 1 = 3
2	CC	0	CA	1	0 + 1 = 1
3	TC	1	AA	2	1 + 2 = 3
4	CT	1	CC	0	1 + 0 = 1
5	TT	2	AC	1	2 + 1 = 3

Similarly, a weighted GRS can be created by including the effect size estimates from the largest GWAS on the topic for each SNP as weight (w): GRS = w_1*SNP_1 + w_2*SNP_2 + ... However, all genetic variants in the GRS need to meet the three aforementioned MR-assumptions (*see* **Note 2**).

3.2 The One-Sample Approach

In this section, we will consider the one-sample approach by analyzing data from the simulated cohort. In traditional observational analyses, a standard regression model (e.g., logistic regression) with adjustments for measured confounders will be run to examine the effect of the exposure (e.g., TL) on the outcome (e.g., AD). However, the result could be biased because of unmeasured confounders not taken into account. We will demonstrate this by running the observational, logistic model: AD ~TL on the simulated data using Stata code below.

```
logit y x
-----------------------------------------------------------------
      y |   Coef.     Std. Err.    z      P>|z|   [95% Conf.   Interval]
 ----+-----------------------------------------------------------
      x | -.6611473   .0069696   -94.86   0.000   -.6748074    -.6474872
  _cons | -3.346124   .0095695  -349.67   0.000   -3.36488     -3.327368
-----------------------------------------------------------------

lincom -1*_b[x], or
-----------------------------------------------------------------
      y | Odds Ratio Std. Err.    z      P>|z|   [95% Conf.   Interval]
 ----+-----------------------------------------------------------
    (1) | 1.937013    .0135001   94.86   0.000   1.910734     1.963655
-----------------------------------------------------------------
```

Thus, a one unit decrease (−1 in **−1*_b[x]** means one unit decrease) in TL is associated with an Odds Ratio (OR) of 1.94 for AD (94% increased odds per additional TL unit decrease) without adjusting for any unmeasured confounder **u**. Thus, the estimate from this model is biased. The true causal Risk Ratio (RR) is 1.5 and the OR is approximately equal to the RR when the outcome is rare, as in this case.

To test if the exposure is causally associated with the outcome using the MR approach, we can run the following model provided the IV assumptions for the genetic variants hold. A significant result for **g** could imply a causal effect from the exposure on the outcome.

```
logit y g
-----------------------------------------------------------------
      y |   Coef.     Std. Err.    z      P >|z|   [95% Conf.   Interval]
 ----+-----------------------------------------------------------
      g |  .0410551   .012362     3.32    0 .001   .016826      .0652842
  _cons | -3.076268   .0099172  -310.20   0.000   -3.095705    -3.056831
-----------------------------------------------------------------
```

The above analysis suggests there is an association between the genetic variant (**g**) and the outcome (**y**). Provided **g** satisfies the IV assumptions, the significant result indicates that the exposure may be causing the outcome.

To obtain the point estimate for the causal effect from the exposure on the outcome, we have to consider another assumption: no effect modification from the genetic variant on the exposure exists (e.g., no interaction between **g** and **x**) (*see* **Note 3**). Hence, we assume this assumption is valid. There are several ways to perform the point estimate analysis for a binary outcome (e.g., AD). We will introduce two estimators: (1) the multiplicative structural mean model (MSMM) estimator [12] and (2) the Wald estimator [13]. The MSMM estimator is calculated by the following code together with the Hansen's J-test, which is used for multiple instruments. A large J-statistics will reject the null hypothesis (that all genetic variants are ok to use) so that at least one instrument might be invalid (*see* **Note 4**).

```
gmm (y*exp(-{ey0} - x*{psi}) - 1), instruments(g1 g2)
-----------------------------------------------------------------
           |             Robust
           |    Coef.   Std. Err.      z   P>|z|   [95% Conf.  Interval]
-----------+-----------------------------------------------------
      /ey0 | -3.339513  .0482258   -69.25  0.000   -3.434033   -3.244992
      /psi | -.3814146  .1241242    -3.07  0.002   -.6246936   -.1381357
-----------------------------------------------------------------

lincom -1*_b[/psi], eform
-----------------------------------------------------------------
           |   exp(b)   Std. Err.      z   P>|z|   [95% Conf.  Interval]
-----------+-----------------------------------------------------
       (1) | 1.464355   .1817618     3.07  0.002   1.148131    1.867674
-----------------------------------------------------------------

estat overid
Test of overidentifying restriction:
Hansen's J chi2(1) = .824692 (p = 0.3638)
```

The above analysis shows that the causal RR for a one unit decrease of TL is 1.46 for AD with a 95% confidence interval (CI) of 1.15–1.87. There is no strong evidence for violations of the nonlinearity assumption for any of the two dummy instruments **g1** and **g2** (*P*-value = 0.36).

Another popular approach for calculating an MR estimate is the Wald ratio estimator [12]. The Wald method is consistent with the above method when the outcome is rare, as in our AD example. The Wald ratio estimator is defined as:

$$\log(\text{RR}) = \frac{\log(\text{RR}_{\text{YG}})}{\beta_{\text{XG}}} \text{ for a causal RR and } \log(\text{OR}) = \frac{\log(\text{OR}_{\text{YG}})}{\beta_{\text{XG}}}$$

for a causal OR, where $\log(RR_{YG})$ or $\log(OR_{YG})$ is the effect size for the association between the genetic variant and the outcome, and β_{XG} is the effect size for the association between the genetic variant and the exposure.

```
reg x g
```

```
------------------------------------------------------------------
       x |    Coef.    Std. Err.    t     P>|t|   [95% Conf. Interval]
---------+--------------------------------------------------------
       g | -.100379    .002984   -33.64   0.000   -.1062275   -.0945305
   _cons |  .0010336   .0023541    0.44   0.661   -.0035803    .0056476
------------------------------------------------------------------
```

```
scalar betaXG = _b[g]
poisson y g
```

```
------------------------------------------------------------------
       y |    Coef.    Std. Err.    z     P>|z|   [95% Conf. Interval]
---------+--------------------------------------------------------
       g |  .0391897   .012075     3.25   0.001    .0155232    .0628562
   _cons | -3.121362   .0096951  -321.95  0.000   -3.140364   -3.10236
------------------------------------------------------------------
```

```
scalar betaYG = _b[g]
dis exp(-1*betaYG/betaXG)
1.4775973
```

Thus, the causal RR is 1.48, which is similar to the MSMM method above which gave a RR of 1.46. The standard error can be obtained either by the bootstrap or by the delta method. Below is a short program in Stata using the bootstrap method; it may take some time to run the **bootstrap** command because it is an iterative process where data are resampled repeatedly.

```
cap program drop myIV
program myIV, rclass
        version 14
        args y x g
        reg `x' `g'
        scalar betaXG = _b["`g'"]
        poisson `y' `g'
        scalar betaYG = _b["`g'"]
        return scalar logRR=-betaYG/betaXG
        scalar list betaXG betaYG logRR
end
bootstrap LOGRR = r(logRR), reps(1000) seed(1234): myIV y x g
```

```
------------------------------------------------------------------
         | Observed    Bootstrap                Normal-based
         |   Coef.    Std. Err.    z    P>|z|   [95% Conf. Interval]
---------+--------------------------------------------------------
```

```
LOGRR |   .3904173        .1188342  3.29  0.001    .1575065    .6233281
---------------------------------------------------------------------
```

estat bootstrap, all eform

```
---------------------------------------------------------------------
         |  Observed              Bootstrap
         |  exp(b)       Bias     Std. Err. [95% Conf. Interval]
---------+-----------------------------------------------------------
   LOGRR | 1.4775973    .005423   .17558913  1.170588   1.865125   (N)
         |                                   1.16809    1.890071   (P)
         |                                   1.158311   1.859608   (BC)
---------------------------------------------------------------------
```

(N)   normal confidence interval
(P)   percentile confidence interval
(BC)   bias-corrected confidence interval

The output shows three different CI's for the bootstrap method. The causal RR is 1.48 with 95% CI being 1.17–1.89 using the percentile method.

3.3   The Two-Sample Approach

In this section, we will consider the two-sample approach by using publically available GWAS summary statistics data. We selected seven SNPs associated with TL, reported to be of genome-wide significance in the ENGAGE Telomere Consortium paper [14]. Again, the MR-assumptions need to hold (*see* **Note 2**). In order to investigate pleiotropy among the chosen SNPs, we performed a heterogeneity test using the Cochran's **Q** statistics with corresponding plot to show this visually (*see* **Note 5**) [15]. The following code will perform this test and create Fig. 4.

```
gen numerator=b*logor*(1/selogor^2)
gen denominator=(b^2)*(1/selogor^2)
sum numerator
   Variable  |  Obs   Mean    Std. Dev.   Min        Max
-------------+---------------------------------------------------
  numerator  |   7   -4.141193  5.114804  -14.0346    .7936
              scalar sum_numerator=r(mean)*r(N)
              sum denominator
   Variable  |  Obs   Mean    Std. Dev.   Min        Max
-------------+---------------------------------------------------
 denominator |   7    13.59267  8.723301  5.928167  29.04013
scalar sum_denominator=r(mean)*r(N)
gen xm2 = (logor/selogor)^2
sum xm2
scalar Xm2 = r(mean)*r(N)
scalar Qrs = Xm2-(abs(-sum_numerator/sum_denominator)/sqrt(1/
sum_denominator))^2
dis "P value for heterogeneity test:" chi2tail(6,Qrs)
P value for heterogeneity test: .26723316
```

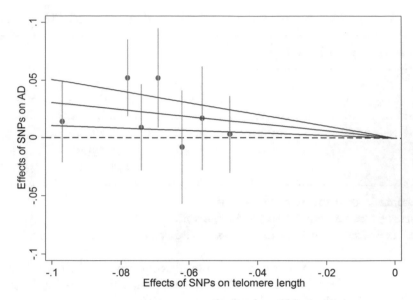

Fig. 4 Heterogeneity test using the Cochran's Q statistics to investigate pleiotropy among the chosen SNPs. The red lines in the plot correspond to the 95% confidence interval, and since no single point (SNP) is located outside of this area, there is no obvious pleiotropic effect detected. Therefore, all SNPs are kept in the analysis, and the effect sizes on AD for these SNPs were extracted from the summary statistics of the IGAP Consortium paper [16]. We then used the inverse-variance weighted method to obtain a causal estimate [17] $\beta = \dfrac{\sum_{i=1}^{m} w\alpha s^{-2}}{\sum_{i=1}^{m} ws^{-2}}$ where m is the number of SNPs, w is effect of SNP on TL, α is the effect of SNP on AD with s being the corresponding standard error

Hence, an insignificant p-value for the heterogeneity test indicates that no SNP effect deviates too much from the other effects.

```
gen hilogor = logor + 1.96*selogor
gen lowlogor = logor - 1.96*selogor
scalar bfit = sum_numerator/sum_denominator
scalar hibfit = bfit + 1.96*sqrt(1/sum_denomina-
tor)
scalar lowbfit = bfit - 1.96*sqrt(1/sum_denomi-
nator)
twoway (scatter logor b) (rspike hilogor low-
logor b) (function y = bfit*x, range(-0.1 0)
lcolor(red)) (function y = hibfit*x, range(-0.1 0)
lcolor(red)) (function y = lowbfit*x, range(-0.1
0) lcolor(red)), xlab(-0.1 -0.08 -0.06 -0.04 -0.02
0) ylab(-0.1 -0.05 0 0.05 0.1) scheme(s1mono)
yline(0, lpattern(dash)) xtitle("Effects of SNPs
on telomere length") ytitle("Effects of SNPs on
AD") legend(off)
```

Table 2
Selected SNPs and their association with telomere length and Alzheimer's disease

Gene	SNP	Risk allele	ENGAGE Telomere Consortium		IGAP Consortium	
			β	se(β)	log(OR)	se(log(OR))
TERC	rs10936599	T	−0.097	0.008	0.014	0.018
TERT	rs2736100	A	−0.078	0.009	0.052	0.017
NAF1	rs7675998	A	−0.074	0.009	0.009	0.019
OBFC1	rs9420907	A	−0.069	0.010	0.052	0.022
ZNF208	rs8105767	A	−0.048	0.008	0.003	0.017
RTEL1	rs755017	A	−0.062	0.011	−0.008	0.025
ACYP2	rs11125529	C	−0.056	0.010	0.017	0.023

OR odds ratio. β denotes the effect size of SNP on telomere length and se(β) is the corresponding standard error. Log(OR) means the effect size of SNP on Alzheimer's disease and se(log(OR)) is the corresponding standard error

The following code performs the analysis for the data shown in Table 2 (*see* **Note 6**).

```
scalar log_or = -sum_numerator/sum_denominator
scalar se_log_or = sqrt(1/sum_denominator)
dis "Odds ratio:" exp(log_or)
Odds ratio: 1.3561689

dis "95% CI:" exp(log_or-1.96*se_log_or)",
"exp(log_or+1.96*se_log_or)
95% CI: 1.1093, 1.6579773

scalar z_statistic=(abs(log_or)/se_log_or)^2
dis "P value:" chi2tail(1,z_statistic)
P value: .00296042
```

The causal OR for one unit decrease of TL is associated with 1.36 (95% CI: 1.11–1.66) odds of AD ($P = 0.003$).

In this chapter, we first briefly introduced the assumptions and materials needed for conducting an MR study, and then presented two practical approaches for how to implement this method. To highlight the technical differences of these approaches, we first applied the method to one simple simulated example and then to one real data example using summary statistics from GWAS studies. These analytical methods can be easily extended to study other risk factors and outcomes as well.

4   Notes

1. Make sure to code the risk allele as the additive effect in the GRS, it is not always the minor allele. When the original SNP is missing in the data, an imputed SNP passing all quality control criteria can be used instead. Alternatively, a proxy can be used where $r^2 > 0.8$ is a common cutoff. Proxies can be found using the SNAP software (http://archive.broadinstitute.org/mpg/snap/ldsearch.php). For the other SNPs included in the GRS, there should be no linkage disequilibrium (LD) between them (r^2 should be very low). In this chapter, the selected SNPs are not correlated (not in LD). However, when multiple SNPs are indeed correlated or in the same LD block, a weighted method can be used to account for these correlations as described by Burgess et al. [18].

2. The first assumption can be tested; if the F-statistic >10 for the association between the genetic variant and the exposure, the IV is usually considered strong [7]. It is easier to achieve a strong IV using a GRS than a single SNP, because multiple variants combined increase the power. The second assumption is more difficult to test, but attempts can be made by testing the association of the IV with other confounders (e.g., GRS ~smoking). The third assumption, concerning pleiotropy, can be tested by alternative strategies. First, associations from the selected SNPs to other outcomes can be analyzed in the data at hand or online (GWAS catalog: http://www.ebi.ac.uk/gwas/ and MR base: http://www.mrbase.org/). Second, outliers in SNP effect sizes can be identified by using the **gtx** package in R software (https://cran.r-project.org/web/packages/gtx/index.html). Finally, a significant intercept using the MR-Egger regression method (https://cran.r-project.org/web/packages/MendelianRandomization/) also indicates that the no-pleiotropy assumption may be violated [19]. However, it is important to keep in mind that although statistical tests are available, the no-pleiotropy assumption is theoretically untestable.

3. The additional assumption, required to assess a point estimate for the causal effect, can be interpreted as there should be a linear association between the exposure and the outcome over the life course, or at least for the age range under study. Using the two-sample approach, with summary statistics from GWAS Consortium data, it may not be possible to examine the nonlinear effect. On the other hand, for the one-sample approach there are methods for this purpose though large sample sizes are required [20].

4. When multiple instruments are used in the MR analysis, the joint validity of the IVs can be tested. The Hansen's J-test performs this test and a large J-statistics may indicate a deviation

from the null where one or several of the IVs are not valid to use in the MR design.

5. A heterogeneity test can be performed using the Cochran's Q statistics which is similar to the methods in the **gtx** package described in **Note 2**. A significant test may imply that not all genetic variants identify the same causal effect. Substantial heterogeneity is an indication of potential violation of the IV assumptions for some SNPs.

6. When performing two-sample analyses, it is of uttermost importance to check that the risk alleles for the exposure are the same in the two different data sets used.

References

1. Needham BL, Rehkopf D, Adler N et al (2015) Leukocyte telomere length and mortality in the National Health and Nutrition Examination Survey, 1999–2002. Epidemiology 26(4):528–535. https://doi.org/10.1097/EDE.0000000000000299

2. Hochstrasser T, Marksteiner J, Humpel C (2012) Telomere length is age-dependent and reduced in monocytes of Alzheimer patients. Exp Gerontol 47(2):160–163. https://doi.org/10.1016/j.exger.2011.11.012

3. Honig LS, Kang MS, Schupf N et al (2012) Association of shorter leukocyte telomere repeat length with dementia and mortality. Arch Neurol 69(10):1332–1339. https://doi.org/10.1001/archneurol.2012.1541

4. Thomas P, NJ OC, Fenech M (2008) Telomere length in white blood cells, buccal cells and brain tissue and its variation with ageing and Alzheimer's disease. Mech Ageing Dev 129(4):183–190. https://doi.org/10.1016/j.mad.2007.12.004

5. Lukens JN, Van Deerlin V, Clark CM et al (2009) Comparisons of telomere lengths in peripheral blood and cerebellum in Alzheimer's disease. Alzheimers Dement 5(6):463–469. https://doi.org/10.1016/j.jalz.2009.05.666

6. Boccardi V, Pelini L, Ercolani S et al (2015) From cellular senescence to Alzheimer's disease: the role of telomere shortening. Ageing Res Rev 22:1–8. https://doi.org/10.1016/j.arr.2015.04.003

7. Lawlor DA, Harbord RM, Sterne JA et al (2008) Mendelian randomization: using genes as instruments for making causal inferences in epidemiology. Stat Med 27(8):1133–1163. https://doi.org/10.1002/sim.3034

8. Zhan Y, Song C, Karlsson R et al (2015) Telomere length shortening and Alzheimer disease—a Mendelian randomization study. JAMA Neurol 72(October):1202–1203

9. Lawlor DA (2016) Commentary: two-sample Mendelian randomization: opportunities and challenges. Int J Epidemiol 45(3):908–915. https://doi.org/10.1093/ije/dyw127

10. Burgess S (2014) Sample size and power calculations in Mendelian randomization with a single instrumental variable and a binary outcome. Int J Epidemiol 43(3):922–929. https://doi.org/10.1093/ije/dyu005

11. Smith GD, Ebrahim S (2003) 'Mendelian randomization': can genetic epidemiology contribute to understanding environmental determinants of disease? Int J Epidemiol 32(1):1–22

12. Palmer TM, Sterne JA, Harbord RM et al (2011) Instrumental variable estimation of causal risk ratios and causal odds ratios in Mendelian randomization analyses. Am J Epidemiol 173(12):1392–1403. https://doi.org/10.1093/aje/kwr026. kwr026 [pii]

13. Fall T, Hagg S, Magi R et al (2013) The role of adiposity in cardiometabolic traits: a Mendelian randomization analysis. PLoS Med 10(6):e1001474. https://doi.org/10.1371/journal.pmed.1001474

14. Codd V, Nelson CP, Albrecht E et al (2013) Identification of seven loci affecting mean telomere length and their association with disease. Nat Genet 45(4):422–427., 427e421-422. https://doi.org/10.1038/ng.2528

15. Johnson T (2013) Gtx: Genetics Toolbox. 0.0.8 edn

16. Lambert JC, Ibrahim-Verbaas CA, Harold D et al (2013) Meta-analysis of 74,046 individuals identifies 11 new susceptibility loci for Alzheimer's disease. Nat Genet 45(12):1452–1458. https://doi.org/10.1038/ng.2802

17. Burgess S, Scott RA, Timpson NJ et al (2015) Using published data in Mendelian randomization: a blueprint for efficient identification of causal risk factors. Eur J Epidemiol 30(7):543–552. https://doi.org/10.1007/s10654-015-0011-z

18. Burgess S, Butterworth A, Thompson SG (2013) Mendelian randomization analysis with multiple genetic variants using summarized data. Genet Epidemiol 37(7):658–665. https://doi.org/10.1002/gepi.21758

19. Bowden J, Davey Smith G, Burgess S (2015) Mendelian randomization with invalid instruments: effect estimation and bias detection through Egger regression. Int J Epidemiol 44(2):512–525. https://doi.org/10.1093/ije/dyv080

20. Burgess S, Davies NM, Thompson SG et al (2014) Instrumental variable analysis with a nonlinear exposure-outcome relationship. Epidimiology 25(6):877–885. https://doi.org/10.1097/EDE.0000000000000161

Chapter 21

Quantifying miRNA Deregulation in Alzheimer's Disease

Ana L. Cardoso and Joana R. Guedes

Abstract

Analysis of miRNA expression in circulating immune cells, such as monocytes, using qRT-PCR arrays, allows the quantification of a wide range of miRNAs in easily accessible biosamples from Alzheimer's disease patients. This technique enables the identification of differentially expressed miRNAs and provides important clues for the discovery of new miRNA-based biomarkers. Here we describe how to isolate a specific lymphocyte population from human blood samples, CD14$^+$ monocytes, and how to extract total RNA, containing short RNAs, from these cells, transcribe the RNA into cDNA and quantify a pre-set of specific miRNAs using customizable PCR plates of 96 or 384 wells.

Key words qRT-PCR arrays, Monocytes, miRNAs, Blood samples, Biomarkers, Alzheimer's disease, Inflammation, Immune cells

1 Introduction

Although high-throughput functional screenings are yet few in the context of neurodegenerative disorders, several interesting reports have been published in the last few years concerning changes in the levels of specific miRNAs in Alzheimer's disease (AD) patients and animal models [1–3]. These changes have been observed both locally, in the brain parenchyma, and peripherally, in biofluids and circulating blood cells, contributing to strengthen the hypothesis that the immune system plays an important role in this disease. These studies also suggest that miRNAs, particularly those in circulating cells or membrane-bound structures, such as exosomes [4], which can be easily quantified in biofluids using standard techniques such as qRT-PCR, can act as potentially interesting biomarkers in the context of dementia. This idea has led to the publication, in the last few years, of several reports describing specific miRNA profiles characteristic of the cerebral spinal fluid (CSF) or plasma of dementia patients [5–7].

Taking into consideration recent reports on the importance of both brain-derived and circulating innate immune cells to the neuroinflammatory events observed in both AD patients and animal

Robert Perneczky (ed.), *Biomarkers for Alzheimer's Disease Drug Development*, Methods in Molecular Biology, vol. 1750, https://doi.org/10.1007/978-1-4939-7704-8_21, © Springer Science+Business Media, LLC 2018

models [2, 8–10], as well as studies concerning the importance of miRNAs to the regulation of the immune response mediated by these cells in both healthy and disease environments [11], circulating immune cells constitute easily accessible cell populations that can be of great interest when searching for new biomarkers of AD. However, it is important to take note that the complexity of the populations of immune cells present in the blood hinders the quantification of cell-specific immune-related miRNAs, a point of great importance since a disease-associated environment can influence the phenotype of some of these subpopulations. When analyzing miRNA levels in peripheral blood mononuclear cells (PBMCs) as a whole, it is easy to find great variability and miss important miRNA fluctuations in specific immune cells subpopulations, since, for example, the same miRNA can be increased or decreased in a specific cell type during the differentiation or activation process [12]. Therefore, it is of crucial importance to perform this kind of analysis, whenever possible, in specific and well-defined immune cell populations.

Here we describe how to isolate monocytes from a human blood samples, collected using venipuncture. We focus our protocol on CD14$^+$ monocytes due to their characteristics as macrophage-precursor cells [13] and their ability to both cross the disrupted blood–brain barrier in AD [14] and to differentiate into microglia/macrophage-like cells capable of interfering with the Aβ levels in the brain. CD14$^+$ monocytes can be separated from other peripheral blood mononuclear cells (PBMCs) employing a gradient centrifugation followed by magnetic-activated cell sorting, and these cells can also be differentiated into monocyte-derived macrophages (MDMs). Both cell types, monocytes and MDMs, can be used to extract total RNA, including short RNA species, such as miRNAs, that can later be transcribed and used for miRNA quantification employing qPCR. In order to analyze the levels of several miRNAs of interest in a single experiment, custom-made PCR plates containing pre-deposited qPCR primers for the selected miRNAs can be prepared, allowing to quantify up to 96 or 384 miRNAs per plate, including reference miRNAs, and to employ the use of interplate calibrators. The levels of these miRNAs can later be compared between samples, in order to identify differentially expressed miRNAs across experimental groups. A later validation of these miRNAs in a larger number of samples, using a single qPCR assay can validate the previous findings, hopefully helping to identify new miRNA-based biomarkers for AD.

2   Materials

Keep all solutions at 4 °C for storage purposes and keep them sterile to avoid contaminations. During the magnetic-activated cell sorting, work fast, keep cells cold, and use pre-cooled solutions. This will prevent capping of antibodies on the cell surface and non-specific cell labeling. RNA extraction and all downstream steps where RNA manipulation is necessary should be performed using RNAse/DNAse-free materials and solutions and in a work surface dedicated to RNA handling, in order to avoid RNA degradation and contamination.

2.1 Sample Collection and Isolation of PBMCs

1. Sterile EDTA-coated tubes (10 mL).
2. Phosphate buffered saline (PBS): 137 mM NaCl, 2.7 mM KCl, 10 mM Na_2HPO_4, 1.8 mM KH_2PO_4 (pH 7.3).
3. Histopaque.
4. Plastic sterile Pasteur pipettes.

2.2 Monocyte Isolation from PBMC Fraction (Magnetic Separation)

1. Beads buffer: PBS, pH 7.3, 0.5% BSA and 2 mM EDTA.
2. CD14 MicroBeads (Miltenyi Biotec).
3. LS Columns (Miltenyi Biotec).
4. MACS Separator (Miltenyi Biotec).
5. 15 mL sterile conical centrifuge tubes.

2.3 Monocyte and Monocyte-derived Maccrophage Culture

1. Cell culture medium: RPMI-1640 with and without 10% FBS (10 mL/L Pen/Strep, 20 mM HEPES, 12 mM $NaHCO_3$, 2 mM L-Glutamine).
2. Macrophage colony stimulating factor human recombinant (M-CSF) dissolved in RPMI-1640 10% FBS at a stock concentration of 10 µg/mL. Keep aliquots of 20 µL at −20 °C and dilute each 10 × with RPMI-1640 10% FBS before addition to the plated CD14+ monocytes.
3. 12-well multiwell plates for adherent cells.

2.4 RNA Extraction and Reverse Transcription

1. miRCURY RNA Isolation Kit—Cell and Plant (Exiqon).
2. β-mercaptoethanol.
3. DNAse I for on-column DNA digestion.
4. DNAse I reaction buffer: 40 mM Tris pH 7.0, 10 mM $MgCl_2$ and 3 mM $CaCl_2$ in RNase-free water.
5. Universal cDNA synthesis kit (Exiqon).
6. 200 µL qPCR grade eppendorf tubes.
7. RNAse-free water.

2.5 qPCR Arrays

1. 96-well Pick-&-Mix microRNA PCR panels with the 92 microRNA × 1 sample layout (Exiqon).
2. ExiLENT SYBR Green Master Mix (Exiqon).
3. Swing bucket centrifuge for 96-well plates.

4. Sealing foils for PCR plates.

5. ROX passive reference dye (if the available real-time PCR cycler requires it).

---

3   Methods

Carry out all procedures at room temperature (RT) unless otherwise specified.

3.1 Sample Collection and Isolation of PBMCs Fraction

1. Collect 40 mL of venous blood through venipuncture to sterile EDTA-coated tubes (4 × 10 mL). The collected blood should be used as soon as possible, but might be stored at 4 °C for 2–3 h (*see* **Note 1**).

2. Dilute each 10 mL of blood in a sterile 50 mL conical centrifuge tube by adding 14 mL RT PBS (use four 50 mL tubes for each patient/control) (*see* **Note 2**).

3. Gently overlay the diluted blood onto 6 mL of Histopaque in another sterile 50 mL conical centrifuge tube, without disturbing the Histopaque surface (use a plastic sterile Pasteur pipette and work quickly but gently, since the Histopaque solution will start to mix with the blood).

4. Centrifuge 20 min at 800 × g, RT, brake off.

5. Dip a glass Pasteur pipette coupled to a rubber pear (you can also use a micropipette with a 1 mL tip) across the layers and suck the cloudy white interface band (which includes the monocytes and lymphocytes - PBMCs) along with no more than 5 mL of fluid above the pellet (without disturbing the red pellet at the bottom of the tube), according to the scheme in Fig. 1. Transfer the PBMC fraction of the same patient/control to a new 50 mL microcentrifuge tube and add PBS up to the 50 mL mark.

6. Centrifuge 10 min, 600 × g, RT, brake on.

7. Aspirate the supernatant and resuspend the pellet with 25 mL RT PBS. At this point you can count the total number of cells and add PBS to the 50 mL mark (if necessary, pass cells through 30 μm nylon mesh filters to remove cell clumps which may clog the columns).

8. Centrifuge 10 min, 600 × g, RT, brake on.

3.2 Monocyte Isolation from PBMCs Fraction (Magnetic Separation): MACS System (Miltenyi Biotec)

1. After estimating the total number of PBMCs and performing the last centrifugation of the PBMC suspension, aspirate the PBS completely, leaving the cell pellet undisturbed.

2. Resuspend the cell pellet in 80 μL of beads buffer per 10^7 total cells and transfer the cells to a 1.5 mL eppendorf per sample.

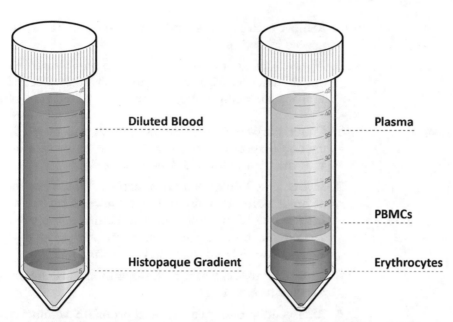

Fig. 1 Representative scheme of the conical centrifuge tube, packed with the diluted blood sample and Histopaque, before and after gradient centrifugation. Following the 20 min centrifugation at 800 × *g*, RT, without break, a yellow cloud should appear in the plasma fraction, above the red blood cell fraction. This cloud corresponds to the PBMC fraction and should be removed carefully, without disturbing the red cell fraction using a glass Pasteur pipette

3. Add 7.5 μL of CD14 MicroBeads per 10^7 total cells.

4. Mix well and incubate for 15 min at 4 °C with continuous mixing (an orbital shaker in a cold room is ideal to keep the cells in suspension).

5. Remove the contents of each eppendorf to a 15 mL microcentrifuge tube and wash the cells by adding 2 mL of beads buffer per 10^7 cells and performing a centrifugation at 300 × *g*, 10 min, break on; aspirate the supernatant completely.

6. Resuspend each PBMC cell pellet in 500 μL of beads buffer.

7. Insert the necessary number of LS Columns (one per sample) with the column wings to the front into an MACS Separator.

8. Prepare the LS Column by rinsing it with beads buffer: apply 3 mL of degassed buffer on the top of the column and let the buffer run through; discard effluent and change collection tube; the LS Column is now ready for magnetic separation.

9. Apply the 500 μL of cell suspension onto the prepared LS Column.

10. If desirable, collect unlabeled cells, which pass through, and wash the LS Column with 3 × 3 mL degassed buffer, adding more buffer only once the column reservoir is empty. This way it is possible to collect the CD14⁻ cell population, which will include mostly lymphocytes.

11. Remove each LS Column from the separator and place it on a new collection tube.

12. Pipette 3 mL buffer onto the LS Column; immediately flush out the fraction with the magnetically labeled cells by firmly applying the plunger supplied with the column (*see* **Note 3**).

3.3 Monocyte Culture

1. Count purified CD14+ monocytes in the magnetic labeled fraction (expect monocyte yield to be ≈10% of total PBMCs and with a purity of ≈95% —*see* **Note 4**).

2. Save at least 2,000,000 cells to extract RNA. Place the volume of beads buffer containing this number of cells in a RNAse/DNAse-free 1.5 mL eppendorf and centrifuge at 4 °C, 400 × *g* for 5 min. Remove the supernatant and keep the pellet at −80 °C until RNA extraction is performed.

3. Centrifuge the remaining cell suspension at 1000 × *g* for 5 min to pellet monocytes.

4. Resuspend monocytes in an appropriate volume of culture medium (RPMI-1640 without FBS), according to your experimental requirements.

5. For MDMs differentiation, plate CD14+ monocytes in 12-well multiwell plates appropriate for adherent cells, at a density of 600,000 cells/well, in 800 μL of RPMI-1640 without serum; leave the cells to adhere overnight (*see* **Note 5**).

6. In the next morning, add a sufficient volume of FBS to achieve 10% FBS in each well (200 μL/800 μL RPMI-1640 without serum) and M-CSF to achieve a final concentration of 50 ng/mL (50 μL of the diluted stock in 1 mL of cell medium).

7. Change the medium with fresh RPMI-1640 10% FBS and add M-CSF (final concentration of 50 ng/mL) every 3 days, in order to remove debris and promote MDMs differentiation (*see* **Note 6**). At day 7, a mature MDMs population should be ready for experiments, such as total RNA extraction (Fig. 2).

3.4 RNA Extraction and Reverse Transcription

1. For total RNA extraction from the isolated monocytes or differentiated macrophages, choose a RNA extraction kit that conserves small RNA species such as the miRCURY RNA Isolation Kit—Cell and Plant (Exiqon—Ref: 300110) and follow the guidelines of the manufacturer. The RNA obtained with these kits can be used for both mRNA and miRNA quantification by qRT-PCR.

2. When employing the miRCURY RNA Isolation Kit—Cell and Plant, start by adding 350 μL of Lysis buffer with 1% β-mercaptoethanol to each eppendorf containing the frozen monocyte cell pellet. If performing RNA extraction from macrophage cultures, divide the 350 μL of Lysis buffer with 1%

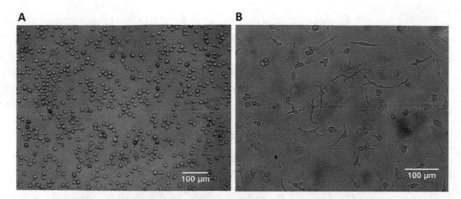

Fig. 2 Morphology of monocytes and MDMs isolated from PBMCs. Representative images showing the morphology of (**A**) monocytes 24 h after isolation and plating, immediately before the addition of M-CSF (50 ng/mL) and (**B**) MDMs obtained following 7 days of differentiation in the presence of M-CSF (50 ng/mL). The images were acquired in a light microscope equipped with the 20× objective

β-mercaptoethanol by all wells containing the same experimental sample and scrap the macrophages with the lysis buffer using a cell scraper, transferring the cell lysate to a 1.5 mL eppendorf tube.

3. Add 200 μL volume of 95–100% ethanol to each 1.5 mL eppendorf tube and mix by vortexing for 10 s. Add the contents of each eppendorf to a single column and collection tube provided in the kit and centrifuge for 1 min at 14,000 × g, RT. Discard the flowthrough and reassemble the spin column with the collection tube. This step will allow the RNA in the sample to bind to the resin matrix in the column.

4. Wash once with 400 μL of Wash solution and centrifuge 2 min at 14,000 × g, RT. Discard the flowthrough and reassemble the spin column with the collection tube.

5. Perform an on-column DNA removal step to improve the purity of your RNA. This is particularly relevant if you also want to use your RNA sample for mRNA quantification. For this purpose prepare a working solution of DNAse I (0.25 Kunitz unit/μL) by diluting the necessary amount of DNAse I reaction buffer (40 mM Tris pH 7.0, 10 mM $MgCl_2$ and 3 mM $CaCl_2$ in RNase-free water) to have 100 μL of solution/column. Apply 100 μL of the DNAse I solution to each column and centrifuge for 2 min at 200 × g to allow the DNAse I solution to penetrate the resin. Incubate for 15 min at 25°–30 °C.

6. Wash twice with 400 μL of Wash solution, centrifuging for 1 min at 14,000 × g, RT and discarding the flowthrough each time.

7. Centrifuge for 2 min at 14,000 × g to completely dry the resin before eluting the RNA. Discard the collection tube and place the column in a new RNAse-free 1.5 mL eppendorf.

8. Add 30 μL of Elution Buffer to the column and centrifuge for 2 min at 200 × *g*, followed by 1 min at 14,000 × *g*. For maximum RNA recovery you can repeat the elution step by placing the eluted volume in the column and repeating the centrifugation. If cDNA synthesis is to be performed immediately after RNA extraction, place the eppendorfs containing the RNA samples on ice or at 4 °C. For long-term storage, before cDNA synthesis, freeze the samples at −80 °C (*see* **Note 7**).

9. Quantify the total RNA in each sample using a NanoDrop or similar device using the minimum sample volume possible.

10. Prepare a dilution of each sample to a concentration of 5 ng/μL using RNAse-free water. Keep both the original samples and the diluted samples on ice at all times to avoid RNA degradation.

11. When using the Universal cDNA synthesis kit (Exiqon—Ref: 203,301) to perform cDNA synthesis, gently thaw the 5× Reaction Buffer and spin both the 5× Reaction Buffer and the Enzyme mix, placing them immediately on ice.

12. Prepare the necessary volume of reverse transcription master mix by mixing (*see* **Note 8**):

    (a) 2 μL of 5× Reaction Buffer/sample.

    (b) 5 μL of RNAse-free water/sample.

    (c) 1 μL Enzyme mix/sample.

13. Add 2 μL of each RNA sample (template RNA at 5 ng/μL) to 8 μL of reverse transcription master mix in qPCR grade 200 μL eppendorf tubes compatible with the available thermocycler. Mix the reaction by gently pipetting and spin down all tubes.

14. Run the reverse transcription reaction in the available thermocycler using the following protocol:

    (a) Incubate for 60 min at 42 °C.

    (b) Heat-inactivate the reverse transcriptase for 5 min at 95 °C.

    (c) Cool immediately and keep at 4 °C.

15. For long-term storage of the cDNA freeze at −20 °C or −80 °C.

3.5 qPCR Arrays

1. Pre-design Pick-&-Mix PCR panels to include primers for your miRNAs of interest. Each plate should contain three wells for interplate calibrators (IPC), in order to facilitate comparisons between different plates. Additionally, RNA spike-in controls (SIC) can be included to assess the quality of the RNA isolation, cDNA synthesis, and PCR reaction, if a synthetic RNA spike-in was previously added to the cDNA synthesis reaction (*see* **Note 9**).

2. When using the ExiLENT SYBR Green Master Mix from Exiqon, place the cDNA samples and the SYBR Green master

mix vial on ice and, if necessary, let the cDNA samples thaw for 15–20 min. Protect the SYBR Green dye from light.

3. Dilute each cDNA sample 100 × with nuclease-free water immediately before preparing the Pick-&-Mix PCR plate. For each 96-well Pick-&-Mix panel, designed to run a single sample, a total volume of 480 μL of cDNA from that sample will be required (*see* **Note 9**). Therefore, 5 μL of cDNA (from the 10 μL RT reaction) should be diluted with 495 μL of nuclease-free water. It is not recommended to store the 100 × cDNA dilution for long periods.

4. Include a passive reference dye, such as ROX, in the cDNA dilution if required by the available real-time PCR cycler. Since the amount of reference dye is instrument-dependent, please follow the recommendations of the manufacturer.

5. Briefly centrifuge each Pick-&-Mix PCR plate in a swing-bucket centrifuge before removing the plate seal.

6. Combine the SYBR Green master mix and the 100 × diluted cDNA (1:1) in a 1.5 mL eppendorf to generate the PCR master mix (e.g., mix 500 μL of cDNA with 500 μL of SYBR Green master mix). Mix by gently inverting the tube and spinning down.

7. Add 10 μL of the PCR master mix to each well of the 96-well Pick-&-Mix PCR plate. Seal the plate with the sealing foil recommended for the available real-time PCR cycler. The plate can be stored at 4 °C, protected from light, for up to 24 h.

8. Spin briefly the plate in a swing-bucket centrifuge (1500 × g for 1 min) to remove air bubbles.

9. Perform real-time PCR amplification followed by melting curve analysis in the available real-time PCR cycler, according to the following protocol:

    (a) Polymerase activation/denaturation – 95 °C, 10 min.

    (b) Amplification (45 cycles) – 10 s at 95 °C followed by 1 min at 60 °C (ramp-rate 1.6 °C/s) with optical read.

    (c) Melting curve analysis protocol with optical read.

3.6 Data Analysis

1. Perform initial data analysis using the software of the available real-time PCR cycler, in order to analyze the melting curves, identify non-detected assays, and obtain raw Ct values for each well. It is not recommended to use auto Ct settings, so set both threshold and baseline manually (*see* **Note 10**).

2. The Ct values can then be analyzed manually or using a dedicated qPCR analysis software, such as GeneEx (Exiqon). Export data from cycler and import it (annotated plates) into GenEx using the Exiqon plate wizard.

3. Perform interplate calibration by subtracting the calibration factor, provided by IPC analysis, to all Ct values of each plate (*see* **Note 11**).

4. Control for SIC values considering exclusion of outlier samples in which SIC values are below or above the expected values.

5. Handle cutoffs and missing data by defining a threshold Ct above which there is no amplification.

6. Choose the best reference gene to normalize all your Ct's from your candidate reference genes. This step can be performed using the NormFinder and/or GeNorm tolls of GenEx, which will give you the miRNA (from your candidate reference genes) that presents less variability across all samples. If all candidate reference genes vary across samples, perform the same analysis and choose a miRNA whose expression does not change significantly (*see* **Note 12**).

7. Perform normalization with the chosen reference miRNA/miRNA and analyze data using GenEx tools. In alternative, Ct values can be obtained with GenEx for each reference miRNA/miRNA and for each sample and analysis can be performed manually.

4 Notes

1. The use of sterile EDTA-coated tubes is important to avoid miRNA loss, since other types of coating, such as heparin, can interfere with miRNA recovery after extraction. In addition, if monocyte differentiation into macrophages is necessary, it is crucial to use sterile tubes, to avoid culture contamination during the differentiation process.

2. Take into consideration that the more the blood is diluted with PBS, before Histopaque gradient centrifugation, the more clear and narrow the PBMC band will be after this step. This will make it easier to remove the PBMC fraction without disturbing the red cell pellet.

3. To increase the purity of the magnetically labeled fraction, this fraction can be passed over a new, freshly prepared LS Column – for up to 10^8 magnetically labeled cells. Although this is usually not necessary for CD14$^+$ monocytes, it may be required for other PBMC populations.

4. The purity of the collected monocyte fraction, or any other cell fraction of interest, should be validated by flow cytometry using specific cell markers. For monocytes, this can be done by incubating the flushed cell population with an anti-CD14 antibody and performing flow cytometry analysis. Expected results should be similar to those presented in Fig. 3.

A

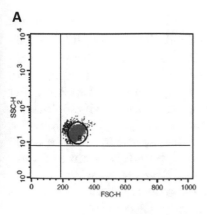

B

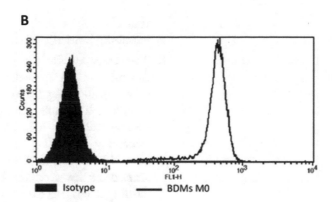

C

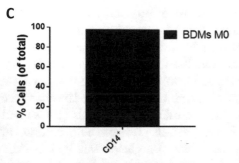

Fig. 3 Characterization of blood-derived CD14+ monocytes by flow cytometry, following isolation by magnetic-activated cell sorting. The expression levels of the CD14+ surface marker were evaluated by flow cytometry, in the FL-1 channel, after magnetic cell sorting using anti-CD14 magnetic beads. (**A**) Representative dot plot of the CD14+ monocyte population. (**B**) Representative histogram of CD14+ surface expression in the analysed population. (**C**) Percentage of analysed cells expressing CD14+. Results are expressed as percentage of total cells

5. The absence of serum overnight in the monocyte culture helps to initiate the differentiation process and to increase the MDM yield. By removing the serum from the culture medium it is possible to mimic what happens when monocytes leave the bloodstream and enter tissues, which, in vivo, is one of the triggers for differentiation.

6. Expect to observe a high number of cell debris and cells in suspension in the first few days of the MDMs differentiation protocol, since not all monocytes will adhere and start the differentiation process. With time and medium changes these cells will be removed and the adherent small round cells will give rise to larger cells with an ameboid or fusiform shape, which correspond to MDMs (Fig. 2).

7. When performing a miRNA or mRNA screening of multiple samples, the cDNA synthesis should be performed simultaneously for all samples, using a common master mix, even if each sample will be run at a different time in a different qPCR plate. This, together with the interplate calibrators and RNA spike-ins

that should be included in each plate, will reduce unspecific variability and allow the direct comparison of all samples.

8. The volumes for the preparation of the RT master mix are optimized for a 96-well Pick-&-Mix PCR panel (Exiqon), with a layout allowing for the evaluation of up to 92 miRNAs per sample. All volumes/sample should be doubled if employing a 384-well Pick-&-Mix PCR panel. If a RNA spike-in control is necessary, 0.5 μL/ sample of the synthetic RNA spike-in should be added to the RT master mix and the volume of water should be lowered to 4.5 μL of RNAse-free water/sample. Adding a 10% excess of each component to the RT master mix is advisable in order to account for pipetting errors.

9. Exiqon provides an extensive list of pre-designed LNA-based primer for miRNA detection. However, custom-designed primer sequences can also be included in the panels. There are different sample layouts available for the 96-well Pick-&-Mix PCR panels, one of which allows the quantification of 92 selected miRNAs in a single sample. In this plate layout, three wells are retained for interplate calibrator controls (IPCs) and one well is used as a RNA spike-in control. The volume of 100 × diluted cDNA necessary for a single 96-well Pick-&-Mix plate was calculated considering the analysis of up to 92 miR-NAs plus controls in a single sample. When using other available Pick-&-Mix plate layouts, the necessary volume of 100 × diluted cDNA may have to be adjusted according to the instructions of the manufacturer.

10. Auto Ct settings performed by the software of real-time PCR cyclers can be set erroneous on non-detected assays, originating false positives, and may also differ from plate to plate, preventing direct comparison of data from different plates. This issue cannot be resolved by interplate calibration, since each well may have a differently calculated baseline and threshold. Therefore, these parameters should be set manually. To do so, the baseline should be set in the cycle interval before the amplification takes-off, while the threshold should be set above background, with the Y-axis in log scale, at a point where all assays with good amplification curves are in the log linear phase.

11. To perform interplate calibration manually, first verify that the IPC wells in each plate have Ct standard deviations within 0.5. If this is not the case, eliminate the outliers, if possible. Next, calculate the average of the IPC replicates for each plate (IPC plate) and the overall IPC average (IPC overall – average of IPC wells from all plates). The plate calibration factor is calculated as the difference between the plate IPC average and the overall IPC average, for each plate (calibration factor = IPC plate – IPC overall).

12. If a good reference gene cannot be identified, Ct values can be normalized to the mean Ct value of each sample (mean Ct of

all genes detected for that sample). This methodology should only be applied when a high number of genes is detected for each sample, which is usually the case when working with miRNA PCR panels.

Acknowledgements

This work was funded by FEDER funds through the Operational Programme Competitiveness Factors – COMPETE 2020 and national funds by FCT – Foundation for Science and Technology under the strategic project with reference from COMPETE: POCI-01-0145-FEDER-007440. Cardoso A.L. is the recipient of a fellowship from FCT with reference SFRH/BPD/108312/2015 and Guedes J.R. is also the recipient of a fellowship from FCT with reference SFRH/BPD/120611/2016.

References

1. Keller A, Backes C, Haas J, Leidinger P, Maetzler W et al (2016) Validating Alzheimer's disease micro RNAs using next-generation sequencing. Alzheimers Dement 12:565–576

2. Guedes JR, Santana I, Cunha C, Duro D, Almeida MR et al (2016) MicroRNA deregulation and chemotaxis and phagocytosis impairment in Alzheimer's disease. Alzheimers Dement 3:7–17

3. Viegas AT, Guedes JR, Oliveira AR, Cardoso AM, Cardoso AL (2017) MiRNAs: new biomarkers and therapeutic targets in dementia. Curr Pharm Des 23:669–692

4. Cheng L, Doecke JD, Sharples RA, Villemagne VL, Fowler CJ et al (2015) Prognostic serum miRNA biomarkers associated with Alzheimer's disease shows concordance with neuropsychological and neuroimaging assessment. Mol Psychiatry 20:1188–1196

5. Kumar P, Dezso Z, MacKenzie C, Oestreicher J, Agoulnik S et al (2013) Circulating miRNA biomarkers for Alzheimer's disease. PLoS One 8:e69807

6. Lugli G, Cohen AM, Bennett DA, Shah RC, Fields CJ et al (2015) Plasma exosomal miRNAs in persons with and without Alzheimer disease: altered expression and prospects for biomarkers. PLoS One 10:e0139233

7. Gui Y, Liu H, Zhang L, Lv W, Hu X (2015) Altered microRNA profiles in cerebrospinal fluid exosome in Parkinson disease and Alzheimer disease. Oncotarget 6:37043–37053

8. Raj T, Rothamel K, Mostafavi S, Ye C, Lee MN et al (2014) Polarization of the effects of autoimmune and neurodegenerative risk alleles in leukocytes. Science 344:519–523

9. Guedes JR, Custodia CM, Silva RJ, de Almeida LP, Pedroso de Lima MC et al (2014) Early miR-155 upregulation contributes to neuroinflammation in Alzheimer's disease triple transgenic mouse model. Hum Mol Genet 23:6286–6301

10. Hong S, Beja-Glasser VF, Nfonoyim BM, Frouin A, Li S et al (2016) Complement and microglia mediate early synapse loss in Alzheimer mouse models. Science 352:712–716

11. Cardoso AL, Guedes JR, de Lima MC (2015) Role of microRNAs in the regulation of innate immune cells under neuroinflammatory conditions. Curr Opin Pharmacol 26:1–9

12. Ponomarev ED, Veremeyko T, Barteneva N, Krichevsky AM, Weiner HL (2011) MicroRNA-124 promotes microglia quiescence and suppresses EAE by deactivating macrophages via the C/EBP-alpha-PU.1 pathway. Nat Med 17:64–70

13. Ginhoux F, Jung S (2014) Monocytes and macrophages: developmental pathways and tissue homeostasis. Nat Rev Immunol 14:392–404

14. Koronyo Y, Salumbides BC, Sheyn J, Pelissier L, Li S et al (2015) Therapeutic effects of glatiramer acetate and grafted CD115+ monocytes in a mouse model of Alzheimer's disease. Brain 138:2399–2422

Part VIII

Preclinical Research

Chapter 22

Imaging of Microglial Activation in Alzheimer's Disease by [11C]PBR28 PET

Cornelius K. Donat, Nazanin Mirzaei, Sac-Pharm Tang, Paul Edison, and Magdalena Sastre

Abstract

Deficits in neuronal function and synaptic plasticity in Alzheimer's disease (AD) are believed to be linked to microglial activation. A hallmark of reactive microglia is the upregulation of mitochondrial translocator protein (TSPO) expression. Positron emission tomography (PET) is a nuclear imaging technique that measures the distribution of trace doses of radiolabeled compounds in the body over time. PET imaging using the 2nd generation TSPO tracer [11C]PBR28 provides an opportunity for accurate visualization and quantification of changes in microglial density in transgenic mouse models of Alzheimer's disease (AD). Here, we describe the methodology for the in vivo use of [11C]PBR28 in AD patients and the 5XFAD transgenic mouse model of AD and compare the results against healthy individuals and wild-type controls. To confirm the results, autoradiography with [3H]PBR28 and immunochemistry was carried out in the same mouse brains. Our data shows that [11C]PBR28 is suitable as a tool for in vivo monitoring of microglial activation and may be useful to assess treatment response in future studies.

Key words TSPO, Microglia, Alzheimer's disease, PET, Autoradiography, Animal mouse model, In vivo imaging

1 Introduction

Inflammatory changes have been firmly linked with deficits in neuronal function and synaptic plasticity in Alzheimer's disease (AD), especially in brain areas controlling memory and cognition, such as hippocampus and cerebral cortex. Imaging studies in our division have detected microglial activation in AD patients at very early clinical stages of the disease [1, 2]. Inflammation is therefore suggested to be an early event, preceding inclusion formation in a number of AD experimental models as well, such as transgenic lines for mutant amyloid precursor protein (APP) [3].

It has been hypothesized that early microglial activation in AD delays disease progression by promoting clearance of Aβ before formation of senile plaques [3]. In addition, microglia

Robert Perneczky (ed.), *Biomarkers for Alzheimer's Disease Drug Development*, Methods in Molecular Biology, vol. 1750, https://doi.org/10.1007/978-1-4939-7704-8_22, © Springer Science+Business Media, LLC 2018

removal of damaged cells is also a very important step in the restoration of the normal brain environment, as if left such cells can become potent inflammatory stimuli, resulting in yet further tissue damage. On the other hand, as we age microglia become steadily less efficient at these processes, tending to become overactivated in response to stimulation and instigating too potent a reaction, which may cause neuronal damage in its own right [4]. Therefore, in later stages, with persistent production of pro-inflammatory cytokines such as IL-1β and TNFα, microglia lose their protective effect [5, 6] and may become detrimental. Recently the debate on microglia function in AD progression has been intensified by reports showing that AD animal models with near complete ablation of proliferating microglia do not display differences in plaque formation but synaptic density [7, 8]. As sustained overproduction of microglial pro-inflammatory mediators is neurotoxic, this raised the question of whether inflammation may have a more relevant effect on neurodegeneration and cognitive decline rather than in Aβ deposition.

The development of new techniques to visualize microgliosis in vivo longitudinally has had the advantage of allowing correlation with changes in behavior and cognition. A technique that may enable such longitudinal in vivo investigations is positron emission tomography (PET) [9]. The development of dedicated PET scanners suitable for imaging animals as small as mice [10–13] has paved the way for researchers to investigate the suitability of PET tracers that could potentially enable visualization of the density of markers associated with neuroinflammation.

The PET tracers for the 18 kDa mitochondrial translocator protein (TSPO), formerly known as the peripheral benzodiazepine receptor (PBR), have been developed in the past decade as a marker for microglia activation [14, 15], although it has also been detected in astrocytoma [16]. TSPO is expressed in the mitochondria membrane of highly proliferating cells and its function was initially associated with the transport of cholesterol, limiting the synthesis of steroid hormones [17]. However, the development of conditional TSPO knockout animals has suggested that TSPO was not required for testosterone production in vivo [18]. TSPO expression is relatively low in the healthy brain compared with other tissues [19], mainly found in the olfactory bulb and non-parenchymal regions such as the ependymal and choroid plexus [20, 21] and its local upregulation at sites of lesions and damage (it increases significantly after brain injury and inflammation) makes it a potentially ideal and sensitive marker for the detection of subtle changes in the region of brain injury [15, 16, 22–25]. In support of this, elevated levels of TSPO expression have been found in the hippocampus, frontal, temporal, and parietal cortices of postmortem AD brains [22, 26, 27].

The prototype TSPO antagonist PK11195 and agonist Ro5-4864 [28] were initially employed to detect the binding site in various tissues. As seen before for other targets, the antagonist showed higher affinity [28] and was then widely employed to detect TSPO as putative biomarker of glial activation and therefore inflammation in vivo. However, accurate quantification of microglial density using [¹¹C]PK11195 has been challenging due to limitations of the ligand including its modest binding affinity, high nonselective binding, and high lipophilicity, yielding a low signal-to-noise ratio [29]. Therefore, the field of TSPO radioligands was rapidly expanding, with several of so-called "second-generation" TSPO ligands translated into in vivo application, including [¹¹C] AC-5216, [¹⁸F]PBR111, both [¹¹C]radiolabeled and [¹⁸F]radiolabeled derivatives of PBR06 and PBR28, [¹⁸F]FEPPA, [¹⁸F]DPA-714, and [¹²³I]CLINDE [30–36]. We recently reported autoradiographic and PET data showing that the binding of [³H] PBR28 in the 5XFAD model of AD coincides with the positive staining of the microglial marker Iba-1 in the same brain areas [37], providing support for the suitability of [¹¹C]PBR28 as a tool for in vivo monitoring of microglial activation. [³H]PBR28 binding was significantly higher in female animals and a significant positive correlation was observed between Aβ plaque load and [³H] PBR28. Similar findings were reported from 16-month-old APP/PS1 mice, another transgenic model of AD with [¹⁸F]E180 [38]. Ex vivo autoradiography with [¹¹C]PBR28 in a rat model of abdominal aortic aneurysm showed a nearly 6 times increased aortic tracer accumulation as compared to controls [39]. In addition, using [¹¹C]PBR28 in healthy rats, in vitro brain autoradiography showed a 19% increase of binding in aged (19.6 months) as compared in young rats (4 months) [40].

In this chapter, we describe the methodology for PET and autoradiography using PBR28 in humans and in mouse models, which have been carried out by us particularly to investigate changes in microglia activation in Alzheimer's disease (*see* **Note 1**).

2 PBR28 PET

2.1 Materials

- Animals: All the animal procedures were approved by the UK Home Office and were in accordance with the Animals (Scientific Procedures) Act of 1986 and the transposed EU directive 2010/63/EU. All the animals were kept in individually ventilated cages in a 12:12-h light-dark cycle with temperature and humidity set to specific ranges, and food and water ad libitum. Six-month-old female 5XFAD (Jax mice, $n = 4$) and four age-matched wild-type female mice (C57Bl6) were used.

- [^{11}C]PBR28 (4.0 ± 2.3 (0.7–8.2) MBq, specific activities 93 ± 54 (8–165) GBq/μmol) for mouse brain.

- Siemens Inveon small animal PET/CT scanner (DPET/MM) at Imanova Ltd.

- Siemens Biograph™ TruePoint™ PET/CT scanner (Siemens, Erlangen, De).

2.2 Methodology for [^{11}C]PBR28 PET in Mice

The mice are maintained under isoflurane anesthesia (1.5–2.5% isoflurane with oxygen flow rate 2–3 L/min) with scavenging for the duration of the scan using an adaptable anesthetic machine (Burton, UK). A needle (size 30G) attached to a length of cannula tubing is inserted and secured into a tail vein (dilated by prior warming the tail) for intravenous administration of [^{11}C]PBR28 (*see* **Note 2**). CT/PET scanners and gamma counters are required to be calibrated in order to ensure correct quantitative output. The CT scanner is calibrated with a water-filled cylinder phantom to generate output in correct Hounsfield units, which can be used for accurate attenuation correction. For the PET scanner, calibration is achieved through scanning a (usually 18F filled) container of accurately known radioactivity concentration. Monitoring the performance of the scanner over time with regular QC scans with a cylinder phantom is essential to ensure that both scanners are functioning correctly and are performing consistently. Each mouse is placed in a Biovet scanning chamber with connection to the anesthetic and scavenging equipment and physiological monitoring system (Biovet, m2m Imaging, USA) for body temperature maintenance (using a heating mat) and respiration rate monitoring (using a respiration pad attached near to the mouse thorax area). The whole body of the mouse is placed in the field of view of the CT scanner and a CT scan (20 min) is acquired for attenuation and scatter correction and to provide structural information. It is important to secure the anesthetized mouse in the chamber (e.g., with tapes) to minimize any movement during scanning and movement of the chamber from one imaging modality to another. Any misalignment between the FOVs is accounted for by the use of a transformation matrix that allows accurate overlay of the PET and CT images. In addition, the alignment of the FOVs is also important for accurate attenuation correction. The mouse chamber is then moved into the field of view of the PET scanner and a 60 min dynamic PET scan can start simultaneously with intravenous administration of [^{11}C] PBR28 into the tail vein. The exact radiotracer dose injected was calculated from the dose in the syringe measured before and after injection using an Isomed 2000 Dose Calibrator (Capintec, Austria), both decay corrected to the time of injection (*see* **Note 3**).

*2.2.1   PET/CT Image
Reconstruction*

The PET images are acquired in list mode and reconstructed with increasing frame times over the duration of the scan to characterize the radiotracer kinetics. 3D histograms with span 3 and maximum ring difference of 79 are used. Fourier rebinning is performed and images are reconstructed using a 2D FBP algorithm and a ramp filter and zoom of 2 to generate images on a 128×128 matrix (Fig. 1, *see* **Note 4**).

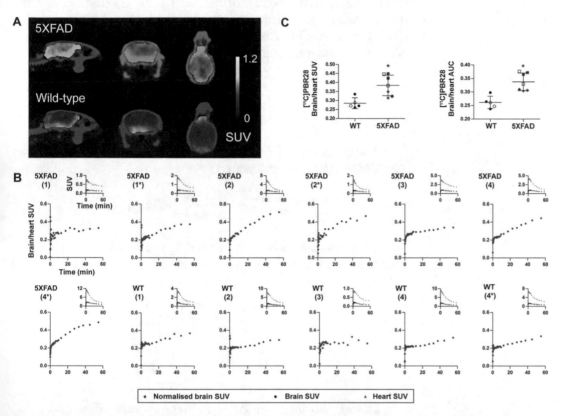

Fig. 1 In vivo PET imaging of TSPO using [¹¹C]PBR28. (**a**) Representative summed images from dynamic reconstruction of simultaneously acquired PET/CT scans from 6-month-old female 5XFAD mice and their age- and gender-matched wild-type littermates ($n = 4$ per group) over 60 min following intravenous injection of [¹¹C]PBR28. Sagittal, coronal, and dorsal orientations of the brain are presented from left to right, showing increased brain [¹¹C]PBR28 retention in the AD mouse model compared with WT controls. SUV scale represents the standardized uptake value. Additionally, a subset of the animals (5XFAD, $n = 3$; WT, $n = 1$) each underwent serial scans (24 h apart) to assess intra-subject test/retest variability (**b**) Brain [¹¹C]PBR28 uptake was normalized to that of the heart. Normalized brain SUV curves for individual scans are shown in red. Brain SUV (black) and heart SUV (gray) curves prior to normalization are also presented as inserts. (**c**) Quantification of [¹¹C]PBR28 uptake detected in the 5XFAD model was significantly higher compared with controls based on measures of brain/heart SUV: 0.376 ± 0.029 vs. 0.287 ± 0.017, 31% higher uptake, $P = 0.035$, and brain/heart area under time-activity curve (AUC): 0.334 ± 0.016 vs. 0.263 ± 0.0127, 27% higher uptake, $P = 0.013$; Test/retest measurements are represented by the same symbols for the animals that underwent serial scans. Average values of serial scans were used for statistical analyses. Data are expressed as mean $\pm$ SEM (Student's t test; *$P < 0.05$) [37]

2.2.2 *Image Analysis*   Image processing and data analysis is performed using an analysis pipeline developed in-house at Imanova Ltd. Briefly, the native DICOM images are converted into Nifti format and the dynamic PET images are visually assessed for motion and aligned to the CT images using a rigid body registration algorithm. PET and CT images are used to define the region of interest (ROI) in the target organ (brain) and reference organ (heart chamber). Time activity curves (TACs) are generated by applying the ROIs to the dynamic PET images. TACs were normalized to the injected activity and body weight, and corrected to the time of radiotracer dosing (decay-corrected) to obtain the standardized uptake value (SUV) as an outcome measure.

$$\mathrm{TAC}_{\mathrm{SUV}}\left(t\right) = \frac{\mathrm{TAC}(t)\left(\frac{\mathrm{kBq}}{\mathrm{mL}}\right)}{\mathrm{Injected\ dose}\left(\mathrm{kBq}\right)/\mathrm{Body\ weight}\left(\mathrm{g}\right)}$$

The average SUV between 30 and 60 min and the area under the TACs (AUC) are calculated.

$$\mathrm{SUV}_{\mathrm{organ}}^{30-60\,\mathrm{min}} = \frac{1}{\mathrm{Nbins}}\sum_{60}^{i=30}\mathrm{TAC}_{\mathrm{SUV}}\left(i\right)$$

To account for changes in radioligand delivery to the brain, the brain SUV and AUC are normalized to the heart SUV and AUC.

$$\mathrm{SUV}_{\mathrm{ratio}}^{30-60\,\mathrm{min}} = \frac{\mathrm{SUV}_{\mathrm{brain}}^{30-60\,\mathrm{min}}}{\mathrm{SUV}_{\mathrm{heart}}^{30-60\,\mathrm{min}}}$$

$$\mathrm{AUC}_{\mathrm{ratio}}^{5-60\,\mathrm{min}} = \frac{\mathrm{AUC}_{\mathrm{brain}}^{5-60\,\mathrm{min}}}{\mathrm{AUC}_{\mathrm{heart}}^{5-60\,\mathrm{min}}}$$

Finally, the intra-subject variability (relative difference, Δ_R) between test–retest is calculated, where D could be either SUV or AUC.

$$\Delta_R\left(\%\right) = 100\times\frac{\left|D_{\mathrm{ratio}}^{\mathrm{test}} - D_{\mathrm{ratio}}^{\mathrm{retest}}\right|}{\left(D_{\mathrm{ratio}}^{\mathrm{test}} + D_{\mathrm{ratio}}^{\mathrm{retest}}\right)/2}$$

2.3 Methodology for Human [¹¹C]PBR28 PET   [¹¹C]PBR28 PET scans should be acquired using a high resolution PET scanner. [¹¹C]PBR28 should be manufactured with high specificity and should conform the QC requirement. A low-dose CT scan was initially acquired to position the patient and to allow attenuation correction. A mean activity of more than 370 MBq of the tracer should be injected followed by a 3D dynamic data acquisition in list mode for 90 min (*see* **Note 5**). A mean activity of 300.3 (±37) MBq of the tracer in 20 mL normal saline was injected

2.3.1 Image Acquisition

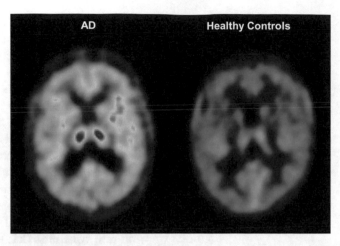

Fig. 2 Illustrative [¹¹C]PBR28 PET imaging. Representative [¹¹C]PBR28 images in a healthy control and in a patient with Alzheimer's disease (AD) dementia. The brain axial view shows increased [¹¹C]PBR28 binding in the AD subject (yellow-red spots) in comparison to the healthy control subject. Of note, both subjects are high-affinity binders. Distribution volume corrected for free fraction of the radio-ligand in plasma (V T/f P) was used for estimating [¹¹C]PBR28 binding values

intravenously over 20 s. 3D dynamic data was acquired in list mode, and reconstruction was performed using standard Siemens software, which included scatter correction and attenuation correction based on 3D ordinary Poisson ordered-subset expectation maximization (OP-OSEM) algorithm. For proper quantification of the tracer, a continuous online sampling should be performed for first 15 min and whole blood activity was measured continuously using online detector. Arterial whole blood activity was measured continuously with an online detector for the first 15 min while discrete blood samples were taken at 5, 10, 20, 30, 50, 70, and 90 min. Samples were centrifuged to detect whole blood and plasma radioactivity and to measure radioactive metabolite levels (Fig. 2).

2.3.2 Image Analysis

[¹¹C]PBR28 dynamic PET should be corrected for head motion using the frame-by-frame realignment tool in statistical parametric mapping (SPM12, Wellcome Trust Centre for Neuroimaging) software. An individualized object map in PET space has to be created for each subject using the following steps: (1) the individual's MRI is co-registered to their native PET space using a PET add image (60–90 min); (2) gray matter, white matter, and CSF maps are generated by segmentation of the co-registered MRI and a binarized gray matter mask was created using a threshold of 0.5; (3) a probabilistic ROI atlas [41] in Montreal Neurologic Institute (MNI) space is transformed into native PET space; (4) the probabilistic atlas in PET space is then applied to the binarized individual gray matter mask to generate individualized gray matter ROIs.

Regional time activity curves are then generated from 0 to 90 min by sampling the dynamic PET scans using the individual's ROIs for the following regions: frontal, temporal, parietal, and occipital cortices and the whole brain (which included all four cortices and subcortical structures). Additional subcortical regions of interest in Alzheimer's disease including posterior cingulate, anterior cingulate, striatum, thalamus, brainstem, and cerebellum are also sampled. As medial temporal lobe is significantly involved in Alzheimer's disease, medial temporal lobe structures are further evaluated in detail by sampling whole medial temporal lobe, hippocampus, parahippocampus, and amygdala. The time-activity curves are created for each region and a metabolite-corrected plasma input function was fitted to a tri-exponential function. Total distribution volume (VT) and rate constants (k1, k2, k3, and k4) for each brain region are calculated using a two-tissue compartmental model with an extravascular compartment in MATLAB (*see* **Notes 6** and **7**).

3   PBR28 Autoradiography

In order to overcome the relatively low effective spatial resolution of PET imaging, especially in relation to the brain size of small animals such as mice, autoradiography assays have been used to evaluate the regional distribution and density of PBR28 binding sites. Autoradiography refers to a bio-analytical technique used to photographically visualize the two-dimensional distribution of radioactive-labeled substance in a biological sample. High-resolution autoradiograms with an intrinsic 0.1–1 μm spatial resolution can be obtained using low-energy radioisotopes such as tritium (^{3}H). Due to the longer half-life of ^{3}H compared with carbon-11, tritiated radioisotopes such as [^{3}H]PBR28 have enabled detection of regions with differential levels of activated microglia in small brain structures and substructures both in the brain of humans and animal models.

Radionuclide imaging or specifically autoradiography, both in vitro and ex vivo, has been a highly useful technique in basic research and applied radioligand development and application. Broken down, in vitro autoradiography refers to radioligand incubation on tissue sections without major metabolic activity. In contrast, ex vivo autoradiography requires injection of the tracer into a living subject, extraction of target tissue, and preparation of sections. In this case, metabolism is an important factor that often seals that fate of a tracer candidate [42].

In both cases, the tissue is then exposed to a detection method such as photosensitive films or emulsion for light- and electron-macro/microscopic detection, phosphor-imaging plates, solid-membrane and particle-counting systems [43].

**3.1 Advantages
and Drawbacks
of Autoradiography**

For targets in the brain, small molecules are primarily employed, due to their superior potential for crossing the blood brain barrier (BBB) [44], synthesis, and radiolabeling strategies.

While molecular imaging, using preclinical and clinical PET and Single-Photon-Emission-Computed Tomography (SPECT) systems, allow longitudinal studies and within-subject comparison, it is restricted in resolution and requires extensive blood-sampling and kinetic modeling for quantification [45].

In contrast, autoradiography offers a number of advantages:

- Wide choice of isotopes, therefore direct applicability of tracers for PET and SPECT but also isotopes with longer half-life, such as tritium (^{3}H), carbon-14 (^{14}C), and iodine-125 (^{125}I).

- Higher resolution in the low micrometer range, especially with tritiated tracers and film but also particle-counting systems (25 μm).

- Easy quantification by using commercially available radioactive standards.

- Application of tracers consisting of high-affinity proteins or antibodies that would normally not cross the BBB or are derived from potent toxins (e.g., frog or snake toxins such as epibatidine or bungarotoxin).

- Absence of major metabolic activity that could interfere with the binding.

- Multi-tracer studies (requiring different isotopes) in the same section when particle counting systems are employed.

- A great advantage of using autoradiography is that the technique allows assessment of the specificity of different TSPO radioligands by comparison with other known markers of microglial activation such as Iba-1, used in immunohistochemical studies to visualize activated microglia [37].

Conversely, autoradiography requires a larger number of subjects in order to be able to show longitudinal changes, it does not allow within-subject comparison, and it requires harvesting of tissue and therefore the death of the subject.

3.2 Materials

1. Hypotonic buffer: 50 mM Tris–HCl, pH 7.4.

2. Isotonic buffer: 50 mM Tris–HCl 140 mM NaCl, 1.5 mM MgCl2, 5 mM KCl, 1.5 mM CaCl2, pH 7.4.

3. Wash buffer: 50 mmol/L Tris Base, 1.5 mmol/L MgCl2, pH 7.4.

4. Microscopic slides (untreated or superfrost).

5. [^{3}H]PBR28 (4 nmol/L).

6. PK11195 (10 μmol/L).

7. Tritium-sensitive film (Kodak BiomaxMR) or phosphor imaging plates (Fuji BAS-TR).

8. Phosphorimager (GE Healthcare Typhoon FLA-7000).

9. [³H]microscale radioactive standards (ART 0123A/B; American Radiolabelled Chemicals, St. Louis, USA).

3.3 Methodology for In Vitro and Ex Vivo Autoradiography Using [³H]PBR28

For rodent brain samples, the technique requires the extraction of brain tissue following transcardial perfusion using 1× PBS to remove excess blood from vessels in order to limit background signal from circulating blood cells, which have been shown by several studies to express TSPO [46, 47]. Freshly extracted brain tissue is snap-frozen by gradual submersion in pre-chilled isopentane on dry ice to prevent protein degradation. Employing a general autoradiography protocol, frozen sections from human or rodent brains cut at a thickness of 10–20 μm are placed on microscopic slides (untreated or Superfrost). Storing these sections for at least 3 days prior to experiments at −80 °C should provide sufficient adhesion. Superfrost plus or polylysine/gelatine treated slides are not required. Slides are then thawed and air-dried for 15–30 min, followed by preincubation in buffer for 15 min at room temperature. Usually, isotonic buffers containing salts are used to mimic in vivo conditions. We have previously compared [³H]PBR28 binding in adjacent human temporal cortex brain sections using a hypotonic buffer with a similar isotonic buffer and could not find a significant difference in total, nonspecific specific binding and ratio of total-to-nonspecific binding. Nonspecific binding and ratio of total-to-nonspecific binding was slightly higher in the hypotonic buffer, which was therefore chosen for all subsequent experiments.

After preincubation, slides are briefly air-dried again. Incompletely dried sections can result in local differences in radioligand binding. This is followed by incubation with the radioligand for 60 min in assay buffer containing [³H]PBR28 (4 nmol/L). The actual concentration of the incubation solution should be checked with liquid scintillation counting, especially when performing a saturation assay. In our hands, [³H]PBR28 shows some surface adherence, which often results in slightly reduced actual concentrations as compared to the calculated concentration. Usually, incubation for 60 min, like with [³H]PBR28, should be sufficient when using high-affinity small molecule tracers, but association and dissociation should be determined with new tracer candidates to ascertain sufficient kinetics for equilibrium binding. An additional set of slides is used to determine the nonspecific binding component, usually by adding an excess (1000× concentration) of a structurally different ligand that binds to the same target. The nonspecific binding component is determined on adjacent sections in the presence of unlabeled PK11195 (10 μmol/L). However in human tissue, we observed a residual binding of [³H]PBR28 in the cortical gray matter (Fig. 3). After incubation, slides are washed twice in ice-cold wash buffer (4 °C; 20 s per wash) followed by a final wash in ice-cold wash buffer (4 °C; 20 s). Note that the number of washing steps and time will have a direct effect on binding, so excessive washing will often reduce specific binding. However, we have also applied a different washing protocol (two times for 60 s in hypotonic buffer (pH 7.4/4 °C), 60 s in ultra-pure water at 4 °C) which works equally well.

Slides are dried in a cool airstream or can then be subjected to PFA vapors, which may reduce contamination of phosphor imaging plates or drying under phosphorous pentoxide. Slides are then exposed for 8 weeks to tritium-sensitive film or 10–14 days to phosphor imaging plates with [³H]-microscale standards in X-ray cassettes at RT.

Images of individual sections are normally acquired with a lightbox and a camera, attached to a microcomputer imaging device analysis software (Microcomputer Imaging Device Core; Interfocus Imaging Ltd., Linton) or a phosphorimager and quantified using various imaging software such as ImageJ, FIJI, or Quantity One. For tissue sections, values are converted to fmol [³H] ligand/mg wet tissue equivalent using the calibrated [3H] microscale radioactive standards (ART 0123A/B; American Radiolabelled Chemicals, St. Louis, USA) for quantification. Specific binding is measured by normalization to background and nonspecific signal for each region of interest (ROI) (Figs. 3 and 4).

Ex vivo autoradiography involves the in vivo injection of [³H] PBR28 or [¹¹C]PBR28 at similar concentrations as the PET. Then,

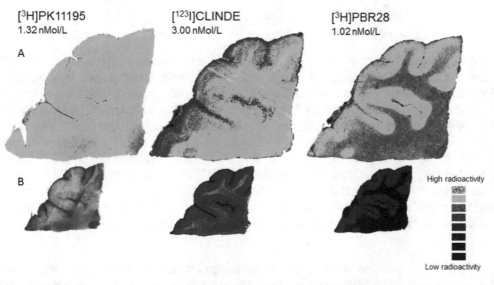

Fig. 3 Representative in vitro autoradiography of total (**a**) and nonspecific binding (**b**, 10 μM PK11195) of three structurally different TSPO radiotracers ([³H]PK11195, [¹²³I]CLINDE, and [³H]PBR28) in a healthy control (53 y, male HAB) from the Stanley Medical Research Institute Neuropathology consortium

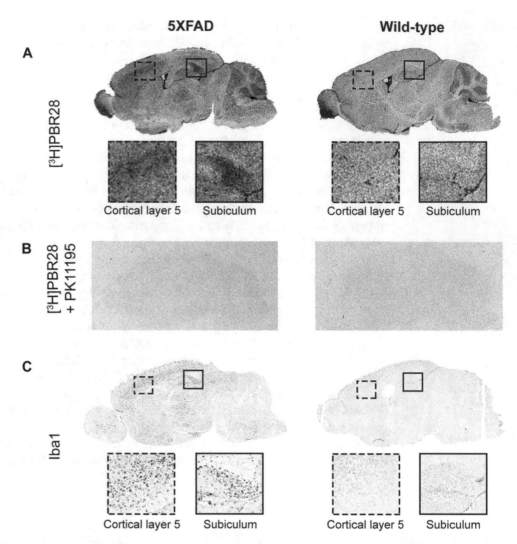

Fig. 4 In vitro characterization of TSPO expression by autoradiography, using [³H]PBR28, coincides with the expression of Iba1, a reactive microglial marker, assessed by immunohistochemistry. (**a**) A representative sagittal brain section from a 6-month-old female 5XFAD mouse showing greater [³H]PBR28 binding compared with that in a wild-type control. Note the considerably higher binding in cortical and hippocampal regions, particularly in the cortical layer 5 and subiculum of the AD mouse model. Similar levels of radioligand binding are observed in the olfactory bulb and cerebellum of both 5XFAD and WT brains. (**b**) Representative images of [³H]PBR28 binding following the displacement of the radioligand by unlabeled PK11195. The pattern and intensity of binding were diminished in both the 5XFAD and WT mice in adjacent sections. (**c**) Representative sections of Iba1 staining in adjacent sections show that areas with higher microglial density coincide with areas of higher [³H]PBR28 binding. (**d**) Representative images showing extensive amyloid deposition, detected by 6C3 staining, in the 5XFAD brain compared with the WT control. From reference [37]

animals are culled and brains extracted and stored at −80 °C. Frozen brains are cut into 10–20 μM sections with a cryostat. Slides are dried in a cool airstream before exposure to tritium-sensitive film (Kodak Biomax MS film, Hemel Hempstead, UK) with [³H] microscale standards in X-ray cassettes at RT (8 weeks).

4   Notes

Although the new generation of TSPO ligands, such as PBR28, seems to have higher specificity than PK11195 for in vivo imaging of activated microglia, there are some limitations and points to have into account:

1. The new generation TSPO tracers are affected by genetic variability of TSPO binding site induced by the rs6971 single-nucleotide polymorphism [48] and recent studies have demonstrated that tracer signal in the high-affinity binders (HAB) is 25–35% higher compared with the mixed affinity (MAB) binders [49, 50]. However, it has been demonstrated that the results from a TSPO subgroup (HAB or MAB) can be translated to the entire AD and MCI population [51]. It is likely that it will hold true for the other tracers. To overcome this complexity when assessing PBR28 radioligand potential in humans, selection of subjects or brain samples from individuals with similar affinity-binding profiles is recommended. This issue is not encountered when using rodent brain tissue.

2. The limitation on dose volume and rate of injection must be taken into consideration for the mouse due to its small size (<5 mL/kg for iv bolus). Typically less than 100 uL total volume is injected slowly with close monitoring of the physiology (respiration rate) during dose injection. This total volume includes any saline used to flush the iv line after tracer injection. In addition, sufficiently high radioactive concentration as part of the radiosynthesis process is required to ensure measurable PET signal.

3. Full quantification of PET data in the mouse is challenging due to its size and limitation of blood volume. If rats or larger animals are used, serial arterial blood samples can be taken during the scan to generate input function for compartmental modeling. An arterial line can be surgically implanted in the tail or femoral artery for collecting blood samples.

4. There are limitations due to the spatial resolution of PET scanners. In practice, the smallest details visible are approximately 2 mm in size; therefore, there is very limited detail within the brain of a mouse. Details at around this scale and smaller will suffer from partial volume averaging, and uptake of radioactivity from these regions will appear to be less intense than they actually are. Blurring outward of intense radioactivity will lead to higher apparent uptake in neighboring regions.

5. The time frames used to create dynamic images from scan data should be chosen as a compromise between the need to get as many counts as possible into each image (this reduces the noise in the image) and the need to have sufficient temporal resolu-

tion to reflect the changing radionuclide distribution in the animal. Additionally, the radioactive decay of [¹¹C] in particular means that fewer decays occur toward the end of a scan than at the beginning—frame times need to be longer in order to gather the same number of counts as earlier in the scan. After 1 h, three [¹¹C] half-lives will have passed, i.e., the decay rate has dropped to just over 10% of its original value.

6. One of the outstanding challenges for TSPO imaging is that no single region is appropriate to serve as the reference region, because TSPO is expressed throughout the brain. Hence, different modeling approaches have been used across different labs leading to discordant results in AD/MCI subjects, and in other neurodegenerative diseases [52–55]. In PET, the mathematical models of the tracer uptake depend on model input and tissue output. Ideally, for a given tracer, we could use (1) plasma input models and (2) reference tissue input models. The parent plasma input function utilizes the activity concentration due to unmetabolized parent compound in plasma, measured by HPLC analysis [56] to configure the kinetic model. The reference tissue input models require a reference region, which should be free of specifically bound tracer. Kinetic compartment modeling provides a particular model to describe the tracer binding properties, and estimate the volume of distribution of the tracer specifically bound in the tissue [57]. The parametric maps can be generated by different modeling approaches, which will allow us to evaluate the data at voxel level. As no specific region of brain is devoid of microglia, arterial input analysis is the gold standard for quantification of [¹¹C]PBR28 PET. In animal models, this has been solved by using the heart as a region of reference [37].

7. It has also been suggested that the extravascular compartment plays a significant role in the quantification of the [¹¹C]PBR28 signal. Due to the high lipophilic feature of the TSPO ligands, the TSPO distribution is heterogeneous in the brain, and a significant proportion of tracer signals were found in the vascular component outside of the brain tissue, such as endothelium and smooth muscle vessel walls, where binding may very much represent the nonspecific binding of the lipids [58]. Thus, one challenge for quantifying TSPO tissue binding is to separate the vast amount of vascular binding. Hence, two tissue-compartmental model with extravascular component (2TCM4k-1K) was proposed, which accounts for the endothelial cells of blood vessels [59]. Recent studies by Veronese et al. further evaluated a validation of the kinetic model with the additional endothelial compartment for [¹¹C]PBR28 through a displacement study using XBD173. The addition of the endothelial component provided a signal compartmentaliza-

tion much more consistent with the underlying biology. Interestingly, the blocking study produced reduction in the tracer concentration of the specific tissue compartment, whereas the non-displaceable compartment remained unchanged. Additionally, it was also demonstrated that TSPO positive vessels account for 30% of the vascular volume in cortical and white matter [60]. While using different methods, the model with lower AIC (Akaike information criterion) is chosen as the preferred model for a predefined ROI. Total volume of distribution (VT) and rate constant (k) parameters will be derived from the kinetic modeling approaches. Kinetic analysis demonstrated that parent fraction of [¹¹C]-PBR28 was reduced from 80 to 5%, and the plasma:blood ratio of tracer concentration increased from 1.1 to 1.4 during a 90 min scan. Based on the AIC, [¹¹C]-PBR28 PET shows preference to 2TCM4k-1 K over 2TCM4k model suggesting the role of extravascular component [59].

References

1. Cagnin A, Brooks DJ, Kennedy AM, Gunn RN, Myers R, Turkheimer FE, Jones T, Banati RB (2001) In-vivo measurement of activated microglia in dementia. Lancet 358:461–467

2. Okello A, Edison P, Archer HA, Turkheimer FE, Kennedy J, Bullock R et al (2009) Microglial activation and amyloid deposition in mild cognitive impairment: a PET study. Neurology 72:56–62

3. Heneka MT, Sastre M, Dumitrescu-Ozimek L, Dewachter I, Walter J, Klockgether T, Leuven V (2005) Focal glial activation coincides with increased BACE1 activation and precedes amyloid plaque deposition in APP(V717I) transgenic mice. J Neuroinflammation 2:22

4. Solito S, Sastre M (2012) Microglia function in Alzheimer's disease. Front Neuropharmacol 3:14

5. Hickman SE, Allison EK, El Khoury J (2008) Microglial dysfunction and defective beta-amyloid clearance pathways in aging Alzheimer's disease mice. J Neurosci 28(33):8354–8360

6. Jimenez S, Baglietto-Vargas D, Caballero C, Moreno-Gonzalez I et al (2008) Inflammatory response in the hippocampus of PS1M146L/APP751SL mouse model of Alzheimer's disease: age-dependent switch in the microglial phenotype from alternative to classic. J Neurosci 28:11650–11661

7. Grathwohl SA, Kälin RE, Bolmont T, Prokop S, Winkelmann G et al (2009) Formation and maintenance of Alzheimer's disease beta-amyloid plaques in the absence of microglia. Nat Neurosci 12:1361–1363

8. Olmos-Alonso A, Schetters ST, Sri S, Askew K, Mancuso R, Vargas-Caballero M, Holscher C, Perry VH, Gomez-Nicola D (2016) Pharmacological targeting of CSF1R inhibits microglial proliferation and prevents the progression of Alzheimer's-like pathology. Brain 139(Pt 3):891–907

9. Matthews PM, Rabiner EA, Passchier J, Gunn RN (2012) Positron emission tomography molecular imaging for drug development. Br J Clin Pharm 73(2):175–186

10. Bao Q, Newport D, Chen M, Stout DB, Chatziioannou AF (2009) Performance evaluation of the inveon dedicated PET preclinical tomography based on the NEMA-NU4 standards. J Nucl Med 50(3):401–408

11. Cherry SR, Gambhir S (2001) Use of positron emission tomography in animal research. ILAR J 42(3):219–232

12. Myers R, Hume SP (2002) Small animal PET. Eur Neuropsychopharmacol 12(6):545–555

13. Tai Y-C, Ruangma A, Rowland et al (2005) Performance evaluation of the inveon dedicated PET preclinical tomograph based on the NEMA-NU4 standards. J Nucl Med 46:455–463

14. Papadopoulos V, Baraldi M, Guilarte TR, Knudsen TB et al (2006) Translocator protein

(18kDa): new nomenclature for the peripheral-type benzodiazepine receptor based on its structure and molecular function. Trends Pharmacol Sci 27(8):402–409

15. Chen MK, Guilarte TR (2008) Translocator protein 18 kDa (TSPO): molecular sensor of brain injury and repair. Pharmacol Ther 118(1):1–17

16. Su Z, Roncaroli F, Durrenberger PF et al (2013) [(1)(1)C]-(R)PK11195 tracer kinetics in the brain of glioma patients and a comparison of two referencing approaches. Eur J Nucl Med Mol Imaging 40(9):1406–1419

17. Rupprecht R, Papadopoulos V, Rammes G, Baghai TC, Fan J, Akula N, Groyer G, Adams D, Schumacher M (2010) Translocator protein (18 kDa) (TSPO) as a therapeutic target for neurological and psychiatric disorders. Nat Rev Drug Discov 9(12):971–988

18. Morohaku K, Pelton SH, Daugherty DJ, Butler WR, Deng W, Selvaraj V (2014) Translocator protein/peripheral benzodiazepine receptor is not required for steroid hormone biosynthesis. Endocrinology 155(1):89–97

19. Banati RB, Newcombe J, Gunn RN, Cagnin A, Turkheimer F, Heppner F, Price G, Wegner F, Giovannoni G, Miller DH (2000) The peripheral benzodiazepine binding site in the brain in multiple sclerosis. Brain 123:2321–2337

20. Benavides J, Quarteronet D, Imbault F, Malgouris C, Uzan A, Renault C et al (1983) Labelling of "peripheral-type" benzodiazepine binding sites in the rat brain by using [3H]PK 11195, an isoquinoline carboxamide derivative: kinetic studies and autoradiographic localization. J Neurochem 41:1744–1750

21. Gehlert DR, Yamamura HI, Wamsley JK (1983) Autoradiographic localization of "peripheral" benzodiazepine binding sites in the rat brain and kidney using [3H]RO5-4864. Eur J Pharmacol 95:329–330

22. Cosenza-Nashat M, Zhao ML, Suh HS, Morgan J, Natividad R, Morgello S, Lee SC (2009) Expression of the translocator protein of 18 kDa by microglia, macrophages and astrocytes based on immunohistochemical localization in abnormal human brain. Neuropathol Appl Neurobiol 35:306–328

23. Scarf AM, Ittner LM, Kassiou M (2009) The translocator protein (18 kDa): central nervous system disease and drug design. J Med Chem 52(3):581–592

24. Dickens AM, Vainio S, Marjamäki P, Johansson J, Lehtiniemi P, Rokka J, Rinne J, Solin O, Haaparanta-Solin M, Jones PA, Trigg W, Anthony DC, Airas L (2014) Detection of microglial activation in an acute model of neuroinflammation using PET and radiotracers 11C-(R)-PK11195 and 18F-GE-180. J Nucl Med 55:466–472

25. Janssen B et al (2016) Imaging of neuroinflammation in Alzheimer's disease, multiple sclerosis and stroke: recent developments in positron emission tomography. Biochim Biophys Acta 1862(3):425–441

26. Venneti S, Lopresti BJ, Wang G, Hamilton RL, Mathis CA, Klunk WE, Apte UM, Wiley CA (2009) PK11195 labels activated microglia in Alzheimer's disease and in vivo in a mouse model using PET. Neurobiol Aging 30:1217–1226

27. Venneti S, Wiley CA, Kofler J (2009) Imaging microglial activation during neuroinflammation and Alzheimer's disease. J Neuroimmune Pharmacol 4:227–243

28. Le Fur G, Vaucher N, Perrier ML, Flamier A, Benavides J, Renault C et al (1983) Differentiation between two ligands for peripheral benzodiazepine binding sites, [3H]RO5-4864 and [3H]PK 11195, by thermodynamic studies. Life Sci 33(5):449–457

29. Guo Q, Colasanti A, Owen DR, Onega M, Kamalakaran A, Bennacef I, Matthews PM, Rabiner EA, Turkheimer FE, Gunn RN (2013) Quantification of the specific translocator protein signal of 18F-PBR111 in healthy humans: a genetic polymorphism effect on in vivo binding. J Nucl Med 54:1915–1923

30. Dupont AC, Largeau B, Santiago Ribeiro MJ, Guilloteau D, Tronel C, Arlicot N (2017) Translocator protein-18 kDa (TSPO) positron emission tomography (PET) imaging and its clinical impact in neurodegenerative diseases. Int J Mol Sci 18(4):pii: E785

31. Tronel C, Largeau B, Santiago Ribeiro MJ, Guilloteau D, Dupont AC, Arlicot N (2017) Molecular targets for PET imaging of activated microglia: the current situation and future expectations. Int J Mol Sci 18(4):pii: E802

32. Holland JP, Liang SH, Rotstein BH, Collier TL, Stephenson NA, Greguric I, Vasdev N (2014) Alternative approaches for PET radiotracer development in Alzheimer's disease: imaging beyond plaque. J Labelled Comp Radiopharm 57:323–331

33. Chauveau F, Van Camp N, Dollé F, Kuhnast B, Hinnen F, Damont A, Boutin H, James M, Kassiou M, Tavitian B (2009) Comparative evaluation of the translocator protein radioligands 11C-DPA-713, 18F-DPA-714, and 11C-PK11195 in a rat model of acute neuroinflammation. J Nucl Med 50:468–476

34. Luus C, Hanani R, Reynolds A, Kassiou M (2010) The development of PET radioligands for imaging the translocator protein (18 kDa): what have we learned? J Lab Comp Radiopharm 53:501–510

35. Owen DR, Matthews PM (2011) Imaging brain microglial activation using positron emission tomography and translocator protein-specific radioligands. Int Rev Neurobiol 101:19–39

36. Jensen P, Feng L, Law I, Svarer C, Knudsen GM, Mikkelsen JD et al (2015) TSPO imaging in glioblastoma multiforme: a direct comparison between 123I CLINDE SPECT, 18F-FET PET, and gadolinium-enhanced MR imaging. J Nucl Med 56(9):1386–1390

37. Mirzaei N, Tang SP, Ashworth S, Coello C, Plisson C, Passchier J et al (2016) In vivo imaging of microglial activation by positron emission tomography with [(11)C]PBR28 in the 5XFAD model of Alzheimer's disease. Glia 64(6):993–1006

38. Liu B, Le KX, Park MA, Wang S, Belanger AP, Dubey S, Frost JL, Holton P, Reiser V, Jones PA, Trigg W, Di Carli MF, Lemere CA (2015) In vivo detection of age- and disease-related increases in neuroinflammation by 18F-GE180 TSPO MicroPET imaging in wild-type and Alzheimer's transgenic mice. J Neurosci 35:15716–15730

39. English SJ, Diaz JA, Shao X, Gordon D, Bevard M, Su G et al (2014) Utility of (18) F-FDG and (11)C-PBR28 microPET for the assessment of rat aortic aneurysm inflammation. EJNMMI Res 4(1):20

40. Walker MD, Dinelle K, Kornelsen R, Lee NV, Miao Q, Adam M et al (2015) [11C]PBR28 PET imaging is sensitive to neuroinflammation in the aged rat. J Cereb Blood Flow Metab 35(8):1331–1338

41. Hammers A, Chen C-H, Lemieux L, Allom R et al (2007) Statistical neuroanatomy of the human inferior frontal gyrus and probabilistic atlas in a standard stereotaxic space. Hum Brain Mapp 28:34–48

42. Giron MC (2009) Radiopharmaceutical pharmacokinetics in animals: critical considerations. Q J Nucl Med Mol Imaging 53(4):359–364

43. Barthe N, Maitrejean S, Cardona A (2012) Handbook of radioactivity analysis, 3rd Revised edn. Academic Press, Oxford

44. Pike VW (2009) PET radiotracers: crossing the blood-brain barrier and surviving metabolism. Trends Pharmacol Sci 30(8):431–440

45. Varnas K, Varrone A, Farde L (2013) Modeling of PET data in CNS drug discovery and development. J Pharmacokinet Pharmacodyn 40(3):267–279

46. Olson JM, Ciliax BJ, Mancini WR, Young AB (1988) Presence of peripheral-type benzodiazepine binding sites on human erythrocyte membranes. Eur J Pharmacol 152:47–53

47. Canat X, Carayon P, Bouaboula M, Cahard D, Shire D, Roque C et al (1993) Distribution profile and properties of peripheral-type benzodiazepine receptors on human hemopoietic cells. Life Sci 52:107–118

48. Owen DR, Yeo AJ, Gunn RN, Song K, Wadsworth G, Lewis A et al (2012) An 18-kDa translocator protein (TSPO) polymorphism explains differences in binding affinity of the PET radioligand PBR28. J Cereb Blood Flow Metab 32:1–5

49. Park E et al (2015) (11)C-PBR28 imaging in multiple sclerosis patients and healthy controls: test-retest reproducibility and focal visualization of active white matter areas. Eur J Nucl Med Mol Imaging 42(7):1081–1092

50. Yoder KK et al (2013) Influence of TSPO genotype on 11C-PBR28 standardized uptake values. J Nucl Med 54(8):1320–1322

51. Fan Z et al (2015) Can studies of neuroinflammation in a TSPO genetic subgroup (HAB or MAB) be applied to the entire AD cohort? J Nucl Med 56(5):707–713

52. Kreisl WC et al (2016) (11)C-PBR28 binding to translocator protein increases with progression of Alzheimer's disease. Neurobiol Aging 44:53–61

53. Kreisl WC et al (2013) In vivo radioligand binding to translocator protein correlates with severity of Alzheimer's disease. Brain 136(Pt 7):2228–2238

54. Nair A et al (2016) Test-retest analysis of a non-invasive method of quantifying [11C]-PBR28 binding in Alzheimer's disease. EJNMMI Res 6(1):72

55. Schuitemaker A et al (2013) Microglial activation in Alzheimer's disease: an (R)-[(1)(1)C]PK11195 positron emission tomography study. Neurobiol Aging 34(1):128–136

56. Shipkova M et al (2000) Determination of the acyl glucuronide metabolite of mycophenolic acid in human plasma by HPLC and emit. Clin Chem 46(3):365–372

57. Innis RB et al (2007) Consensus nomenclature for in vivo imaging of reversibly binding radioligands. J Cereb Blood Flow Metab 27(9):1533–1539

58. Hinz R, Boellaard R (2015) Challenges of quantification of TSPO in the human brain. Clin Transl Imaging 3(6):403–416

59. Rizzo G et al (2014) Kinetic modeling without accounting for the vascular component impairs the quantification of [(11)C]PBR28 brain PET data. J Cereb Blood Flow Metab 34(6):1060–1069

60. Veronese M et al (2017) Kinetic modelling of [11C]PBR28 for 18 kDa translocator protein PET data: a validation study of vascular modelling in the brain using XBD173 and tissue analysis. J Cereb Blood Flow Metab:271678X17712388

Chapter 23

In Vivo Two-Photon Calcium Imaging of Hippocampal Neurons in Alzheimer Mouse Models

Marc Aurel Busche

Abstract

The use of in vivo two-photon microscopy in mouse models of Alzheimer's disease (AD) has propelled studies of disease mechanisms and treatments. For instance, this approach allowed for the first time to study in the intact brain the dynamics of individual amyloid plaques, and the effects of anti-amyloid therapies on plaque formation and growth. Moreover, by combining two-photon microscopy with fluorescent calcium indicators, an amyloid-dependent abnormal hyperactivity of cortical and hippocampal neurons was revealed as a primary neuronal impairment, which was not predicted from previous in vitro analyses. Here, a method for in vivo two-photon calcium imaging with single-cell and single-action potential accuracy in the hippocampus of Alzheimer mouse models is presented.

Key words Alzheimer's disease, Mouse models, Amyloid-β, Two-photon microscopy, Calcium imaging, In vivo imaging, Hippocampus, Neuronal hyperactivity

1 Introduction

Alzheimer's disease (AD) impairs memory and other cognitive functions and causes dementia. The symptomatic phase of AD is preceded by a very long clinically silent period, which is characterized by the abnormal aggregation of amyloid-β (Aβ) and tau in the brain [1, 2]. Why it takes many years or even decades until cognitive impairments manifest is still mysterious, but several aspects of this process are now being unraveled. Clinical and preclinical evidence suggest that during the silent period of AD, individual neurons and large-scale networks become dysfunctional and that the symptomatic phase is initiated when the pathophysiological alterations progress and compensatory mechanisms fail [3, 4]. For instance, human studies using functional magnetic resonance imaging (fMRI) have demonstrated that several years prior to cognitive decline there is a profound impairment of the so-called default-mode network, which is typically more active during rest

Robert Perneczky (ed.), *Biomarkers for Alzheimer's Disease Drug Development*, Methods in Molecular Biology, vol. 1750, https://doi.org/10.1007/978-1-4939-7704-8_23, © Springer Science+Business Media, LLC 2018

than during cognitive tasks and is thought to mediate internal mental activity [5–7]. Furthermore, fMRI studies have established that the hippocampus, which is critical for learning and memory functions, is abnormally hyperactive before cognitive impairments are apparent, and becomes hypoactive after symptoms emerge [8–10]. Remarkably, the degree of hippocampal hyperactivity was found to be directly correlated with the speed of cognitive decline [11], making it a possible biomarker for drug development. Indeed, in people at the earliest symptomatic stage of AD, called mild cognitive impairment, treatment with the antiepileptic drug levetiracetam reduced hippocampal hyperactivity and improved the performance in a hippocampus-dependent memory task [12, 13]. To reveal the underlying neuronal mechanisms, our group developed an approach for in vivo two-photon calcium imaging of the hippocampus in transgenic mouse models of AD [14]. The method allows functional, cellular-resolution imaging of neuronal populations in the hippocampus with single-action potential accuracy, which is not possible with the available human neuroimaging techniques. We revealed in an Alzheimer mouse model (the APP23xPS45 model) that hyperactivity of CA1 hippocampal neurons is directly due to the actions of soluble Aβ species, and precedes the deposition of amyloid plaques as well as the development of spatial memory impairments. Intriguingly, at later disease stages, that is after plaque formation, many neurons in the hippocampus become functionally silent. Figure 1 shows schematically the method of hippocampal imaging in the intact brain in vivo using two-photon microscopy.

2 Materials

1. Mice, wild-type and transgenic (e.g., the APP23xPS45 model of AD [15])

   All animal studies should be carried out according to the guidelines and regulations of the relevant authorities. In APP23xPS45 mice, hyperactive neurons are present in the hippocampus already at ~1.5 months of age. While these young mice already overproduce Aβ in their brains, they do not yet exhibit amyloid plaques (Fig. 2a).

2. Anesthesia unit (e.g., isoflurane applied through a vaporizer)

   Anesthesia should be performed in accordance with the relevant animal care regulations.

3. Heating pad

   Keeping the body temperature of the mouse at ~37–38 °C throughout the entire experiment is critical for accurate neuronal activity recordings.

4. Animal monitoring system to control body temperature, breathing and heart rate as well as blood pressure.

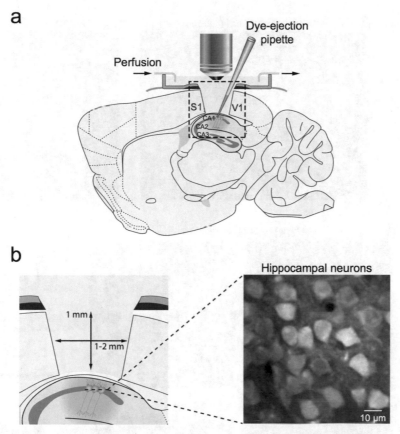

Fig. 1 Schematic illustration of the in vivo approach for hippocampal imaging. (**a**) Side view of the brain after removal of cortical tissue overlying the hippocampus. A recording chamber is glued to the skull to allow head fixation and perfusion with warm standard external saline. CA1 hippocampal neurons, shown in green, are stained by pressure injection of calcium indicator via a glass pipette. (**b**) Left, Detailed view of the hippocampal imaging window (from boxed region in **a**). Right, Representative in vivo image of hippocampal neurons stained with the calcium indicator Fluo-8 AM and imaged with two-photon microscopy. Adapted from [14]

5. Lubricant ophthalmic ointment.

6. Local anesthetic (e.g., 2% lidocaine).

7. Standard external saline for mouse.

8. Device for skull immobilization during surgery, staining, and imaging (e.g., stereotaxic apparatus).

    Our group, for example, used a custom-made recording chamber with central access opening that is glued to the skull with cyanoacryl glue (Fig. 1a). The chamber is fixed in a holder to immobilize the skull and perfused with warm (37 °C) standard external saline [16].

9. Dissecting stereomicroscope.

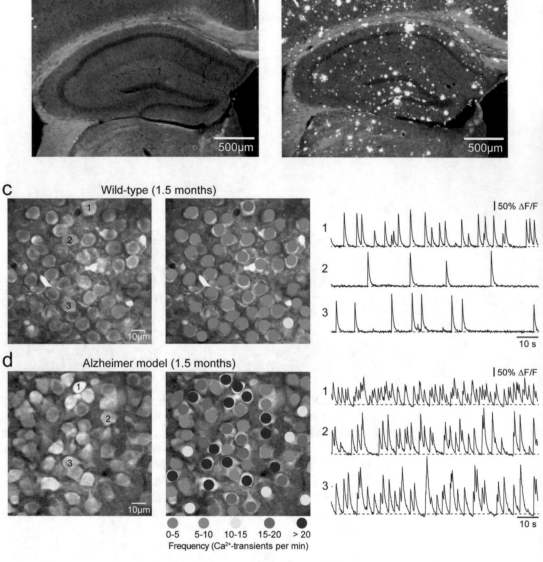

Fig. 2 Increased fractions of hyperactive neurons in the hippocampus before plaque formation. (**a, b**) Representative hippocampal sections from a young (left) and an old (right) APP23xPS45 mouse, respectively, stained with thioflavin-S to visualize amyloid plaques. Note that there are no plaques in the young mouse. (**c, d**) Left, Hippocampal neurons in a wild-type (**c**) and an APP23xPS45 (**d**) mouse stained with the calcium indicator Fluo-8 AM and imaged with in vivo two-photon microscopy. Middle, Activity maps of neurons shown in left panel. Hue is determined by the frequency of spontaneous calcium transients. Right, Example activity traces of neurons indicated in left panel. Adapted from [14]

10. Dissecting instruments.

11. High-speed dental drill.

12. Cut needles, 27-gauge.

13. Pump for aspiration of cortical tissue above hippocampus.

14. Membrane-permeant fluorescent calcium indicator (e.g., Fluo-8 AM).

15. Centrifugal filters.

16. Glass capillaries.

17. Pipette puller.

18. Motorized x–y–z micromanipulator.

19. Pressure application system.

20. Low-melting-point agarose.

    The agarose solution should be freshly prepared before every experiment.

21. Glass coverslips.

22. Two-photon microscope for in vivo imaging.

    This can be a commercially available microscope or a custom-built design. It requires a mode-locked Ti:sapphire pulsing laser (e.g., from Coherent or Spectra-Physics) and a water-immersion, high-numerical-aperture (N.A.) objective.

3 Method

3.1 Hippocampal Cranial Window Preparation

1. All experiments should comply with institutional and national animal care guidelines. Anesthetize the mouse (e.g., with the volatile anesthetic isoflurane) and continuously monitor the depth of anesthesia by testing the animal's reflexes during the surgery. Note that the sensitivity towards anesthetic agent can vary between wild-type and transgenic animals.

2. Place the anesthetized animal on a heating pad to maintain the body temperature at ~37–38 °C. Continuous monitoring of body temperature, heart and breathing rate, and blood pressure is required. Lubricate the eyes with ophthalmic ointment.

3. After application of a local anesthetic (e.g., 2% lidocaine), carefully remove the skin and clean the exposed cranial bone. Dry the bone (e.g., with compressed air).

4. Skull immobilization (e.g., with stereotaxic apparatus or using perfusable, custom-made chamber system (Fig.1)) is critical to avoid movement artifacts during the following surgery, staining, and imaging.

5. Localize the hippocampal region using stereotactic coordinates, and label it with a marker pen.

6. Under a dissecting microscope, perform a craniotomy above the hippocampus using a dental drill.

7. Remove the dura and gently aspirate the overlying cortical tissue using a cut needle (e.g., 27 gauge) connected to a pump until the external capsule becomes visible. The cortex and top-most layers of the external capsule are peeled away so that the deeper layers of the external capsule and the alveus are not damaged (*see* **Note 1**).

8. During the cortical removal, continuously rinse with standard external saline.

3.2 Calcium Indicator Labeling In Vivo

1. Carefully transfer the mouse from the surgery table to the two-photon microscope stage.

2. Prepare the membrane-permeant calcium indicator (e.g., Fluo-8 AM). We typically dissolve Fluo-8 AM in DMSO plus 20% Pluronic F-127, and dilute this solution with a standard pipette solution to a final concentration of 0.5–1 mM. Filter dye solution directly before application (e.g., through centrifugal filter).

3. Fill a glass micropipette (~3–5 MΩ resistance) with dye solution and place pipette directly over the hippocampal surface using a micromanipulator.

4. Advance dye-containing pipette slowly into the hippocampal tissue (~200–250 μm below the surface) and pressure-inject the dye for 1 min at ~10PSI. Pull the pipette slowly back to ~100–150 μm below the surface and apply another pressure pulse to eject the dye. Slowly remove the pipette.

5. Fill the cortical opening with 2% low-melting-point agarose in standard external saline and put a glass coverslip on top (*see* **Notes 2** and **3**).

6. Depending on the calcium indicator used, wait for about 45 min to obtain a stable maximal fluorescence level in labeled neurons.

3.3 Two-Photon Imaging of CA1 Neurons In Vivo

1. Tune the two-photon microscope to the appropriate wavelength (e.g., 920 nm for Fluo-8 AM)

2. Use a high N.A. water-immersion objective (e.g., Nikon 40×, 0.8 N.A., working distance 3.5 mm). The objective lens should remain immersed in external standard saline at all times during imaging.

3. Start the two-photon imaging. To minimize phototoxicity, the laser intensity under the objective should not exceed 70 mW. To resolve the time course of neuronal calcium transients, use a recording speed of at least 10 Hz.

4. Monitor spontaneous activity of CA1 hippocampal neurons. We try to image as many neurons as possible. We typically record neurons for 3–5 min. Note that activity levels in the

hippocampus are markedly higher than in layer 2/3 of the cerebral cortex, where neuronal activity is sparse [15, 17]. At ~0.8% isoflurane, the median frequency of CA1 neurons in wild-type mice is 4.5 calcium transients per min, whereas the frequency is 12.4 calcium transients per min in transgenic mice [14] (*see* **Note 4**).

5. We have defined the "hyperactive" CA1 neurons as those neurons with activity levels above 20 calcium transients per min (based on a 3–5 min continuous recording) [14].

6. Figure 2c, d shows representative examples of the activity status of hippocampal neurons in the APP23xPS45 model and a wild-type control mouse, respectively.

4 Notes

1. An outstanding preparation is crucial for successful recordings of hippocampal activity. Any preparation that shows blood, edema, and/or tissue damage prevents adequate visualization of the neurons. Thus, great care should be taken while aspirating the cortex, and the deeper layers of the external capsule should not be physically touched.

2. Brain movement must be minimized in order to obtain stable recordings. It is important to let the agarose cool down before filling the cortical opening to avoid tissue damage from the heat. The coverslip should be placed when the agarose is still liquid. Avoid any cracks and bubbles in the agarose.

3. When electrode access to the hippocampus is needed (e.g., to perform electrical recordings of the stained neurons or to locally infuse drugs) do not place the coverslip but fill the cortical opening with an extra-thick layer of agarose for mechanical stabilization.

4. It is critical to monitor the vital parameters throughout the entire experiment. Keep the breathing rate at 90–120 breaths per min by adjusting the isoflurane level. Maintain the body temperature at 37–38 °C.

5. Depending on the age of the transgenic animal, the fluorescent calcium indicator (e.g., Fluo-8 AM) will also stain amyloid plaques (in the APP23xPS45 model first plaques start to appear at ~3 months of age). The plaques appear as large and bright spheres, which are surrounded by darker areas. As an independent control, we typically stain the plaques in the area of interest after the neuronal recordings with thioflavin-S, which is a selective marker [18]. Thioflavin-S can be delivered in a similar way as the calcium indicator, namely via pressure application from a glass micropipette (*see* [14] for detailed description). Alternatively, intravenous injections of the fluorescent dye methoxy-X04 have

been used by several groups to acutely stain plaques [19]. If plaques are stained, the fluorescence of the plaque indicator (e.g., thioflavin-S or methoxy-X04) and the calcium indicator (e.g., Fluo-8 AM) must be split using an adequate beam splitter. Figure 3 illustrates the activity status of neurons in the vicinity of an amyloid plaque (blue) in aged APP23xPS45 mice; quantitative analyses showed that hyperactive neurons are located primarily near amyloid plaques (Fig. 3c) [15].

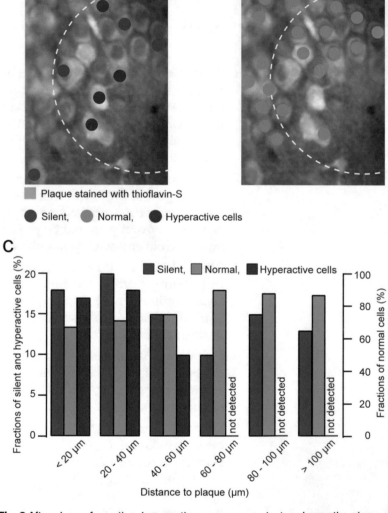

Fig. 3 After plaque formation, hyperactive neurons are clustered near the plaques. (**a**, **b**) Spatial distribution of silent (blue), normal (green), and hyperactive (red) neurons around an amyloid plaque in an old APP23xPS45 mouse (*see* **Note 5**). (**c**) Summary graph shows the abundance of silent, normal, and hyperactive neurons at different distances from the border of the nearest plaque. Adapted from [14]

5   Discussion

In vivo two-photon calcium imaging of the hippocampus is a method that allows to directly assess the effects of Alzheimer's pathology, such as amyloid plaques, on the function of local neuronal circuits that are relevant for learning and memory. The method provides an ideal functional in vivo assay to test new therapeutic approaches for AD [17]. Our group, for example, demonstrated that the acute reduction of soluble Aβ species by a gamma secretase inhibitor (GS-inhibitor) can rescue neuronal hyperactivity in APP23xPS45 mice [14] (Fig. 4). While two-photon microscopy was initially limited to the superficial brain areas such as the upper layers of the cerebral cortex [15, 18], the development of the "hippocampal window procedure" allowed for the first time cellular-resolution functional imaging of deeper brain areas. In recent years, this approach has been employed, for example, to study hippocampal place cells [20, 21], basic electrical patterns of hippocampal neurons [22], the activity of hippocampal neurons during memory tasks [23] and at rest [24], the activity of interneurons [25], the activity of dendrites during spatial navigation [26], and dendritic inhibition during fear learning [27]. Importantly, these and many other studies have not found that the hippocampal cranial

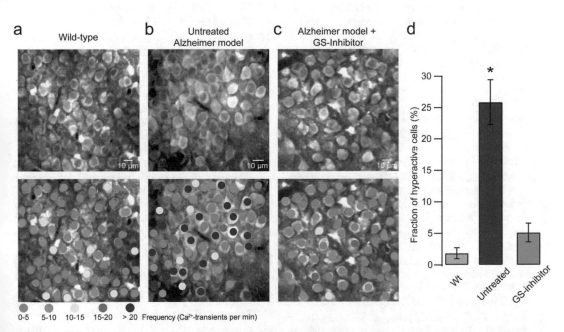

Fig. 4 Treatment with a gamma secretase inhibitor rescues neuronal hyperactivity. (**a–c**) Top panel, Hippocampal neurons imaged in vivo from a wild-type mouse (**a**), an untreated APP23xPS45 mouse (**b**) and an APP23xPS45 mouse treated with a gamma secretase inhibitor (GS-inhibitor, **c**). Bottom panel, Activity maps of neurons shown in top panel. (**d**) Summary graph shows the relative fractions of hyperactive neurons in wild-type (Wt) as well as untreated and treated APP23xPS45 mice, respectively. Adapted from [14]

window alters the basic patterns of hippocampal activity, which have traditionally been recorded electrically through the intact cortex [28–30]. As an alternative approach to the hippocampal cranial window procedure the implantation of microendoscopes into the brain has been introduced and used, for example, to study glioma growth and angiogenesis [31] and plasticity of hippocampal dendrites [32]. In conclusion, in vivo two-photon calcium imaging of the hippocampus provides an excellent opportunity to better understand how hippocampal neurons operate, interact, and control behaviors, and how disease affects all these normal functions.

Acknowledgement

This work was supported by the Alzheimer Forschung Initiative.

References

1. Ossenkoppele R, Jansen WJ, Rabinovici GD et al (2015) Prevalence of amyloid PET positivity in dementia syndromes: a meta-analysis. JAMA 313(19):1939–1949. https://doi.org/10.1001/jama.2015.4669

2. Jansen WJ, Ossenkoppele R, Knol DL et al (2015) Prevalence of cerebral amyloid pathology in persons without dementia: a meta-analysis. JAMA 313(19):1924–1938. https://doi.org/10.1001/jama.2015.4668

3. Busche MA, Konnerth A (2016) Impairments of neural circuit function in Alzheimer's disease. Philos Trans R Soc Lond B Biol Sci 371(1700):pii: 20150429. https://doi.org/10.1098/rstb.2015.0429

4. De Strooper B, Karran E (2016) The cellular phase of Alzheimer's disease. Cell 164(4):603–615. https://doi.org/10.1016/j.cell.2015.12.056

5. Sperling RA, Laviolette PS, O'Keefe K et al (2009) Amyloid deposition is associated with impaired default network function in older persons without dementia. Neuron 63(2):178–188. https://doi.org/10.1016/j.neuron.2009.07.003

6. Hedden T, Van Dijk KR, Becker JA et al (2009) Disruption of functional connectivity in clinically normal older adults harboring amyloid burden. J Neurosci 29(40):12686–12694. https://doi.org/10.1523/JNEUROSCI.3189-09.2009

7. Sheline YI, Raichle ME, Snyder AZ et al (2010) Amyloid plaques disrupt resting state default mode network connectivity in cognitively normal elderly. Biol Psychiatry 67(6):584–587. https://doi.org/10.1016/j.biopsych.2009.08.024

8. Dickerson BC, Salat DH, Greve DN et al (2005) Increased hippocampal activation in mild cognitive impairment compared to normal aging and AD. Neurology 65(3):404–411. https://doi.org/10.1212/01.wnl.0000171450.97464.49

9. Bookheimer SY, Strojwas MH, Cohen MS et al (2000) Patterns of brain activation in people at risk for Alzheimer's disease. N Engl J Med 343(7):450–456. https://doi.org/10.1056/NEJM200008173430701

10. Quiroz YT, Budson AE, Celone K et al (2010) Hippocampal hyperactivation in presymptomatic familial Alzheimer's disease. Ann Neurol 68(6):865–875. https://doi.org/10.1002/ana.22105

11. O'Brien JL, O'Keefe KM, LaViolette PS et al (2010) Longitudinal fMRI in elderly reveals loss of hippocampal activation with clinical decline. Neurology 74(24):1969–1976. https://doi.org/10.1212/WNL.0b013e3181e3966e

12. Bakker A, Albert MS, Krauss G et al (2015) Response of the medial temporal lobe network in amnestic mild cognitive impairment to therapeutic intervention assessed by fMRI and memory task performance. NeuroImage Clin 7:688–698. https://doi.org/10.1016/j.nicl.2015.02.009

13. Bakker A, Krauss GL, Albert MS et al (2012) Reduction of hippocampal hyperactivity improves cognition in amnestic mild cognitive impairment. Neuron 74(3):467–474. https://doi.org/10.1016/j.neuron.2012.03.023

14. Busche MA, Chen X, Henning HA et al (2012) Critical role of soluble amyloid-beta for early hippocampal hyperactivity in a mouse model of Alzheimer's disease. Proc Natl Acad Sci U S A 109(22):8740–8745. https://doi.org/10.1073/pnas.1206171109

15. Busche MA, Eichhoff G, Adelsberger H et al (2008) Clusters of hyperactive neurons near amyloid plaques in a mouse model of Alzheimer's disease. Science 321(5896):1686–1689. https://doi.org/10.1126/science.1162844

16. Stosiek C, Garaschuk O, Holthoff K et al (2003) In vivo two-photon calcium imaging of neuronal networks. Proc Natl Acad Sci U S A 100(12):7319–7324. https://doi.org/10.1073/pnas.1232232100

17. Busche MA, Grienberger C, Keskin AD et al (2015) Decreased amyloid-beta and increased neuronal hyperactivity by immunotherapy in Alzheimer's models. Nat Neurosci 18(12):1725–1727. https://doi.org/10.1038/nn.4163

18. Eichhoff G, Busche MA, Garaschuk O (2008) In vivo calcium imaging of the aging and diseased brain. Eur J Nucl Med Mol Imaging 35(Suppl 1):S99–106. https://doi.org/10.1007/s00259-007-0709-6

19. Kuchibhotla KV, Wegmann S, Kopeikina KJ et al (2014) Neurofibrillary tangle-bearing neurons are functionally integrated in cortical circuits in vivo. Proc Natl Acad Sci U S A 111(1):510–514. https://doi.org/10.1073/pnas.1318807111

20. Dombeck DA, Harvey CD, Tian L et al (2010) Functional imaging of hippocampal place cells at cellular resolution during virtual navigation. Nat Neurosci 13(11):1433–1440. https://doi.org/10.1038/nn.2648

21. Danielson NB, Zaremba JD, Kaifosh P et al (2016) Sublayer-specific coding dynamics during spatial navigation and learning in hippocampal area CA1. Neuron 91(3):652–665. https://doi.org/10.1016/j.neuron.2016.06.020

22. Grienberger C, Chen X, Konnerth A (2014) NMDA receptor-dependent multidendrite Ca(2+) spikes required for hippocampal burst firing in vivo. Neuron 81(6):1274–1281. https://doi.org/10.1016/j.neuron.2014.01.014

23. Rajasethupathy P, Sankaran S, Marshel JH et al (2015) Projections from neocortex mediate top-down control of memory retrieval. Nature 526(7575):653–659. https://doi.org/10.1038/nature15389

24. Villette V, Malvache A, Tressard T et al (2015) Internally recurring hippocampal sequences as a population template of spatiotemporal information. Neuron 88(2):357–366. https://doi.org/10.1016/j.neuron.2015.09.052

25. Kaifosh P, Lovett-Barron M, Turi GF et al (2013) Septo-hippocampal GABAergic signaling across multiple modalities in awake mice. Nat Neurosci 16(9):1182–1184. https://doi.org/10.1038/nn.3482

26. Sheffield ME, Dombeck DA (2015) Calcium transient prevalence across the dendritic arbour predicts place field properties. Nature 517(7533):200–204. https://doi.org/10.1038/nature13871

27. Lovett-Barron M, Kaifosh P, Kheirbek MA et al (2014) Dendritic inhibition in the hippocampus supports fear learning. Science 343(6173):857–863. https://doi.org/10.1126/science.1247485

28. Hahn TT, Sakmann B, Mehta MR (2007) Differential responses of hippocampal subfields to cortical up-down states. Proc Natl Acad Sci U S A 104(12):5169–5174. https://doi.org/10.1073/pnas.0700222104

29. Harvey CD, Collman F, Dombeck DA et al (2009) Intracellular dynamics of hippocampal place cells during virtual navigation. Nature 461(7266):941–946. https://doi.org/10.1038/nature08499

30. Mizuseki K, Diba K, Pastalkova E et al (2011) Hippocampal CA1 pyramidal cells form functionally distinct sublayers. Nat Neurosci 14(9):1174–1181. https://doi.org/10.1038/nn.2894

31. Barretto RP, Ko TH, Jung JC et al (2011) Time-lapse imaging of disease progression in deep brain areas using fluorescence microendoscopy. Nat Med 17(2):223–228. https://doi.org/10.1038/nm.2292

32. Attardo A, Fitzgerald JE, Schnitzer MJ (2015) Impermanence of dendritic spines in live adult CA1 hippocampus. Nature 523(7562):592–596. https://doi.org/10.1038/nature14467

Part IX

Related Concepts: Cognitive Testing and Advanced Analytics

Chapter 24

Cognitive Assessment in Alzheimer's Disease Clinical Trials

Geraint Price

Abstract

Many tests are available for the assessment of cognitive function. This chapter describes the common features and practical requirements of test administration, key considerations in the selection and interpretation of tests, and their application in Alzheimer's disease drug development.

Key words Neuropsychological assessment, Cognitive assessment, Methods, Alzheimer's disease, Drug development

1 Introduction

Cognitive (or neuropsychological) assessment may range from brief screening to detect cognitive impairment, to comprehensive measurement of general intellectual ability or "IQ," the assessment of specific functions such as memory or language, or their more specific subcategories (e.g., episodic memory, language fluency). A wide range of different instruments for conducting cognitive assessments is available, and each has its own manual which must be consulted in order to administer the test. This chapter does not describe the administration of specific tests but, instead, provides an overview of key common features that they share.

The chapter will describe the general principles of cognitive assessment for clinical practice or research purposes, followed by discussion of considerations of particular relevance to Alzheimer's disease and drug development.

Clinical diagnosis of cognitive impairment requires detailed history-taking, behavioral observation, and (often) informant interview [1]. In some cases clinicians may obtain sufficient diagnostic information by interweaving cognitive tasks flexibly into their clinical interview, without the need for formal cognitive test administration. This chapter, by contrast, describes the processes to be followed in situations where a formal, standardized neuropsychological assessment is required.

Robert Perneczky (ed.), *Biomarkers for Alzheimer's Disease Drug Development*, Methods in Molecular Biology, vol. 1750, https://doi.org/10.1007/978-1-4939-7704-8_24, © Springer Science+Business Media, LLC 2018

The added value of undertaking a formal cognitive assessment, over and above clinical interview and observation, is the ability to quantify the level of cognitive functioning, by obtaining objective numerical measures of performance which can be compared with established cutoff scores (in order to categorize subjects as impaired or unimpaired) or a normative distribution (to yield a percentile or standardized score), and analyzed statistically for research purposes.

Cognitive assessment involves *selection* and *administration* of the tests, and *interpretation* of the results. The "Materials" and "Methods" sections below concern the middle stage, test administration. This is a technical skill which usually requires a relevant undergraduate degree followed by specific training in psychometric test administration.

2   Materials

Test administration requires a suitable **room** (*see* **Notes 1** and **2**), quiet and free from disturbance (i.e., with suitable soundproofing, "do not disturb" notice, and telephones switched off), with a suitable desk (*see* **Note 3**).

Subjects must have any **reading glasses or hearing aids** required to functionally correct their vision and hearing.

1. **Computer-administered tests** (which are becoming increasingly available, but not yet commonplace) may require no further equipment other than the computer and any response keys provided.

2. Traditional "paper and pencil" tests will generally require:

    (a) **Administrator's record form** (*see* **Note 4**).

    (b) **Subject's response form**, if needed (*see* **Note 5**).

    (c) **Pens and pencils** for administrator and participant.

    (d) **Stopwatch** (for tests requiring the timing of subject's responses).

    (e) **Clock or watch** visible to the administrator (for memory tests with delayed-recall conditions).

    (f) **Test-specific stimulus materials** as specified in the test manual (*see* **Note 6**).

3   Methods

Before starting, check (via questioning and observation) for any issues which may compromise test performance, e.g., tiredness, illness, significant anxiety, lack of motivation, and sensory or motor disabilities. Continue to observe throughout (*see* **Note 7**).

Explain to the subject the purpose of the assessment and the potential outcomes, in order to obtain informed consent to proceed (*see* **Note 8**).

Explain the process of the assessment (duration, opportunities for breaks), and pre-empt demoralization by explaining that the test will include some tasks that most subjects find difficult.

For standardization purposes, task instructions to the *subject* are usually written on the record form for the administrator to read out verbatim. Instructions to be followed by the *administrator* are generally described in the manual or record form in specific detail: for example, "The words should be read aloud at a rate of approximately one word every 1.5 seconds" [2], "If response is very brief, say *Tell me more*" [3], or an instruction to allow at least 25 min to elapse between Immediate and Delayed Recall trials [4].

For scoring purposes, the manual or record form will either indicate the precise responses that may be considered correct (e.g., "*police* is required"), or will specify if credit may be given for equivalent or approximate alternatives (e.g., "a word or phrase signifying one or more members of the police department" [5] (*see* **Note 9**).

During test administration, general encouragement is given as required but, unless specifically instructed otherwise in the manual, feedback on performance is not given.

4 Notes

1. A few tests explicitly require a different setting, e.g., the Multiple Errands Test [6] which is conducted in a "real-world" setting such as a shopping precinct.

2. Some tests (or research protocols) may have additional testing-room requirements. For example, tests including clock-drawing (drawing a clock-face from memory) or orientation to time ("Without looking at a watch, can you tell me what the time is now?") will specify that no clock must be visible to the participant in the testing room.

3. Some test manuals or research protocols will make specific requirements, e.g., for a visuospatial task such as copying a figure, the examiner may be required to sit opposite the participant across a square table, in order to standardize the alignment of the presented stimulus and the copy.

4. The administrator's form must be concealed from subjects, e.g., using a screen or clipboard, to prevent them from seeing the correct answers printed on the form and/or the marks being awarded for their responses.

5. Subject response forms are required for tests in which the participant must write or draw their responses, for example, the

Trail Making Test [7] or Digit Symbol Substitution Tests such as the Coding subtest of the WAIS-IV [8].

6. Some tests (e.g., the Naming items of the MMSE) [9] require the use of commonly available items (e.g., a pen and a watch). Most tests include stimulus booklets incorporating all the visual stimuli to be displayed during test administration, e.g., figures to be copied, or pictures to be named or memorized. Some tests require (and provide) additional items of equipment, for example, the Block Design subtest of the WAIS-IV [8].

7. If a temporary compromising issue is identified, it will usually be preferable to defer the assessment to another occasion. If this is not practical (e.g., if the subject is not available to return on another occasion, if the issue comes to light after part of the test has already been administered, or if the compromising issue is permanent, e.g., chronic tremor or speech impediment), it will be necessary to consider whether a compromised test result is better (or worse) than no result at all, in order to decide whether to continue with the assessment.

8. For subjects with already-established cognitive impairment, an evaluation of their mental capacity to decide whether or not to participate in the assessment will be required. Irrespective of capacity considerations, an explanation of any potential adverse outcomes (in particular the possibility that the assessment may give rise to unwelcome news) is an ethical requirement.

9. In some tests it is difficult or impossible to anticipate all potential responses (for example, in a semantic fluency test in which the subject must generate a list of items of furniture, it would be impractical for the manual to list every conceivable correct answer), so the test administrator must sometimes exercise judgment in deciding whether to award credit (if the participant gives a response whose acceptability is unclear, such as "washbasin"). Nevertheless, test manuals often provide highly detailed instructions, in an attempt to keep this to a minimum.

5   Test Selection and Interpretation

The selection and interpretation of tests require clinical expertise in neuropsychology as well as technical expertise in psychometrics, and are generally undertaken by clinicians with relevant doctoral level qualifications.

Test selection must take into account a range of factors including the particular cognitive function to be assessed (based on clinical or theoretical considerations), the psychometric properties of available tests, and the time available to administer the assessment. There may be a tension between these considerations. Typically, broad composite indices of general cognitive ability derived from lengthy well-normed tests such as the WAIS [8] offer the most robust psychometric properties, whereas the pragmatics and specific hypotheses of a study may instead require briefer tests, and/or tests which precisely target a particular function of interest, and these are less likely to achieve the gold standard psychometric properties. Relevant psychometric properties include the reliability of the obtained data, and the potential for ceiling or floor effects. For example, if the assessor wishes to track subtle cognitive changes in high-functioning subjects, then it will be important to choose a highly reliable test with a high ceiling.

Consequently, the interpretation of test results must always take into account the limitations of the tests that were selected. A particular danger is that a numerical test result may give a spurious sense of precision. For example, reporting an IQ score as 113 gives an entirely false impression that IQ can be measured accurately to three significant figures. Well-normed tests will provide confidence intervals around the obtained result, thus permitting the result to be reported with appropriate degree of confidence (for example, "with 90% confidence, this subject's IQ falls between 101 and 125").

Similarly, there is a danger that numerical cognitive test results may be perceived as more objective than other sources of information, whereas in reality the different sources of information are complementary and must be considered together. Cognitive test scores should be questioned, or interpreted cautiously, if they are inconsistent with behavioral or clinical observations.

Cognitive assessment is subject to practice effects whereby if participants repeat the same test on multiple occasions, their performance will tend to improve [10]. It is therefore important to obtain an accurate measurement at the first attempt if at all possible, since a repeat attempt following an erroneous or discontinued administration may give an overestimate of the true level of function. While some tests provide alternate forms to mitigate against practice effects, practice may still be evident across alternate forms [11]. If it is necessary to repeat the same test on two or more occasions (for example, in order to monitor cognitive change over time), then the presence of a practice effect should be presumed and taken into account in the interpretation of the results.

6   Cognitive Assessment in Alzheimer's Disease Drug Development

Perhaps because neuropsychological assessment is an explicit requirement in research criteria for a clinical diagnosis of Alzheimer's disease [12, 13], the use of cognitive assessments in

Alzheimer's disease research is ubiquitous. There is, however, a consequent risk that cognitive assessments may be simply included in Alzheimer's research protocols by default, without clear consideration of how (or even whether) they serve the purposes of the research. For example, the Mini Mental State Examination [9] is used so universally in dementia research that it may be included as a standard fixture of Alzheimer's research protocols even though, for studies of milder or preclinical stages of the disease, ceiling effects may render it insensitive [14].

Clearly, the qualities required of a cognitive assessment will depend on its purpose and function within the research protocol. Scores on cognitive tests may be used for *participant selection*, with particular cognitive score profiles specified as inclusion/exclusion criteria; as *outcome measures* (either as the determinants of categorical endpoints, or as continuous data for the analysis of change from baseline); or as *contributors to diagnostic decisions* in study designs where inclusion criteria, endpoints, or other required data are based on diagnostic judgments which are, in turn, informed by cognitive assessment. They may also be used for *screening*: for example, where studies lack the resources for a comprehensive clinical assessment of every participant, but cognitive test administrators are more readily available, it may be efficient for the cognitive assessment to be undertaken for all participants, with prespecified profiles defined as triggers for further comprehensive assessment, adjudication, or full clinical evaluation.

Tests which are suitable for one purpose may be less suitable for others. For example, in a trial of the effectiveness of a treatment for Alzheimer's disease, the MMSE may be suitable for participant selection but insufficiently sensitive to serve as an outcome measure. Of the various purposes above, the use of cognitive assessments as outcome measures probably carries the greatest potential for misinterpretation. Not only must ceiling, floor, and practice effects be taken into account but, in addition, the trade-off between sensitivity and specificity will apply. Tests which are sufficiently sensitive to detect small changes in cognition will also be sensitive to extraneous or confounding influences, such as time of day, distraction, hunger, fatigue, mood, illness, or medications. Despite best efforts to predict and control such factors, a degree of measurement error is unavoidable, due to imperfect control of the wide range of extraneous (and sometimes subtle or unknown) factors which may affect test performance.

This measurement error is not a sign of a poorly designed cognitive test, but a reflection of the reality of human cognition and its sophisticated sensitivity to all aspects of the environment. A hallmark of a well-validated test is that it has anticipated and quantified this measurement error, by providing details of test-retest reliability in validation samples. Test validation is however a lengthy and resource-intensive process, and while some relatively novel test batteries (such as the ADCS-PACC: [15]) may hold the promise of high sensitivity to subtle change, they may not yet have established the level of test-retest reliability data which is available for older tests.

An important consideration in interpreting cognitive changes is the extent to which they match the expected profiles of cognitive change in Alzheimer's disease. For example, do the treatment and control groups differ specifically with respect to episodic memory, word-finding, and executive functioning? Or do they, instead, differ with respect to alertness, attention, and cognitive speed? Considerations of this type may be important in judging whether the difference represents an impact on the progression of the underlying cognition or, instead, simply a general cognition-enhancing effect. Here again, some novel and potentially sensitive tests (for example, computerized tests) may have the disadvantage that they are less familiar to clinicians or researchers and thus more difficult to interpret.

For these reasons, if novel or clinically unfamiliar tests (such as the ADCS-PACC [15] or CANTAB [16]) are chosen on the basis of their potential sensitivity to change, it is advisable to use them in combination with more thoroughly validated or clinically well-understood tests (such as the Wechsler tests [5, 8], RBANS [2], or Harrison neuropsychological test battery [17]), to permit robust interpretation of the findings and greater scope to evaluate alternative possible explanations of changes.

References

1. Kipps CM, Hodges JR (2005) Cognitive assessment for clinicians. J Neurol Neurosurg Psychiatry 76(Suppl I):i22–i30

2. Randolph C (1998) Repeatable battery for the assessment of neuropsychological status: manual. Pearson, Bloomington

3. Stern RA, White T (2003) Neuropsychological assessment battery: administration, scoring, and interpretation manual. PAR, Inc., Lutz, FL

4. Benedict R, Brandt J (1997) Brief visuospatial memory test—revised (BVMT-R). PAR, Inc., Lutz, FL

5. Wechsler D (1997) Wechsler memory scale—third edition (WMS–III) administration and scoring manual. The Psychological Corporation, San Antonio, TX

6. Knight C, Alderman N, Burgess PW (2002) Development of a simplified version of the multiple errands test for use in hospital settings. Neuropsychol Rehabil 12(3):231–255

7. Reitan RM, Wolfson D (1985) The Halstead–Reitan neuropsychological test battery: theory and clinical interpretation. Neuropsychological Press, Tucson, AZ

8. Wechsler D (2008) Wechsler adult intelligence scale—fourth edition (WAIS-IV) administration and scoring manual. The Psychological Corporation, San Antonio, TX

9. Folstein M, Folstein SE, McHugh PR (1975) "Mini-mental state". A practical method for grading the cognitive state of patients for the clinician. J Psychiatr Res 12(3):189–198

10. Bartels C, Wegrzyn M, Wiedl A, Ackermann V, Ehrenreich H (2010) Practice effects in healthy adults: a longitudinal study on frequent repetitive cognitive testing. BMC Neurosci 11:118

11. Beglinger LJ, Gaydos B, Tangphao-Daniels O et al (2005) Practice effects and the use of alternate forms in serial neuropsychological testing. Arch Clin Neuropsychol 20(4):517–529

12. McKhann G, Drachman D, Folstein M et al (1984) Clinical diagnosis of Alzheimer's disease: report of the NINCDS-ADRDA work group under the auspices of Department of Health and Human Services Task Force on Alzheimer's disease. Neurology 34(7):939–944

13. Dubois B, Feldman HH, Jacova C et al (2007) Research criteria for the diagnosis of Alzheimer's

disease: revising the NINCDS-ADRDA criteria. Lancet Neurol 6(8):734–746

14. Simard M (1998) The mini-mental state examination: strengths and weaknesses of a clinical instrument. Can Alzheimer Dis Rev 12:10–12

15. Donohue MC, Sperling RA, Salmon DP et al (2014) The preclinical Alzheimer cognitive composite: measuring amyloid-related decline. JAMA Neurol 71(8):961–970

16. Fray PJ, Robbins TW, Sahakian BJ (1996) Neuropsychiatric applications of CANTAB. Int J Geriatr Psychiatry 11:329–336

17. Harrison J, Minassian SL, Jenkins L, Black RS, Koller M, Grundman M (2007) A neuropsychological test battery for use in Alzheimer disease clinical trials. Arch Neurol 64(9):1323–1329

Chapter 25

Data Mining and Machine Learning Methods for Dementia Research

Rui Li

Abstract

Patient data in clinical research often includes large amounts of structured information, such as neuroimaging data, neuropsychological test results, and demographic variables. Given the various sources of information, we can develop computerized methods that can be a great help to clinicians to discover hidden patterns in the data. The computerized methods often employ data mining and machine learning algorithms, lending themselves as the computer-aided diagnosis (CAD) tool that assists clinicians in making diagnostic decisions. In this chapter, we review state-of-the-art methods used in dementia research, and briefly introduce some recently proposed algorithms subsequently.

Key words Data mining, Machine learning, Computer-aided diagnosis, Alzheimer, Classification, Pattern mining, Multi-view, Clustering

1 Introduction

Alzheimer's disease (AD) is a progressive, degenerative, and incurable disease of the brain and the main cause of dementia. The number of people suffering from dementia is expected to grow rapidly in the next decades due to increasing life expectancy, which will have a major negative impact on healthcare systems worldwide. Despite technological progress, the correct diagnosis of AD is still a challenging clinical task, in particular in the early disease stages. From a data analysis point of view, we need to develop reliable statistical methods that can act as helpful computer-aided diagnosis (CAD) tools to arrive at the correct diagnosis.

A part of the patient data from medical applications is stored in a structured manner. This data can come from different sources, such as brain scans (for example, positron emission tomography (PET)), demographic information, and neuropsychological tests. Clinicians use diverse information to arrive at a diagnosis; however, they may have difficulties in diagnosing some patients whose symptoms are ambiguous. Furthermore, disagreement among clinicians

Robert Perneczky (ed.), *Biomarkers for Alzheimer's Disease Drug Development*, Methods in Molecular Biology, vol. 1750, https://doi.org/10.1007/978-1-4939-7704-8_25, © Springer Science+Business Media, LLC 2018

also appears often. Therefore, gaining better insight into data not only helps clinicians in improving diagnostic accuracy, but also assists them in making medical decisions. In general, for our purposes we divide patient data into two categories, imaging data (e.g., PET scans) and non-imaging data (e.g., demographic information, neuropsychological tests), and we need to develop algorithms to discover hidden information in both data sources. Data mining and machine learning methods are valuable tools in this regard. Over the past several decades, many algorithms have been proposed and have demonstrated good performance in mining medical data. Decision tree and support vector machines (SVM) are well-known algorithms (for an overview of these methods, please *see* [1]). Since the year 2006, deep learning has been applied successfully in many applications. Deep learning is regarded as the new generation of the neural networks that was very popular in the early 1990s. At present, medical data analysis faces a new exciting era, in which big data, deep learning, and significant computational power meet. First, various types of data can be collected and stored in a big data architecture such as NoSQL or Hadoop. Second, deep learning can benefit from the large amounts of data by its deep architecture which is able to capture complex patterns. Third, the computer cluster (CPU or graphic processing unit (GPU)) is becoming easier to access and the cost is constantly decreasing. However, the amount of data may still be small in some medical domains due to different reasons; for example, it is challenging to collect large amounts of data in dementia due to reasons such as high costs and high drop-out rates in clinical trials. Hence, we still need to develop other methods that can help us discover patterns in the data.

The aim of this chapter is to offer an overview of the state-of-the-art methods in mining medical data relevant for AD research, followed by some recently proposed algorithms.

2 Overview of State-of-the-Art Methods

Medical image analysis is of great interest in diverse medical fields. It not only helps clinicians to make critical diagnostic decisions, but may also discover interesting patterns in the available data. Medical data can be divided into two groups, namely the imaging and non-imaging data. For example, MRI (magnetic resonance imaging) and PET are commonly used imaging techniques. MRI is a favored imaging technique in diagnosing AD, since it provides robust information about general atrophy as well as atrophy of certain regions of interest, such as the hippocampus. Fluorodeoxyglucose-PET (FDG-PET), on the other hand, is a noninvasive technique which is able to measure brain metabolic activity quantitatively, and which has consistently been shown to assist in diagnosing AD in early clinical stages [2]. The conventional approaches in analyzing MRI and PET images can be roughly categorized as voxel-based morphometry (VBM) and statistical approaches. VBM applies simple statistical tests, such as the t-test, across different groups of subjects to discover discriminative voxels. Voxels are considered independently, which can be seen as the univariate method. Some other statistical approaches employ more advanced algorithms to perform multivariate analysis. For example, principal component analysis (PCA) has been used to extract features, which are then fed into a classifier [3]. PCA is a popular method in many different fields. It converts the data into different principal components, capturing the variances in the data so that the characteristics of the data are learned. Following the line of advanced algorithms (such as Gaussian mixture model (GMM)), we can develop powerful methods that can discover meaningful patterns in the data. GMM differs from PCA in that it is essentially a clustering method that groups similar data together. The data in one group (cluster) have similar statistical characteristics compared to the data in another group. Thus, interesting patterns may be discovered by comparing these groups of data. Recently, there is also a great interest in applying deep learning methods in the analysis of medical data. One study, for example, [4] applied the stacked auto-encoder to learn a feature representation to differentiate the mild cognitive impairment (MCI) from AD dementia. The authors claimed that the nonlinear relations can be captured by the proposed deep learning model. As we collect increasing amounts of medical data, we believe that the deep learning method should lend itself as a helpful tool.

Compared to the mining of imaging data, the mining of non-imaging data appears to be very limited. An exemplary work [5] applied the subgroup discovery algorithm to interpret structured patient data, revealing some interesting rules that help clinicians gain deep insights into the data.

Combining various sources of data is very popular in the dementia domain. For example, multi-modality image analysis makes use of MRI and PET for a more reliable analysis, building on the complementary information. To combine various sources of information, multiple kernel learning [6] offers a framework to train a model that can benefit from the diverse information. Stacked generalization [7] is another approach to benefiting a model from the various sources of information, which will be explained in the consecutive section. Having introduced some of the state-of-the-art methods in analyzing the imaging and non-imaging data, we will briefly introduce some recently proposed algorithms.

We summarize the commonly used data mining and machine learning algorithms in mining the medical data in Table 1 to gain a clear overview. Supervised algorithms differ from unsupervised algorithms in that the former requests labels of the data. Label

Table 1
Commonly used data mining and machine learning algorithms in medical data mining

Supervised algorithms	Unsupervised algorithms
Support vector machines (SVM)	Gaussian mixture model
k-nearest neighbor (KNN)	k-means clustering
Naïve Bayes	Principal component analysis (PCA)
Random forest	Independent component analysis (ICA)

means a data record may be annotated as, for example, NC (normal control) or MCI. The choice of algorithms often depends on the underlying applications and practical concerns.

3   Introduction to Relevant Algorithms

3.1   Mining PET Imaging Data

PET gives us detailed insights into molecular processes occurring in tissues. It is a three-dimensional medical imaging technology based on the detection of positrons. A healthy brain should reveal a good activity level, indirectly measured by quantifying glucose metabolism (FDG-PET). By investigating the activity reflected by the PET, we are able to distinguish NC, MCI, and AD images. Prior to the image analysis, PET images are usually pre-processed by spatial normalization and smoothing, in appropriate software packages such as SPM [8]. The spatial normalization ensures the processed image to be the same size, so that images can be directly compared. Smoothing can increase the signal-to-noise ratio. In addition, intensity normalization is also of great importance, eliminating the impact of different amounts of injected tracers, for example. Normalization can be achieved in relation to the metabolism of the entire brain (grand mean) or select brain regions (cerebellum, primary sensorimotor cortex, etc.) [9].

The work [10] introduced a Gaussian mixture model and model selection approach to automatically extract features from PET scans and further build a predictive model for classification. GMM [11] is a popular clustering method that assumes the data is generated by more than one Gaussian distribution. It assigns a data point to a class label to which the point belongs with the largest probability. The solution of GMM can be achieved by the Expectation Maximization (EM), which is guaranteed to converge, so that a locally optimal solution is always assured. However, the number of clusters must be defined in advance, which can be a great practical concern. Therefore, the Bayesian Information

Criterion (BIC) [12] was employed to choose the optimal number of clusters. The BIC is frequently used for model selection, trading off the model fitness and model complexity. The experimental results on two independent datasets demonstrate good performance in particular for the MCI versus AD dementia classification. The good performance is credited to the proposed GMM and model selection approach that extracts discriminative features from the PET scans. Especially, the model selection (BIC) plays a crucial role, because it can avoid overfitting and underfitting of the data. Overfitting and underfitting are related to the number of clusters in this application. It is worth mentioning that another clustering algorithm, such as k-means, requires a pre-defined number of clusters k, which is challenging to determine in advance. The practical problem is handled by the model selection in the proposed method. Thus, mining the PET scans by a clustering method combined with a model selection approach demonstrates promising results. The implementation of the MATLAB code is publicly available at: https://github.com/RuiLiDMML/GMMMS.

3.2 Mining Non-imaging Data

Clinical data also contain non-imaging data, such as demographic information and neuropsychological tests. It is of great medical interest to reveal hidden patterns that may help clinicians gain new insights. A pattern may simply be a rule, for example, "IF age greater than 70, THEN chance of suffering from AD is high." In data mining, subgroup discovery [13] is a powerful tool in discovering interesting variable combinations pointing to a particular target class. The target class may be the people who suffer from AD, and the variables of interest can be age, gender, genetic information, etc. A particular combination of these variables may suggest a higher probability of being an AD patient. In Fig. 1, 50% of the entire population has a disease, but the percentage dramatically increases to 90% in a subgroup "age >65 and gender = male." Thus, we may be interested in such a subgroup representing an obvious contrast to the whole population. Quantitatively, the interestingness of a subgroup can be measured by a quality function, whose definition is referred to in the work CN2 [14]. In a high-dimensional database, the search for all possible combinations of variables grows exponentially. Therefore, the work SDVQP [15] proposed an optimization-based approach to coping with the extensive search space problem while still yielding high-quality rules. The key idea is to preselect promising features for subgroup discovery, so that the search space is kept small but still fruitful. The experiment was conducted on the ADNI dataset. The discovered rules include "If MMSE >25 AND ApoE = E3/E3 THEN non-AD ($\rho = 0.07$)." ρ can be interpreted as a confidence score, the higher the more confident. The rules can be ranked by the confidence score, so that medical experts may only need to interpret the top ones to avoid looking at all the rules.

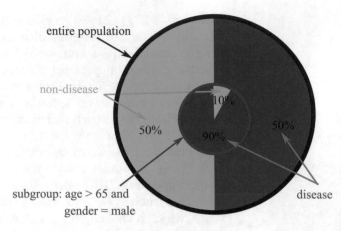

Fig. 1 Pie chart illustration of subgroup discovery

The pattern mining, subgroup discovery as a subfield, can be a great tool to gain better understanding of the data. Compared to the black-box algorithms, such as SVM, the pattern mining may yield interesting knowledge that can be digested and interpreted by humans. Therefore, pattern mining (a subfield of data mining) will likely gain in popularity in the field of medical applications.

3.3 Mining Multi-View Data

Clinical data include imaging and non-imaging data, and using the complementary information effectively may result in better diagnostic results. Majority voting is a simple method combining the decisions from different sources to make a final decision. However, the interdependency among various sources cannot be discovered. Stacking [7] has been proposed as an approach to learning the interdependency among different sources so that a better decision can be made based on the learned decision behaviors. A stacked multi-view learning [16] was suggested to make good use of the complementary information contained in several types of clinical data. The experiments showed a better result than using any information source alone. In this study, the predictions from different views (sources) were stacked to perform a meta-level learning. One view can be the imaging data and another view can be the demographic information. The meta-level learning is supposed to be trained by the class probability yielded from the base level views. In such a manner, the final classifier is able to learn the interdependency among various views to make a more reliable prediction. The performance of multi-view stacking is analyzed by a regression analysis. It reveals that a medium meta-level correlation of the views and the relatively high base-level correlation of the views may indicate good performance. The Fig. 2 demonstrates the workflow of the stacked multi-view learning. A base classifier (e.g., SVM [1]) is applied to the training data to yield the class probability estimates for both classes (assume two classes problem) using a tenfold cross-validation. The meta-level features are in fact the yielded class probability estimates, building the meta-level training model.

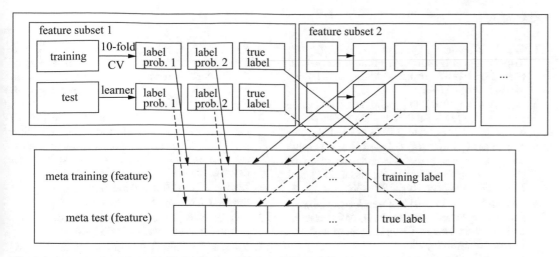

Fig. 2 Demonstration of stacking. *CV* cross-validation. Feature subset: view, i.e., information source

Similarly, the meta-level test features are constructed by applying the same base classifier to the test data. The true labels (if available) of the test data are reserved only for validating the final result. The goal of such a model is to learn the relationship between true decisions and the decisions made by various base classifiers.

4 Discussions and Outlook

CAD is increasingly recognized as a potentially helpful tool in assisting clinicians in establishing more accurate diagnoses. Computerized methods should therefore be further explored and developed to improve our ability to effectively mine medical data. In this chapter, we have briefly introduced some of the state-of-the-art methods for data mining in dementia research. We also shed some light on the current popular deep learning and big data topics. Subsequently, we introduced three recently proposed algorithms in mining of imaging data, non-imaging data, and the use of both data types. As more and more data is collected and intelligent algorithms are developed, CAD should be a great help to clinicians in making better diagnostic decisions. Finally, the mining of genetic information may also help us find interesting patterns and gain deep insights into the disease.

Acknowledgments

Some of the proposed methods were developed during the author's appointment at Technische Universität München (TUM), Munich, Germany. The author thanks Prof. Dr. Stefan Kramer for his academic guidance during the PhD study at Technische Universität München and Johannes Gutenberg-Universität Mainz.

References

1. Wu X, Kumar V, Quinlan JR et al (2007) Top 10 algorithms in data mining. Knowl Inf Syst 14(1):1–37. https://doi.org/10.1007/s10115-007-0114-2

2. Drzezga A (2009) Diagnosis of Alzheimer's disease with [18F]PET in mild and asymptomatic stages. Behav Neurol 21(1):101–115

3. López MM, Ramírez J, Górriz JM et al (2009) SVM-based cad system for early detection of the Alzheimer's disease using kernel PCA and LDA. Neurosci Lett 464:233–238

4. Suk H-I, Shen D (2013) Deep learning-based feature representation for AD/MCI classification. Med Image Comput Comput Assist Interv 16(2):583–590

5. Schmidt J, Hapfelmeier A, Müller M et al (2010) Interpreting PET scans by structured patient data: a data mining case study in dementia research. J Knowl Inf Syst 24:149–170

6. Bach FR, Lanckriet GRG, Jordan MI (2004) Multiple kernel learning, conic duality, and the SMO algorithm. Paper presented at the proceedings of the twenty-first international conference on machine learning, Banff, AB, Canada

7. Wolpert D (1992) Stacked generalization. Neural Netw 5(2):241–259

8. SPM (2005) Statistical parametric mapping. http://www.filionuclacuk/spm/software/spm5/

9. Yakushev I, Landvogt C, Buchholz HG et al (2008) Choice of reference area in studies of Alzheimer's disease using positron emission tomography with fluorodeoxyglucose-F18. Psychiatry Res 164(2):143–153

10. Li R, Perneczky R, Drzezga A et al (2015) Gaussian mixture models and model selection for [18F] fluorodeoxyglucose positron emission tomography classification in Alzheimer's disease. PLoS One 10(4):e0122731

11. Bishop CM (2006) Pattern recognition and machine learning. Springer, New Delhi

12. Schwarz GE (1978) Estimating the dimension of a model. Ann Stat 6(2):461–464

13. Klösgen W (1996) A multipattern and multistrategy discovery assistant. Advances in knowledge discovery and data mining. 249–271

14. Lavrac N, Kavsek B, Flach P et al (2004) Subgroup discovery with CN2-SD. J Mach Learn Res 5:153–188

15. Li R, Perneczky R, Drzezga A et al (2015) Efficient redundancy reduced subgroup discovery via quadratic programming. J Intell Inf Syst 44(2):271–288

16. Li R, Hapfelmeier A, Schmidt J et al (2011) A case study of stacked multi-view learning in dementia research

INDEX

Robert Perneczky (ed.), *Biomarkers for Alzheimer's Disease Drug Development*, Methods in Molecular Biology, vol. 1750, https://doi.org/10.1007/978-1-4939-7704-8, © Springer Science+Business Media, LLC 2018

Printed in the United States
By Bookmasters

04231370-01065529